Essentials of

DIAGNOSIS & TREATMENT

Essentials of
DIAGNOSIS & TREATMENT

Second Edition

a LANGE medical book

Lawrence M. Tierney, Jr., MD
Professor of Medicine
University of California, San Francisco
Associate Chief of Medical Services
Veterans Affairs Medical Center
San Francisco, California

Sanjay Saint, MD, MPH
Assistant Professor of Medicine
Division of General Medicine
University of Michigan Medical School
Research Scientist
Ann Arbor Veterans Affairs Medical Center
Ann Arbor, Michigan

Mary A. Whooley, MD
Assistant Professor of Medicine
University of California, San Francisco
Section of General Internal Medicine
Veterans Affairs Medical Center
San Francisco, California

Lange Medical Books/McGraw-Hill
Medical Publishing Division

New York   Chicago   San Francisco   Lisbon   London   Madrid
Mexico City   Milan   New Delhi   San Juan   Seoul   Singapore
Sydney   Toronto

McGraw-Hill

A Division of The McGraw·Hill Companies

Essentials of Diagnosis & Treatment, Second Edition

5   6   7   8   9   0   DOCDOC   0   9   8   7   6   5   4   3

ISSN: 97-70188
ISBN: 0-07-137826-X

The book was set in Times Roman by Circle Graphics.
The editors were Shelley Reinhardt, Jim Ransom, and Karen Davis.
The production supervisor was Phil Galea.
The cover designer was Mary McKeon.
The index was prepared by Pat Perrier.
R. R. Donnelley/Crawfordsville was the printer and binder.

This book was printed on acid-free paper.

To Camilla Payne

Contents

Contributors

Brendan T. Campbell, MD
Research Fellow, Robert Wood Johnson Clinical Scholars Program,
University of Michigan Medical School, Ann Arbor
btcamp@umich.edu
Common Surgical Disorders

Aaron E. Carroll, MD
Pediatric Resident, Department of Pediatrics, University of
Washington School of Medicine, Seattle
acarro@u.washington.edu
Common Pediatric Disorders

Harold R. Collard, MD
Chief Medical Resident, University of California, San Francisco
collard@itsa.ucsf.edu
References

Mark D. Eisner, MD, MPH
Assistant Professor of Medicine, Division of Occupational &
Environmental Medicine and Division of Pulmonary & Critical
Care Medicine, Department of Medicine, University of California,
San Francisco
eisner@itsa.ucsf.edu
Pulmonary Diseases

Neal Fischbach, MD
Clinical Fellow, Division of Hematology and Oncology, University
of California, San Francisco
fischba@itsa.ucsf.edu
Hematologic Diseases; Oncologic Diseases

Rebecca Ann Jackson, MD
Assistant Professor, Department of Obstetrics, Gynecology, and
Reproductive Sciences, University of California, San Francisco;
Medical Director, Gynecologic Ambulatory Services,
San Francisco General Hospital
jacksonr@obgyn, ucsf.edu
Gynecologic, Obstetric, & Breast Disorders

Ashish K. Jha, MD
Chief Medical Resident, University of California, San Francisco; San
    Francisco Veterans Affairs Medical Center
ashish@itsa.ucsf.edu
References

Jacob Johnson, MD
Resident, Department of Otolaryngology, University of California,
    San Francisco
jacobj@itsa.ucsf.edu
Common Disorders of the Ear, Nose, & Throat

Catherine Bree Johnston, MD, MPH
Assistant Clinical Professor of Medicine, Division of Geriatrics,
    Department of Medicine, University of California, San Francisco;
    Program Director, Geriatric Fellowship, San Francisco Veterans
    Affairs Medical Center
bree526@itsa.ucsf.edu
Geriatric Disorders

S. Claiborne Johnston, MD, PhD
Assistant Professor, Department of Neurology, University of
    California, San Francisco
clayj@itsa.ucsf.edu
Neurologic Diseases

Daniel R. Kaul, MD
Fellow, Division of Infectious Diseases, University of Michigan
    Medical School, Ann Arbor
kauld@med.umich.edu
Infectious Diseases

Kewchang Lee, MD
Assistant Clinical Professor of Psychiatry, University of California,
    San Francisco; Chief of Psychiatry Consultation, San Francisco
    Veterans Affairs Medical Center
kewlee@itsa.ucsf.edu
Psychiatric Disorders

Joan Chia-Mei Lo, MD
Assistant Professor of Medicine, University of California, San
    Francisco; Staff Physician, San Francisco General Hospital
jlo@itsa.ucsf.edu
Endocrine Disorders

Rajesh S. Mangrulkar, MD
Lecturer, Division of General Medicine, Department of Internal
    Medicine, University of Michigan Health System, Ann Arbor, and
    Ann Arbor Veterans Affairs Medical Center
rajm@umich.edu
Fluid, Acid-Base, & Electrolyte Disorders

V. Raman Muthusamy, MD
Assistant Clinical Professor of Medicine, Division of
   Gastroenterology, University of California, San Francisco
Gastrointestinal Diseases; Hepatobiliary Disorders

Brahmajee Nallamothu, MD, MPH
Fellow, Division of Cardiovascular Disease, University of Michigan
   Health System, Ann Arbor
bnallamo@umich.edu
Cardiovascular Diseases

Kurt Robert Oelke, MD
Rheumatology Fellow, Department of Rheumatology, University of
   Michigan Medical School, Ann Arbor
koelke@med.umich.edu
Rheumatologic & Autoimmune Disorders

Stephanie T. Phan, MD
Ophthalmology Resident, University of California, San Francisco
steph_phan@yahoo.com
Common Disorders of the Eye

Jack Resneck, Jr., MD
Chief Resident, Department of Dermatology, University of
   California, San Francisco
resneck@itsa.ucsf.edu
Dermatologic Disorders

Sanjay Saint, MD, MPH
Assistant Professor of Medicine, Division of General Medicine,
   University of Michigan Medical School; Research Scientist, Ann
   Arbor Veterans Affairs Medical Center, Ann Arbor, Michigan
saint@umich.edu
Common Genetic Disorders

Stephen M. Schenkel, MD, MPP
Resident, Department of Emergency Medicine, University of
   Michigan Health System and St. Joseph Mercy Hospital,
   Ann Arbor
sschenke@umich.edu
Poisoning

Lawrence M. Tierney, Jr., MD
Professor of Medicine, University of California, San Francisco;
   Associate Chief of Medical Services, Veterans Affairs Medical
   Center, San Francisco, California
Lawrence.Tierney@med.va.gov
Pearls

Louise C. Walter, MD
Geriatrics Fellow, University of California, San Francisco
louisew@itsa.ucsf.edu
Geriatric Disorders

Suzanne Watnick, MD
Nephrology Fellow, Robert Wood Johnson Clinical Scholar, Yale
    University, Yale-New Haven Hospital, New Haven, Connecticut
suzanne.watnick@yale.edu
Genitourinary & Renal Disorders

Preface

This second edition of *Essentials of Diagnosis Treatment* adds a feature which we believe is unique in medical texts—a Clinical Pearl for each main entity. The Pearl as it has come to be known in medical parlance is a brief aphorism or maxim capsulizing and emphasizing some important principle of diagnosis, treatment, or prognosis—often adorned with intended humor and expressed in colloquial idiom. A Pearl should if possible be "pithy" and memorable, thus expressed sometimes with more certainty than perhaps is warranted by the facts of every case. Some Pearls are truly unforgettable, such as, "A stroke is never a stroke until it's had 50 of D50." One of the authors was offered this Pearl over 30 years ago by an older doctor, and what it means is that focal neurologic deficits may be due to metabolic abnormalities—in particular, severe hypoglycemia—and that appropriate interventions may therefore restore normal nervous system function. While all the Pearls in this book are not as catchy or compelling as that one, they are nonetheless useful teaching aids and we hope the reader enjoys picking them and looking at them. We should be grateful if our readers would send us Pearls of their own for possible inclusion in subsequent editions—and if any of ours seem off the point or unclear, we want to know that, too.

Our modest goal has been to provide a slim volume summarizing the crucial points in diagnosis, differential diagnosis, and treatment of selected diseases. One clinical reference is provided in each case as a starting point for further study.

We want to thank our editor at Lange/McGraw-Hill, Shelley Reinhardt, for support, encouragement, and exhortation without limit in the development of this book.

Lawrence M. Tierney, Jr., MD
Sanjay Saint, MD, MPH
Mary A. Whooley, MD

San Francisco
Ann Arbor
October, 2001

Cardiovascular Diseases

Aortic Dissection

- **Essentials of Diagnosis**
  - Most patients between age 50 and age 70; risks include hypertension, Marfan's syndrome, bicuspid aortic valve, coarctation of the aorta, and pregnancy
  - Type A involves the ascending aorta or arch; type B does not
  - Sudden onset of chest pain with interscapular radiation in at-risk patient
  - Unequal blood pressures in upper extremities; new diastolic murmur of aortic insufficiency occasionally seen in type A
  - Chest x-ray nearly always abnormal; ECG unimpressive unless right coronary artery compromised
  - CT, transesophogeal echocardiography, MRI, or aortography usually diagnostic

- **Differential Diagnosis**
  - Acute myocardial infarction
  - Angina pectoris
  - Acute pericarditis
  - Pneumothorax
  - Pulmonary embolism
  - Boerhaave's syndrome

- **Treatment**
  - Nitroprusside and beta-blockers to lower systolic blood pressure to approximately 100 mm Hg, pulse to 60/min
  - Emergent surgery for type A dissection; medical therapy for type B is reasonable, with surgery or percutaneous intra-aortic stenting reserved for high-risk patients

- **Pearl**

Severe hypertension in a patient appearing to be in shock is aortic dissection until proved otherwise.

Reference

Pretre R et al: Aortic dissection. Lancet 1997;349:1461. [PMID: 9461334]

Pulmonary Stenosis

- **Essentials of Diagnosis**
  - A congenital disorder causing symptoms only when transpulmonary valve gradient is > 50 mm Hg
  - Exertional dyspnea and chest pain due to right ventricular ischemia; sudden death occurs in severe cases
  - Jugular venous distention, parasternal lift, systolic ejection murmur, delayed and soft pulmonary component of S_2
  - Right ventricular hypertrophy on ECG; poststenotic dilation of the main and left pulmonary arteries on chest x-ray
  - Echo-doppler is diagnostic

- **Differential Diagnosis**
  - Left ventricular failure due to any cause
  - Left-sided valvular disease
  - Primary pulmonary hypertension
  - Chronic pulmonary embolism
  - Sleep apnea
  - Chronic obstructive pulmonary disease
  - Eisenmenger's syndrome

- **Treatment**
  - All patients require endocarditis prophylaxis
  - Symptomatic patients with gradients > 50 mm Hg: percutaneous balloon or surgical valvuloplasty; asymptomatic patients with gradients > 75 mm Hg and right ventricular hypertrophy: evaluate for treatment
  - Prognosis for those with mild disease is good

- **Pearl**

Flushing with the murmur as described raises the issue of carcinoid syndrome.

Reference

Gibbs JL: Interventional catheterisation. Opening up I: the ventricular outflow tracts and great arteries. Heart 2000;83:111. [PMID: 10618351]

Aortic Coarctation

- ■ Essentials of Diagnosis
  - Elevated blood pressure in the aortic arch and its branches with reduced blood pressure distal to the left subclavian artery
  - Lower extremity claudication or leg weakness with exertion in young adults is characteristic
  - Systolic blood pressure is higher in the arms than in the legs, but diastolic pressure is similar compared with radial
  - Femoral pulses delayed and decreased, with pulsatile collaterals in the intercostal areas; a harsh, late systolic murmur may be heard in the back; an aortic ejection murmur suggests concomitant bicuspid aortic valve
  - Electrocardiography with left ventricular hypertrophy; chest x-ray may show rib notching inferiorly due to collaterals
  - Transesophageal echo with doppler or MRI is diagnostic; angiography confirms gradient across the coarctation

- ■ Differential Diagnosis
  - Essential hypertension
  - Renal artery stenosis
  - Renal parenchymal disease
  - Pheochromocytoma
  - Mineralocorticoid excess
  - Oral contraceptive use
  - Cushing's syndrome

- ■ Treatment
  - Surgery is the mainstay of therapy; balloon angioplasty in selected patients
  - All patients require endocarditis prophylaxis even after correction
  - Twenty-five percent of patients remain hypertensive after surgery

- ■ Pearl

Hypertension in a patient with a bicuspid aortic valve raises concern about coarctation.

Reference

Ovaert C et al: Balloon angioplasty of native coarctation: clinical outcomes and predictors of success. J Am Coll Cardiol 2000;36;988. [PMID: 10732899]

Atrial Septal Defect

■ **Essentials of Diagnosis**

- Patients with small defects are usually asymptomatic and have a normal life span
- Large shunts symptomatic by age 40, including exertional dyspnea, fatigue, and palpitations
- Paradoxical embolism may occur (ie, upper or lower extremity thrombus embolizing to brain or extremity rather than lung), more typically after shunt reversal
- Right ventricular lift, widened and fixed splitting of S_2, and systolic flow murmur in the pulmonary area
- Electrocardiography may show right ventricular hypertrophy and right axis deviation (in ostium secundum defects), left anterior hemiblock (in ostium primum defects); complete or incomplete right bundle branch block in 95%
- Atrial fibrillation commonly complicates
- Echo-doppler with agitated saline contrast injection is diagnostic; radionuclide angiogram or cardiac catheterization estimates ratio of pulmonary flow to systemic flow (PF:SF)

■ **Differential Diagnosis**

- Left ventricular failure
- Left-sided valvular disease
- Primary pulmonary hypertension
- Chronic pulmonary embolism
- Sleep apnea
- Chronic obstructive pulmonary disease
- Eisenmenger's syndrome
- Pulmonary stenosis

■ **Treatment**

- Small defects do not require surgical correction
- Surgery or percutaneous closure devices indicated for patients with PF:SF > 1.7 or even smaller PF:SF shunts if there is evidence of right ventricular failure
- Surgery is contraindicated in patients with pulmonary hypertension and right-to-left shunting

■ **Pearl**

Endocarditis is rare given low interatrial gradient, and endocarditis prophylaxis is thus unnecessary.

Reference

Meisner H et al: Atrioventricular septal defect. Pediatr Cardiol 1998;19:276. [PMID: 9636249]

Ventricular Septal Defect

- ■ Essentials of Diagnosis
  - Symptoms depend on the size of the defect and the magnitude of the left-to-right shunt
  - Many congenital ventricular septal defects close spontaneously during childhood
  - Small defects in adults are usually asymptomatic except for complicating endocarditis
  - Large defects usually associated with a loud pansystolic murmur along the left sternal border, a systolic thrill, and a loud P_2
  - Echo-doppler diagnostic; radionuclide angiogram or cardiac catheterization quantifies the ratio of pulmonary flow to systemic flow (PF:SF)

- ■ Differential Diagnosis
  - Mitral regurgitation
  - Aortic stenosis
  - Cardiomyopathy due to various causes

- ■ Treatment
  - Small shunts in asymptomatic patients may not require surgery
  - Mild dyspnea can be treated with diuretics and preload reduction
  - PF:SF shunts over 2 are repaired to prevent irreversible pulmonary vascular disease
  - Surgery if patient has developed shunt reversal (Eisenmenger's syndrome) without fixed pulmonary hypertension
  - Prophylaxis for infective endocarditis

- ■ Pearl

The smaller the defect, the more likely that it is endocarditis.

Reference

Belli E et al: Transaortic closure of residual intramural ventricular septal defect. Ann Thorac Surg 2000;69:1496. [PMID: 10881829]

Patent Ductus Arteriosus

- **Essentials of Diagnosis**
  - Caused by failure of closure of embryonic ductus arteriosus with continuous blood flow from aorta to pulmonary artery
  - Symptoms are those of left ventricular failure or pulmonary hypertension; many complaint-free
  - Widened pulse pressure, a loud S_2, and a continuous, "machinery" murmur loudest over the pulmonary area but heard posteriorly
  - Echo-doppler helpful, but contrast or MR aortography is the study of choice

- **Differential Diagnosis**

  In patients presenting with left heart failure:
  - Mitral regurgitation
  - Aortic stenosis
  - Ventricular septal defect

  If pulmonary hypertension dominates the picture, consider:
  - Primary pulmonary hypertension
  - Chronic pulmonary embolism
  - Eisenmenger's syndrome

- **Treatment**
  - Pharmacologic closure in premature infants, using indomethacin or aspirin
  - Surgical or percutaneous closure in patients with large shunts or symptoms; efficacy in the presence of moderate pulmonary hypertension is debated
  - Prophylaxis for infective endocarditis

- **Pearl**

  Patients usually remain asymptomatic as adults if problems have not developed by age 10.

Reference

Rao PS:Transcatheter occlusion of patent ductus arteriosus: which method to use and which ductus to close. Am Heart J 1996;132:905. [PMID: 8831389]

Mitral Stenosis

■ Essentials of Diagnosis

- Always caused by rheumatic heart disease, but 30% of patients have no history of that disorder
- Dyspnea, orthopnea, paroxysmal nocturnal dyspnea, even hemoptysis—often precipitated by volume overload (pregnancy, salt load) or tachycardia
- Right ventricular lift in many; opening snap occasionally palpable
- Crisp S_1, increased P_2, opening snap; these sounds often easier to appreciate than the characteristic low-pitched apical diastolic murmur
- Electrocardiography shows left atrial abnormality and, commonly, atrial fibrillation; echo confirms diagnosis, quantifies severity

■ Differential Diagnosis

- Left ventricular failure due to any cause
- Mitral valve prolapse (if systolic murmur present)
- Pulmonary hypertension due to other cause
- Left atrial myxoma
- Cor triatriatum (in patients under 30)
- Tricuspid stenosis

■ Treatment

- Heart failure symptoms may be treated with diuretics and sodium restriction
- With atrial fibrillation, ventricular rate controlled with beta-blockers, calcium channel blockers such as verapamil, or digoxin; long-term anticoagulation instituted with warfarin
- Valvuloplasty or valve replacement in symptomatic patients with mitral orifice of less than 1.2 cm^2; valvuloplasty preferred in non-calcified valves
- Prophylaxis for beta-hemolytic streptococcal infections until age 25 and for infective endocarditis for lifetime

■ Pearl

Occasional patients have hoarseness due to recurrent laryngeal nerve compression between aorta and pulmonary artery.

Reference

Bruce CJ et al: Clinical assessment and management of mitral stenosis. Cardiol Clin 1998;16:375. [PMID: 9742320]

1

Mitral Regurgitation

- **Essentials of Diagnosis**
  - Causes include rheumatic heart disease, infectious endocarditis, mitral valve prolapse, ischemic papillary muscle dysfunction, torn chordae tendineae
  - Acute: immediate onset of symptoms of pulmonary edema
  - Chronic: asymptomatic for years, then exertional dyspnea and fatigue
  - S_1 usually reduced; a blowing, high-pitched pansystolic murmur increased by finger squeeze over the apex is characteristic; S_3 commonly seen in chronic regurgitation; murmur is not pansystolic and less audible in acute
  - Left atrial abnormality and often left ventricular hypertrophy on ECG; atrial fibrillation typical in chronic cases
  - Echo-doppler confirms diagnosis, estimates severity

- **Differential Diagnosis**
  - Aortic stenosis or sclerosis
  - Tricuspid regurgitation
  - Hypertrophic obstructive cardiomyopathy
  - Atrial septal defect
  - Ventricular septal defect

- **Treatment**
  - Acute mitral regurgitation due to endocarditis or torn chordae may require immediate surgical repair
  - Prophylaxis for infective endocarditis in chronic cases; surgical repair for severe symptoms or for left ventricular dysfunction (eg, ejection fraction < 55%) or for enlargement by echo
  - Mild to moderate symptoms can be treated with diuretics, sodium restriction, and afterload reduction (eg, ACE inhibitors); digoxin, beta-blockers, and calcium channel blockers control ventricular response with atrial fibrillation, and warfarin anticoagulation should be given

- **Pearl**

An overlooked physical sign in mitral regurgitation is a rapid up-and-down carotid pulse.

Reference

Cooper HA et al: Treatment of chronic mitral regurgitation. Am Heart J 1998;135(6 Part 1):925. [PMID: 9630095]

Aortic Stenosis

- **Essentials of Diagnosis**
  - Causes include congenital bicuspid valve and progressive senile calcification of a normal three-leaflet valve; rheumatic fever rarely, if ever, causes isolated aortic stenosis
  - Dyspnea, angina, and syncope singly or in any combination; sudden death in less than 1% of asymptomatic patients
  - Weak and delayed carotid pulses; a soft, absent, or paradoxically split S_2; a harsh diamond-shaped systolic ejection murmur to the right of the sternum, often radiating to the neck
  - Electrocardiography shows left ventricular hypertrophy, and x-ray may show calcification in the aortic valve
  - Echo confirms diagnosis and estimates valve area and gradient; cardiac catheterization confirms severity, documents concomitant coronary atherosclerotic disease, present in 50%

- **Differential Diagnosis**
  - Mitral regurgitation
  - Hypertrophic obstructive or even dilated cardiomyopathy
  - Atrial or ventricular septal defect
  - Syncope due to other causes, eg, ventricular tachycardia

- **Treatment**
  - Surgery is indicated for all symptomatic patients, ideally before heart failure develops
  - Asymptomatic patients with declining left ventricular function considered for surgery if echo-doppler demonstrates a very high aortic valve gradient (> 80 mm Hg) or severely reduced valve areas (≤ 0.7 cm^2)
  - Percutaneous balloon valvuloplasty for temporary (6 months) relief of symptoms in poor surgical candidates

- **Pearl**

Galliverden's phenomenon is the auscultatory finding of an aortic stenosis murmur at both the aortic area and the apex, with no murmur at the left lower sternal border.

Reference

Otto CM: Timing of aortic valve surgery. Heart 2000;84:211. [PMID: 10908267]

Aortic Regurgitation

- **Essentials of Diagnosis**
  - Causes include congenital bicuspid valve, endocarditis, rheumatic heart disease, Marfan's syndrome, aortic dissection, ankylosing spondylitis, reactive arthritis, and syphilis
  - Acute aortic regurgitation: acute onset of pulmonary edema
  - Chronic aortic regurgitation: asymptomatic until middle age, when chest pain or symptoms of left heart failure develop
  - Acute aortic regurgitation: reduced S_1 and an S_3 along with signs of acute pulmonary edema
  - Chronic aortic regurgitation: reduced first heart sound, wide pulse pressure, water-hammer pulse, subungual capillary pulsations (Quincke's sign), rapid rise and fall of pulse (Corrigan's pulse), and a diastolic murmur over a partially compressed femoral artery (Duroziez's sign)
  - Soft, high-pitched, decrescendo diastolic murmur in chronic aortic regurgitation; occasionally, an accompanying apical low-pitched diastolic rumble (Austin Flint murmur) in nonrheumatic patients; in acute aortic regurgitation, the diastolic murmur can be short
  - ECG shows left ventricular hypertrophy, and x-ray shows left ventricular dilation
  - Echo-doppler confirms diagnosis, estimates severity

- **Differential Diagnosis**
  - Pulmonary hypertension with Graham Steell murmur
  - Mitral or, rarely, tricuspid stenosis
  - Left ventricular failure due to other cause
  - Dock's murmur of left anterior descending artery stenosis

- **Treatment**
  - Vasodilators (eg, nifedipine and ACE inhibitors) delay the progression to valve replacement
  - In chronic aortic regurgitation, surgery reserved for patients with symptoms of mild left ventricular dysfunction or enlargement on echocardiography
  - Acute regurgitation caused by aortic dissection or endocarditis requires surgical replacement of the valve

- **Pearl**

The Key-Hodgkin murmur of aortic regurgitation is harsh and raspy and caused by leaflet eventration.

Reference

Bonow RO: Chronic aortic regurgitation. Role of medical therapy and optimal timing for surgery. Cardiol Clin 1998;16:449. [PMID: 9742324]

Tricuspid Stenosis

- ■ Essentials of Diagnosis
  - • Usually rheumatic in origin; rarely, seen in carcinoid heart disease
  - • Almost always associated with mitral stenosis when rheumatic
  - • Evidence of right-sided failure: hepatomegaly, ascites, peripheral edema, jugular venous distention with prominent *(a)* wave
  - • A diastolic rumbling murmur along the left sternal border, increasing with inspiration
  - • Echo-doppler is diagnostic

- ■ Differential Diagnosis
  - • Aortic regurgitation
  - • Mitral stenosis
  - • Pulmonary hypertension due to any cause with right heart failure

- ■ Treatment
  - • Valve replacement in severe cases
  - • Balloon valvuloplasty may prove to be useful in many patients

- ■ Pearl

Three percent of cases of left-sided rheumatic heart disease are associated with tricuspid stenosis.

Reference

Blaustein AS et al: Tricuspid valve disease. Clinical evaluation, physiopathology, and management. Cardiol Clin 1998;16:551. [PMID: 9742330]

1

Tricuspid Regurgitation

- **Essentials of Diagnosis**
  - Causes include infective endocarditis, right ventricular heart failure, carcinoid syndrome, systemic lupus erythematosus, and Ebstein's anomaly
  - Most cases secondary to dilation of the right ventricle from left-sided heart disease
  - Edema, abdominal discomfort, anorexia; otherwise, symptoms of associated disease
  - Prominent *(v)* waves in jugular venous pulse; pulsatile liver, abdominojugular reflux
  - Characteristic high-pitched blowing holosystolic murmur along the left sternal border increasing with inspiration
  - Echo-doppler is diagnostic

- **Differential Diagnosis**
  - Mitral regurgitation
  - Aortic stenosis
  - Pulmonary stenosis
  - Atrial septal defect
  - Ventricular septal defect

- **Treatment**
  - Diuretics and dietary sodium restriction in patients with evidence of fluid overload
  - If symptoms are severe and tricuspid regurgitation is primary, valve repair, valvuloplasty, or removal is preferable to valve replacement

- **Pearl**

Over 90% of apparently isolated right heart failure is caused by left-sided failure.

Reference

Waller BF et al: Pathology of tricuspid valve stenosis and pure tricuspid regurgitation—Part II. Clin Cardiol 1995;18:167. [PMID: 7743689]

Angina Pectoris

- ■ Essentials of Diagnosis
  - Pressure-like episodic precordial chest discomfort, precipitated by exertion or stress, relieved by rest or nitrates
  - Generally caused by atherosclerotic coronary artery disease; cigarette smoking, diabetes, hypertension, hypercholesterolemia, and family history are established risk factors
  - S_4, S_3, mitral murmur may occur transiently with pain
  - Electrocardiography usually normal between episodes (or may show evidence of old infarction); electrocardiography with pain usually shows evidence of ischemia, classically ST depression
  - Diagnosis from history and stress tests; confirmed and staged by coronary arteriography

- ■ Differential Diagnosis
  - Other coronary syndromes (myocardial infarction, unstable angina, vasospasm)
  - Tietze's syndrome (costochondritis)
  - Intercostal neuropathy, especially caused by herpes zoster
  - Cervical radiculopathy
  - Peptic ulcer disease
  - Esophageal spasm or reflux disease
  - Cholecystitis
  - Pneumothorax
  - Pulmonary embolism
  - Pneumonia

- ■ Treatment
  - Address reversible risk factors (smoking, hypertension, hypercholesterolemia, hyperglycemia)
  - Sublingual nitroglycerin as needed for individual episodes
  - Ongoing treatment includes aspirin, long-acting nitrates, beta-blockers, and calcium channel blockers
  - Angioplasty with or without stenting considered in patients with anatomically suitable stenoses who remain symptomatic on medical therapy
  - Bypass grafting for patients with refractory angina on medical therapy, three-vessel disease (or two-vessel disease with proximal left anterior descending artery disease) and decreased left ventricular function, or left main coronary artery disease

- ■ Pearl

Up to 20% of patients with ischemic episodes do not show electrocardiographic changes with pain.

Reference

Lee TH et al: Evaluation of the patient with acute chest pain. N Engl J Med 2000;342:1187. [PMID: 10770985]

Prinzmetal's Angina

- ■ Essentials of Diagnosis
  - Caused by intermittent focal spasm of an otherwise normal coronary artery
  - The chest pain resembles typical angina; often more severe and occurs at rest
  - Affects women under 50, occurs in the early morning, and typically involves the right coronary artery
  - Electrocardiography shows ST elevation, but enzyme studies are normal
  - Diagnosis can be confirmed by ergonovine challenge during cardiac catheterization

- ■ Differential Diagnosis
  - Typical angina pectoris
  - Myocardial infarction
  - Unstable angina
  - Tietze's syndrome (costochondritis)
  - Cervical radiculopathy
  - Peptic ulcer disease
  - Esophageal spasm or reflux disease
  - Cholecystitis
  - Pericarditis
  - Pneumothorax
  - Pulmonary embolism
  - Pneumonia

- ■ Treatment
  - Nitrates and calcium channel blockers effective acutely
  - Long-acting nitrates and calcium channel blockers are the mainstay of chronic therapy
  - Stenting in affected coronary artery (usually right) in some, but prognosis excellent given absence of atherosclerosis

- ■ Pearl

Cocaine use can lead to myocardial ischemia or infarction from vasospasm.

Reference

Yasue H et al: Coronary spasm: clinical features and pathogenesis. Intern Med 1997;36:760. [PMID: 9392345]

Unstable Angina

- **Essentials of Diagnosis**
  - Spectrum of illness between chronic stable angina and acute myocardial infarction
  - Characterized by accelerating angina, pain at rest, or pain that is less responsive to medications
  - Usually due to atherosclerotic plaque rupture, spasm, hemorrhage, or thrombosis
  - Chest pain resembles typical angina but is more severe and lasts longer (up to 30 minutes)
  - ECG may show dynamic ST depression or T wave changes during pain but normalizes when symptoms abate; a normal ECG, however, does not rule out unstable angina

- **Differential Diagnosis**
  - Typical angina pectoris
  - Myocardial infarction
  - Coronary vasospasm
  - Aortic dissection
  - Tietze's syndrome (costochondritis)
  - Cervical radiculopathy
  - Peptic ulcer disease
  - Esophageal spasm or reflux disease
  - Cholecystitis
  - Pericarditis
  - Pneumothorax
  - Pulmonary embolism
  - Pneumonia

- **Treatment**
  - Hospitalization with bed rest, telemetry, and exclusion of myocardial infarction
  - Low-dose aspirin (81–325 mg) should be given immediately on admission and every day thereafter; intravenous heparin is of benefit in some
  - Beta-blockers to keep heart rate and blood pressure in the low-normal range
  - In high-risk patients, glycoprotein IIb/IIIa inhibitors shown to be of benefit, especially if percutaneous intervention likely
  - Nitroglycerin, either in paste or intravenously
  - Cardiac catheterization and consideration of revascularization in appropriate candidates

- **Pearl**

Aortic dissection should be considered in any chest pain syndrome for which aggressive anticoagulation is being contemplated.

Reference

Ambrose JA et al: Unstable angina: current concepts of pathogenesis and treatment. Arch Intern Med 2000;160:25. [PMID: 10632302]

1

Acute Myocardial Infarction

- **Essentials of Diagnosis**
  - Prolonged (> 30 minutes) chest pain, associated with shortness of breath, nausea, left arm or neck pain, and diaphoresis; can be painless in diabetics
  - S_4 common; S_3, mitral insufficiency on occasion
  - Cardiogenic shock, ventricular arrhythmias may complicate
  - Electrocardiography shows ST elevation or depression, T wave inversion, or evolving Q waves; however, can be normal or unchanged in up to 10%
  - Elevated cardiac enzymes (troponin, CKMB)
  - Regional wall motion changes by echo
  - Non-Q wave infarct may mean additional jeopardized myocardium

- **Differential Diagnosis**
  - Stable or unstable angina
  - Tietze's syndrome (costochondritis)
  - Aortic dissection
  - Cervical radiculopathy
  - Carpal tunnel syndrome
  - Esophageal spasm or reflux
  - Pulmonary embolism
  - Cholecystitis
  - Pericarditis
  - Pneumothorax
  - Pneumonia

- **Treatment**
  - Monitoring, aspirin, and analgesia for all; heparin for most
  - Reperfusion by thrombolysis or angioplasty in selected patients with either ST segment elevation or new left bundle branch block on ECG
  - Glycoprotein IIb/IIIa inhibitors considered in non-Q wave infarcts
  - Beta-blockers for heart rate and blood pressure control, and survival advantage when given chronically
  - Nitroglycerin for recurrent ischemic pain; also useful for relieving pulmonary congestion and reducing blood pressure
  - ACE inhibitor may confer survival benefit

- **Pearl**

Monitoring for prompt treatment of ventricular fibrillation remains the most cost-effective intervention to prolong life.

Reference

Maynard S et al: Management of acute coronary syndromes. BMJ 2000;321:220. [PMID: 10903658]

Atrial Fibrillation

- ■ Essentials of Diagnosis
  - • The most common chronic arrhythmia
  - • Causes include mitral valve disease, hypertensive and ischemic heart disease, dilated cardiomyopathy, alcohol use, hyperthyroidism, pericarditis, cardiac surgery; many are idiopathic ("lone" atrial fibrillation)
  - • Complications include precipitation of cardiac failure, arterial embolization
  - • Palpitations, shortness of breath, chest pain common
  - • Irregularly irregular heartbeat, variable intensity S_1, occasional S_3; S_4 absent in all
  - • Electrocardiography shows ventricular rate of 80–170/min in untreated patients; if associated with an accessory pathway, the ventricular rate can be > 200/min with wide QRS and antegrade conduction through the pathway

- ■ Differential Diagnosis
  - • Multifocal atrial tachycardia
  - • Atrial flutter or tachycardia with variable block
  - • Sinus arrhythmia
  - • Normal sinus rhythm with multiple premature contractions

- ■ Treatment
  - • Control ventricular response with digoxin, beta-blocker, calcium channel blocker—choice depending upon contractile state of left ventricle
  - • Cardioversion with countershock in unstable patients with acute atrial fibrillation; elective countershock or antiarrhythmic agents (eg, ibutilide, procainamide, amiodarone, sotalol) in stable patients once a left atrial thrombus has been ruled out or effectively treated
  - • Chronic warfarin or aspirin in all patients not cardioverted
  - • With elective cardioversion, anticoagulation for 4 weeks prior to and 4 weeks after the procedure unless transesophageal echocardiography excludes a left atrial thrombus

- ■ Pearl

Atrial fibrillation is a relatively uncommon rhythm in acute myocardial infarction and implies the presence of pericarditis.

Reference

Prystowsky EN: Management of atrial fibrillation: therapeutic options and clinical decisions. Am J Cardiol 2000;85:3D. [PMID: 10822035]

1

Atrial Flutter

- **Essentials of Diagnosis**
  - Especially common in COPD; also seen in dilated cardiomyopathy, especially in alcoholics
  - Atrial rate between 250 and 350 beats/min with every second, third, or fourth impulse conducted by the ventricle
  - Patients may be asymptomatic, complain of palpitations, or have evidence of congestive heart failure
  - Flutter *(a)* waves visible in the neck in occasional patients
  - Electrocardiography shows "sawtooth" P waves in V_1 and the inferior leads; ventricular response usually regular; less commonly, irregular due to variable atrioventricular block

- **Differential Diagnosis**
  With regular ventricular rate:
  - Automatic atrial tachycardia
  - Atrioventricular nodal reentry tachycardia
  - Sinus tachycardia
  With irregular ventricular rate:
  - Atrial fibrillation
  - Multifocal atrial tachycardia

- **Treatment**
  - Often spontaneously converts to atrial fibrillation
  - Electrical cardioversion is reliable and safe
  - Conversion may also be achieved by drugs (eg, ibutilide)
  - Risk of embolization is lower than for atrial fibrillation, but anticoagulation still recommended
  - Amiodarone in patients with chronic atrial flutter
  - Consider radiofrequency ablation in patients with chronic atrial flutter refractory to medical therapy

- **Pearl**
  A regular heart rate of 140–150 in a patient with COPD is flutter until proved otherwise.

Reference

Campbell, RW: Atrial flutter. Eur Heart J 1998;19(Suppl E):E37. [PMID: 9717023]

Multifocal Atrial Tachycardia

- ■ Essentials of Diagnosis
  - • Classically seen in patients with severe COPD; electrolyte abnormalities (especially hypomagnesemia or hypokalemia) may also be responsible
  - • Symptoms those of the underlying disorder, but some may complain of palpitations
  - • Irregularly irregular heart rate
  - • Electrocardiography shows at least three different P wave morphologies with varying P–P intervals
  - • Ventricular rate usually between 100 and 140 beats/min; if less than 100, rhythm is wandering atrial pacemaker

- ■ Differential Diagnosis
  - • Normal sinus rhythm with multiple premature atrial contractions
  - • Atrial fibrillation
  - • Atrial flutter with variable block
  - • Reentry tachycardia with variable block

- ■ Treatment
  - • Treatment of the underlying disorder is most important
  - • Verapamil particularly useful for rate control; digitalis ineffective
  - • Intravenous magnesium and potassium administered slowly may convert some patients to sinus rhythm even if serum levels are within normal range
  - • Medications causing atrial irritability, such as theophylline, should be avoided
  - • Atrioventricular nodal ablation with permanent pacing is used in rare cases that are refractory to pharmacologic therapy

- ■ Pearl

Irregularly irregular rhythm in COPD is more commonly multifocal atrial tachycardia than atrial fibrillation.

Reference

McCord J et al: Multifocal atrial tachycardia. Chest 1998;113:203. [PMID: 9440591]

| 1 | **Paroxysmal Supraventricular Tachycardia (PSVT)** |

■ Essentials of Diagnosis

- A group of arrhythmias including supraventricular reentrant tachycardia (over 90% of cases), automatic atrial tachycardia, and junctional tachycardia
- Attacks usually begin and end abruptly, last seconds to hours
- Patients often asymptomatic but occasionally complain of palpitations, mild shortness of breath, or chest pain
- Electrocardiography between attacks normal unless the patient has Wolff-Parkinson-White syndrome
- Unless aberrant conduction occurs, the QRS complexes are regular and narrow; the location of the P wave helps determine the origin of the PSVT
- Electrophysiologic study establishes the exact diagnosis

■ Differential Diagnosis

No P:
- Atrioventricular nodal reentry tachycardia

Short RP:
- Atrioventricular reentrant tachycardia
- Intra-atrial reentry tachycardia

Long RP:
- Atrial tachycardia
- Some atrioventricular nodal reentry tachycardia
- Permanent junctional reciprocating tachycardia

■ Treatment

- Many attacks resolve spontaneously; if not, first try vagal maneuvers such as carotid sinus massage
- Prevention of frequent attacks can be achieved by digoxin, calcium channel blockers, beta-blockers, or antiarrhythmics such as procainamide or sotalol; many believe electrophysiologic study and ablation of the abnormal reentrant circuit or focus, when available, is the treatment of choice (> 90% success rate)

■ Pearl

In Q-wave infarct computer readouts with short PR intervals, look carefully for a delta wave.

Reference

Basta M et al: Current role of pharmacologic therapy for patients with paroxysmal supraventricular tachycardia. Cardiol Clin 1997;15:587. [PMID: 9403162]

Ventricular Tachycardia

- **Essentials of Diagnosis**
  - Three or more consecutive premature ventricular beats; non-sustained (lasting < 30 seconds) or sustained
  - Mechanisms are reentry or automatic focus; may occur spontaneously or with myocardial infarction
  - Other causes include acute or chronic ischemia, cardiomyopathy, and drugs (eg, antiarrhythmics)
  - Most patients symptomatic; syncope, palpitations, shortness of breath, and chest pain are common
  - S_1 of variable intensity; S_3 present
  - Electrocardiography shows a regular, wide-complex tachycardia (usually between 140 and 220 beats/min); between attacks, the ECG often shows evidence of prior myocardial infarction

- **Differential Diagnosis**
  - Any cause of supraventricular tachycardia with aberrant conduction (but a history of myocardial infarction or low ejection fraction indicates ventricular tachycardia until proved otherwise)
  - Atrial flutter with aberrant conduction

- **Treatment**
  - Depends upon whether the patient is stable or unstable
  - If stable: intravenous lidocaine, procainamide, or amiodarone can be used initially
  - If unstable (hypotension, congestive heart failure, or angina): immediate synchronized cardioversion
  - For chronic, recurrent, sustained ventricular tachycardia, either automatic implantable cardiac defibrillator placement or suppressive treatment guided by electrophysiologic studies should be considered
  - Treatment of recurrent asymptomatic, nonsustained ventricular tachycardia is controversial; in a patient with ischemic heart disease and a low left ventricular ejection fraction (<35%), an implantable cardiac defibrillator or electrophysiologic study should be considered

- **Pearl**

The first 60 beats may be slightly irregular and misdiagnosed as atrial fibrillation with aberrant conduction.

Reference

Doherty JU et al: Ventricular arrhythmias. Preventing sudden death with drugs and ICD devices. Geriatrics 2000;55:26. [PMID: 10953684]

Sudden Cardiac Death

- **Essentials of Diagnosis**
  - Death in a well patient within 1 hour of symptom onset
  - Sudden death can be due to cardiac or noncardiac disease
  - Most common cause (over 80% of cases) is ventricular fibrillation or tachycardia in the setting of coronary artery disease
  - Ventricular fibrillation is almost always the terminal rhythm

- **Differential Diagnosis**

  Noncardiac causes of sudden death:
  - Pulmonary embolism
  - Asthma
  - Aortic dissection
  - Ruptured aortic aneurysm
  - Intracranial hemorrhage
  - Tension pneumothorax
  - Anaphylaxis

- **Treatment**
  - If sudden cardiac death occurs in the setting of acute myocardial infarction, long-term management is no different from that of other patients with myocardial infarction
  - In the absence of myocardial infarction, the recurrence rate of sudden cardiac death in ischemic disease is 50% in 2 years; therefore, an aggressive approach (cardiac catheterization, revascularization) to prevent another event is warranted
  - Electrolyte abnormalities, digitalis toxicity, pacemaker malfunction can be the cause and are treated accordingly
  - Without an obvious cause, echocardiography and cardiac catheterization indicated; electrophysiologic studies in patients with normal echo-doppler and coronary anatomy
  - A transvenous cardiac defibrillator is strongly considered in all patients surviving an episode of sudden cardiac death secondary to ventricular fibrillation or tachycardia without a transient or reversible cause

- **Pearl**

  In sudden cardiac death in adults, if myocardial infarction is ruled out, the prognosis is paradoxically worse than if ruled in—it suggests that active ischemia is still ongoing, and urgent cardiac catheterization is obligatory.

Reference

Goldberger JJ: Treatment and prevention of sudden cardiac death: effect of recent clinical trials. Arch Intern Med 1999;159:1281. [PMID: 10386504]

Atrioventricular Block

1

- **Essentials of Diagnosis**
  - First-degree block: delayed conduction at the level of the atrioventricular node; PR interval > 0.20 s
  - Second-degree block; Mobitz I–progressive prolongation of the PR interval and decreasing R–R interval prior to a blocked sinus impulse; Mobitz II shows fixed PR intervals before a beat is dropped
  - Third-degree block is due to complete block at or below the node; P waves and QRS complexes occur independently of one another, both at fixed rates
  - Clinical manifestations of third-degree block include chest pain, syncope, and shortness of breath; cannon *(a)* waves in neck veins; first heart sound varies in intensity

- **Differential Diagnosis**

  Causes of first-degree and Mobitz I atrioventricular block:
  - Increased vagal tone
  - Drugs that prolong atrioventricular conduction

  Causes of Mobitz II and third-degree atrioventricular block:
  - Chronic degenerative conduction system disease (Lev's and Lenegre's syndromes)
  - Acute myocardial infarction; inferior myocardial infarction causes complete block at the node, anterior myocardial infarction below it
  - Acute myocarditis (eg, Lyme disease, viral myocarditis)
  - Digitalis toxicity
  - Congenital

- **Treatment**
  - In symptomatic patients with Mobitz I, permanent pacing
  - For those with Mobitz II or infranodal third-degree atrioventricular block, permanent pacing unless a reversible cause (eg, drug toxicity, inferior myocardial infarction, Lyme disease) is present

- **Pearl**

  A "circus of atrial sounds" may be created by atrial contractions at different rates than ventricular, eg, in complete heart block.

Reference

Hayes DL: Evolving indications for permanent pacing. Am J Cardiol 1999; 83(5B):161D. [PMID: 10089860]

1

Congestive Heart Failure

- **Essentials of Diagnosis**
  - Two pathophysiologic categories: systolic dysfunction and diastolic dysfunction
  - Systolic: the ability to pump blood is compromised; ejection fraction is decreased; causes include coronary artery disease, dilated cardiomyopathy, myocarditis, "burned-out" hypertensive heart disease, and valvular heart disease
  - Diastolic heart unable to relax and allow adequate diastolic filling; normal ejection fraction; causes include ischemia, hypertension with left ventricular hypertrophy, aortic stenosis, hypertrophic cardiomyopathy, restrictive cardiomyopathy, and small vessel disease (eg, diabetes mellitus)
  - Evidence of both common, but up to 20% of patients will have isolated diastolic dysfunction
  - Symptoms and signs can result from left-sided failure, right-sided failure, or both
  - Left ventricular failure: exertional dyspnea, orthopnea, paroxysmal nocturnal dyspnea, pulsus alternans, rales, gallop rhythm; pulmonary venous congestion on chest x-ray
  - Right ventricular failure: fatigue, malaise, elevated venous pressure, hepatomegaly, and dependent edema
  - Diagnosis confirmed by echo or pulmonary capillary wedge measurement

- **Differential Diagnosis**
  - Pericardial disease
  - Nephrosis or cirrhosis
  - Hypothyroidism

- **Treatment**
  - Systolic dysfunction: vasodilators (ACE inhibitors or combination of hydralazine and isosorbide dinitrate), beta-blockers, spironolactone, and low-sodium diet; for symptoms, use diuretics and digoxin; anticoagulation advocated by many in high-risk patients
  - Diastolic dysfunction: a negative inotrope (beta-blocker or calcium channel blocker), low-sodium diet, and diuretics for symptoms

- **Pearl**

Ninety-five percent of right heart failure is caused by left heart failure.

Reference

Watson RD et al: ABC of heart failure. Clinical features and complications. BMJ;2000;320:236. [PMID: 10642237]

Myocarditis

- ■ Essentials of Diagnosis
  - • Focal or diffuse inflammation of the myocardium due to various infections, toxins, drugs, or immunologic reactions; viral infection, particularly with coxsackieviruses, is the most common cause
  - • Other infectious causes include Rocky mountain spotted fever, Q fever, Chagas' disease, Lyme disease, AIDS, trichinosis, toxoplasmosis, and acute rheumatic fever
  - • Symptoms include fever, fatigue, palpitations, chest pain, or symptoms of congestive heart failure, often following an upper respiratory tract infection
  - • Electrocardiography may reveal ST–T wave changes, conduction blocks
  - • Echocardiography shows diffusely depressed left ventricular function and enlargement
  - • Routine myocardial biopsy usually not recommended since inflammatory changes are often focal and nonspecific

- ■ Differential Diagnosis
  - • Acute myocardial ischemia or infarction due to coronary artery disease
  - • Pneumonia
  - • Congestive heart failure due to other causes

- ■ Treatment
  - • Bed rest
  - • Specific antimicrobial treatment if an infectious agent can be identified
  - • Immunosuppressive therapy is controversial
  - • Appropriate treatment of the systolic dysfunction that may develop: vasodilators (ACE inhibitors or combination of hydralazine and isosorbide dinitrate), beta-blockers, spironolactone, digoxin, low-sodium diet, and diuretics

- ■ Pearl

"Rule of thirds" for patients with viral myocarditis: one-third return to normal, one-third have stable left ventricular dysfunction, and one-third have a rapidly deteriorating course.

Reference

Pisani B et al: Inflammatory myocardial diseases and cardiomyopathies. Am J Med 1997;102:459. [PMID: 9217643]

1

Dilated Cardiomyopathy

■ Essentials of Diagnosis

- A cause of systolic dysfunction, this represents a group of disorders that lead to congestive heart failure
- Symptoms and signs of congestive heart failure: exertional dyspnea, cough, fatigue, paroxysmal nocturnal dyspnea, cardiac enlargement, rales, gallop rhythm, elevated venous pressure, hepatomegaly, and dependent edema
- Electrocardiography may show nonspecific repolarization abnormalities and atrial or ventricular ectopy but is not diagnostic
- Echocardiography reveals depressed contractile function and cardiomegaly
- Cardiac catheterization useful to exclude ischemia as a cause

■ Differential Diagnosis

Causes of dilated cardiomyopathy:
- Alcoholism
- Post viral myocarditis
- Sarcoidosis
- Postpartum
- Doxorubicin toxicity
- Endocrinopathies (thyroid disease, acromegaly, pheochromocytoma)
- Hemochromatosis
- Idiopathic

■ Treatment

- Treat the underlying disorder when identifiable
- Abstention from alcohol
- Routine management of systolic dysfunction, including with vasodilators (ACE inhibitors or a combination of hydralazine and isosorbide dinitrate), beta-blockers, spironolactone, and low-sodium diet; digoxin and diuretics for symptoms

■ Pearl

Causes of death: one-third pump failure, one-third arrhythmia, one-third stroke, of which the latter is most preventable.

Reference

Elliott P: Cardiomyopathy. Diagnosis and management of dilated cardiomyopathy. Heart 2000;84:106. [PMID: 20321212]

Hypertrophic Obstructive Cardiomyopathy (HOCM)

- **Essentials of Diagnosis**
  - Asymmetric myocardial hypertrophy causing dynamic obstruction to left ventricular outflow below the aortic valve
  - Sporadic or dominantly inherited
  - Obstruction is worsened by increasing left ventricular contractility or decreasing filling
  - Symptoms are dyspnea, chest pain, and syncope; a subgroup of younger patients is at high risk for sudden cardiac death (1% per year), especially with exercise
  - Sustained, bifid (rarely trifid) apical impulse, S_4
  - Electrocardiography shows exaggerated septal Q waves suggestive of myocardial infarction; supraventricular and ventricular arrhythmias may also be seen
  - Echocardiography with hypertrophy, evidence of dynamic obstruction from abnormal systolic motion of the anterior mitral valve leaflet

- **Differential Diagnosis**
  - Hypertensive heart disease
  - Restrictive cardiomyopathy (eg, amyloidosis)
  - Aortic stenosis
  - Ischemic heart disease
  - Athlete's heart

- **Treatment**
  - Beta-blockers are the initial drug of choice in symptomatic patients, especially those with evidence of dynamic obstruction
  - Calcium channel blockers may also be useful
  - Otherwise, surgical myectomy, percutaneous transcoronary septal reduction with alcohol, or dual-chamber pacing are considered; automatic implantable cardiac defibrillator, amiodarone in patients at high risk for sudden death is controversial
  - Natural history is unpredictable; sports requiring high cardiac output should be discouraged
  - All first-degree relatives evaluated with echocardiography
  - Prophylaxis for infective endocarditis is required

- **Pearl**

Hypertrophic cardiomyopathy is the pathologic feature most frequently associated with sudden death in athletes.

Reference

Spirito P et al: Perspectives on the role of new treatment strategies in hypertrophic obstructive cardiomyopathy. J Am Coll Cardiol 1999;33:1071. [PMID: 10091838]

1

Restrictive Cardiomyopathy

- **Essentials of Diagnosis**
  - Characterized by impaired diastolic filling with preserved left ventricular function
  - Causes include amyloidosis, sarcoidosis, hemochromatosis, scleroderma, carcinoid syndrome, endomyocardial fibrosis, and post-radiation or postsurgical fibrosis
  - Clinical manifestations are those of the underlying disorder; congestive heart failure with right-sided symptoms and signs usually predominates
  - Electrocardiography may show low voltage and nonspecific ST–T wave abnormalities; supraventricular and ventricular arrhythmias may also be seen
  - Echo-doppler shows increased wall thickness with preserved contractile function and mitral and tricuspid inflow velocity patterns consistent with impaired diastolic filling

- **Differential Diagnosis**
  - Constrictive pericarditis
  - Hypertensive heart disease
  - Hypertrophic obstructive cardiomyopathy
  - Aortic stenosis
  - Ischemic heart disease

- **Treatment**
  - Sodium restriction and diuretic therapy for patients with evidence of fluid overload; diuresis must be cautious, as volume depletion may worsen this disorder
  - Digitalis is not indicated unless systolic function becomes impaired or atrial fibrillation occurs
  - Treatment of underlying disease causing the restriction if possible

- **Pearl**

Hemochromatosis is characterized by diagnostic T2-weighted images of the heart and other involved organs; one-third of patients have whiter right upper quadrants on plain chest films.

Reference

Kushwasha SS et al: Restrictive cardiomyopathy. N Engl J Med 1997;336:267. [PMID: 8995091]

Acute Rheumatic Fever

- **Essentials of Diagnosis**
  - A systemic immune process complicating group A beta-hemolytic streptococcal pharyngitis
  - Usually affects children between the ages of 5 and 15; rare after 25
  - Occurs 1–5 weeks after throat infection
  - Diagnosis based on Jones criteria (two major or one major and two minor) and confirmation of recent streptococcal infection
  - Major criteria: erythema marginatum, migratory polyarthritis, subcutaneous nodules, carditis, and Sydenham's chorea; the latter is the most specific, least sensitive
  - Minor criteria: fever, arthralgias, elevated erythrocyte sedimentation rate, elevated C-reactive protein, PR prolongation on ECG, and history of rheumatic fever

- **Differential Diagnosis**
  - Juvenile or adult rheumatoid arthritis
  - Endocarditis
  - Osteomyelitis
  - Systemic lupus erythematosus
  - Lyme disease
  - Disseminated gonococcal infection

- **Treatment**
  - Bed rest until vital signs and ECG become normal
  - Salicylates and nonsteroidal anti-inflammatory drugs reduce fever and joint complaints but do not affect the natural course of the disease; rarely, corticosteroids may be used
  - If streptococcal infection is still present, penicillin is indicated
  - Prevention of recurrent streptococcal pharyngitis in patients less than 25 years old (a monthly injection of benzathine penicillin is most commonly used)

- **Pearl**

Inappropriate tachycardia in a child with a recent sore throat suggests rheumatic fever.

Reference

da Silva NA et al: Rheumatic fever. Still a challenge. Rheum Dis Clin North Am 1997;23:545. [PMID: 9287377]

1

Acute Pericarditis

- **Essentials of Diagnosis**
  - Inflammation of the pericardium due to viral infection, drugs, myocardial infarction, autoimmune syndromes, renal failure, cardiac surgery, trauma, or neoplasm
  - Common symptoms include pleuritic chest pain radiating to the shoulder (trapezius ridge) and dyspnea; pain improves with sitting up and expiration
  - Examination may reveal fever, tachycardia, and an intermittent friction rub; clinical manifestations of cardiac tamponade may occur in any patient
  - Electrocardiography usually shows PR depression, diffuse ST segment elevation followed by T wave inversions
  - Echocardiography may reveal pericardial effusion

- **Differential Diagnosis**
  - Acute myocardial infarction
  - Aortic dissection
  - Pulmonary embolism
  - Pneumothorax
  - Pneumonia
  - Cholecystitis

- **Treatment**
  - Aspirin or nonsteroidal anti-inflammatory agents such as ibuprofen or indomethacin to relieve symptoms; rarely, steroids for recurrent cases
  - Hospitalization for patients with symptoms suggestive of significant effusions or cardiac tamponade

- **Pearl**

Patients with uremic pericarditis characteristically are afebrile, and many lack ST segment elevation.

Reference

Oakley CM: Myocarditis, pericarditis and other pericardial diseases. Heart 2000;84:449. [PMID: 10995424]

Cardiac Tamponade

- **Essentials of Diagnosis**
  - Life-threatening disorder occurring when pericardial fluid accumulates under pressure; effusions increasing rapidly in size may cause an elevated intrapericardial pressure (> 15 mm Hg), leading to impaired cardiac filling and decreased cardiac output
  - Common causes include metastatic malignancy, uremia, viral or idiopathic pericarditis, and cardiac trauma; however, any cause of pericarditis can cause tamponade
  - Clinical manifestations include dyspnea, cough, tachycardia, hypotension, pulsus paradoxus, jugular venous distention, and distant heart sounds
  - Electrocardiography usually shows low QRS voltage and occasionally electrical alternans; chest x-ray shows an enlarged cardiac silhouette with a "water-bottle" configuration if a large (> 250 mL) effusion is present—which it need not be if effusion develops rapidly
  - Echocardiography delineates effusion and its hemodynamic significance, eg, atrial collapse; cardiac catheterization confirms the diagnosis if equalization of diastolic pressures in all four chambers occurs and there is loss of the normal y-descent

- **Differential Diagnosis**
  - Tension pneumothorax
  - Right ventricular infarction
  - Severe left ventricular failure
  - Constrictive pericarditis
  - Restrictive cardiomyopathy
  - Pneumonia with septic shock

- **Treatment**
  - Immediate pericardiocentesis
  - Volume expansion until pericardiocentesis is performed
  - Definitive treatment for reaccumulation may require surgical anterior and posterior pericardiectomy or percutaneous balloon pericardiotomy

- **Pearl**

Pulsus paradoxus is useful only in regular rhythms.

Reference

Tsang TS: Diagnosis and management of cardiac tamponade in the era of echocardiography. Clin Cardiol 1999;22:446. [PMID: 10410287]

1

Constrictive Pericarditis

- **Essentials of Diagnosis**
  - A thickened fibrotic pericardium impairing cardiac filling and decreasing cardiac output
  - May follow tuberculosis, cardiac surgery, radiation therapy, or viral, uremic, or neoplastic pericarditis
  - Symptoms include gradual onset of dyspnea, fatigue, weakness, pedal edema, and abdominal swelling; right-sided heart failure symptoms often predominate, with ascites sometimes disproportionate to pedal edema
  - Physical examination reveals tachycardia, elevated jugular venous distention with rapid y-descent, Kussmaul's sign, hepatosplenomegaly, ascites, "pericardial knock" following S_2, and peripheral edema
  - Pericardial calcification on chest film in less than half; electrocardiography may show low QRS voltage; liver function tests abnormal from passive congestion
  - Echocardiography can demonstrate a thick pericardium and normal left ventricular function; CT or MRI is more sensitive in revealing pericardial pathology; cardiac catheterization demonstrates dip-and-plateau pattern to left and right ventricular diastolic pressure tracings with a prominent y-descent (in contrast to restrictive cardiomyopathy)

- **Differential Diagnosis**
  - Cardiac tamponade
  - Right ventricular infarction
  - Restrictive cardiomyopathy
  - Cirrhosis with ascites (most common misdiagnosis)

- **Treatment**
  - Acute treatment usually includes gentle diuresis
  - Definitive therapy is surgical stripping of the pericardium
  - Evaluation for tuberculosis

- **Pearl**

Constriction should be excluded in a patient with new onset ascites felt due to cirrhosis.

Reference

Myers RB et al: Constrictive pericarditis: clinical and pathophysiologic characteristics. Am Heart J 1999;138(2 Part 1):219. [PMID: 10426832]

Cor Pulmonale

- **Essentials of Diagnosis**
  - Heart failure resulting from pulmonary disease
  - Most commonly due to COPD; other causes include pulmonary fibrosis, pneumoconioses, recurrent pulmonary emboli, primary pulmonary hypertension, sleep apnea, and kyphoscoliosis
  - Clinical manifestations are due to both the underlying pulmonary disease and the right ventricular failure
  - Chest x-ray reveals an enlarged right ventricle and pulmonary artery; electrocardiography may show right axis deviation, right ventricular hypertrophy, and tall, peaked P waves (P pulmonale) in the face of low QRS voltage
  - Pulmonary function tests usually confirm the presence of underlying lung disease, and echocardiography will show right ventricular dilation but normal left ventricular function and elevated right-ventricular systolic pressures

- **Differential Diagnosis**
  Other causes of right ventricular failure:
  - Left ventricular failure (due to any cause)
  - Pulmonary stenosis
  - Left-to-right shunt causing Eisenmenger's syndrome

- **Treatment**
  - Treatment is primarily directed at the pulmonary process causing the right heart failure (eg, oxygen if hypoxia is present)
  - In frank right ventricular failure, include salt restriction, diuretics, and oxygen
  - For primary pulmonary hypertension, cautious use of vasodilators (calcium channel blockers) or continuous infusion prostacyclin may benefit some patients

- **Pearl**
  Oxygen is the furosemide of the right ventricle.

Reference

Auger WR: Pulmonary hypertension and cor pulmonale. Curr Opin Pulm Med 1995;1:303. [PMID: 9363069]

Hypertension

■ **Essentials of Diagnosis**

- In most patients (95% of cases), no cause can be found
- Chronic elevation in blood pressure (> 140/90 mm Hg) occurs in 15% of white adults and 30% of black adults in the United States; onset usually between ages 20 and 55
- The pathogenesis is multifactorial: a combination of environmental, dietary, genetic, and neurohormonal factors all contribute
- Most patients are asymptomatic; some, however, complain of headache, epistaxis, or blurred vision if hypertension is severe
- Most diagnostic study abnormalities are referable to "target organ" damage: heart, kidney, brain, retina, and peripheral arteries

■ **Differential Diagnosis**

Secondary causes of hypertension:
- Coarctation of the aorta
- Renal insufficiency
- Renal artery stenosis
- Pheochromocytoma
- Cushing's syndrome
- Primary hyperaldosteronism
- Chronic use of oral contraceptive pills or alcohol

■ **Treatment**

- Decrease blood pressure with a single agent (if possible) while minimizing side effects
- Many recommend diuretics and beta-blockers as initial therapy, but considerable latitude is allowed for individual patients
- Other agents useful either alone or in combination include ACE inhibitors, angiotensin II receptor blockers, and calcium channel blockers; α_1-blockers are considered second-line agents
- If hypertension is unresponsive to medical treatment, evaluate for secondary causes

■ **Pearl**

A disease without a pearl—30 million Americans have it, and no clinical feature is characteristic, either symptomatically or on examination.

Reference

Carretero OA et al: Essential hypertension. Part I: definition and etiology. Circulation 2000;101:3295. [PMID: 10645931]

Deep Venous Thrombosis

■ Essentials of Diagnosis

- Dull pain or tight feeling in the calf or thigh
- Up to half of patients are asymptomatic in the early stages
- Increased risk: congestive heart failure, recent major surgery, neoplasia, oral contraceptive use by smokers, prolonged inactivity, varicose veins, hypercoagulable states (eg, protein C deficiency, nephrotic syndrome)
- Physical signs unreliable
- Doppler ultrasound and impedance plethysmography are initial tests of choice (less sensitive in asymptomatic patients); venography is definitive
- Pulmonary thromboembolism, especially with proximal, above-the-knee deep vein thrombosis

■ Differential Diagnosis

- Calf strain or contusion
- Cellulitis
- Ruptured Baker cyst
- Lymphatic obstruction
- Congestive heart failure, especially right-sided

■ Treatment

- Anticoagulation with intravenous heparin (goal PTT twice normal) for 5 days followed by oral warfarin for 3–6 months; thrombolytics in acute phlebitis may prevent valvular damage and postphlebitic syndrome
- Subcutaneous low-molecular-weight heparin may be substituted for intravenous heparin
- NSAIDs for associated pain and swelling
- For idiopathic and recurrent cases, hypercoagulable conditions should be considered, although factor V Leiden should be sought on a first episode without risk factors in patients of European ethnicity
- Postphlebitic syndrome (chronic venous insufficiency) is common following an episode of deep venous thrombosis and should be treated with graduated compression stockings, local skin care, and, in many, chronic warfarin administration

■ Pearl

The left lower extremity is 1 cm greater in circumference that the right in 90% of the population at any point of measurement.

Reference

Gorman WP et al: ABC of arterial and venous disease. Swollen lower limb–1: general assessment and deep vein thrombosis. BMJ 2000;320:1453. [PMID: 10837054]

1

Atrial Myxoma

- **Essentials of Diagnosis**
  - Most common cardiac tumor, usually originating in the interatrial septum, with 80% growing into the left atrium; 5–10% bilateral
  - Symptoms fall into one of three categories: (1) systemic—fever, malaise, weight loss; (2) obstructive—positional dyspnea and syncope; and (3) embolic—acute vascular or neurologic deficit
  - Diastolic "tumor plop" or mitral stenosis-like murmur; signs of congestive heart failure and systemic embolization in many
  - Episodic pulmonary edema, classically when patient assumes an upright position
  - Leukocytosis, anemia, accelerated erythrocyte sedimentation rate
  - MRI or echocardiogram demonstrates tumor

- **Differential Diagnosis**
  - Subacute infective endocarditis
  - Lymphoma
  - Autoimmune disease
  - Mitral stenosis
  - Cor triatriatum
  - Parachute mitral valve
  - Other causes of congestive heart failure

- **Treatment**
  - Surgery usually curative (recurrence rate is approximately 5%)

- **Pearl**

The diagnosis may be made by retrieval of embolic material by Fogarty catheter.

Reference

Reynen K: Cardiac myxomas. N Engl J Med 1995;333:1610. [PMID: 7477198]

2

Pulmonary Diseases

Acute Respiratory Distress Syndrome (ARDS)

- **Essentials of Diagnosis**
  - Rapid onset of dyspnea and respiratory distress, commonly in setting of trauma, shock, or sepsis
  - Tachypnea, fever; crackles or rhonchi by auscultation
  - Arterial hypoxemia refractory to supplemental oxygen; hypercapnia and respiratory acidosis in impending respiratory failure
  - Diffuse alveolar and interstitial infiltrates by radiography, often sparing costophrenic angles
  - Normal pulmonary capillary wedge pressure
  - Acute lung injury defined by a PaO_2/FIO_2 ratio < 300; ARDS is defined by PaO_2/FIO_2 ratio < 200

- **Differential Diagnosis**
  - Cardiogenic pulmonary edema
  - Primary pneumonia due to any cause
  - Diffuse alveolar hemorrhage
  - Bronchiolitis obliterans with organizing pneumonia

- **Treatment**
  - Mechanical ventilation with supplemental oxygen; positive end-expiratory pressure often required
  - Low tidal volume ventilation, using 6 mL/kg predicted body weight, may reduce mortality but very uncomfortable
  - Supportive therapy including adequate nutrition, vigilance for other organ dysfunction, and prevention of nosocomial complications (eg, catheter-related infection, venous thromboembolism)
  - Mortality rate is 40–60%

- **Pearl**

When in doubt, run the patient dry; it works in both cardiogenic and noncardiogenic pulmonary edema.

Reference

Ware LB et al: The acute respiratory distress syndrome. N Engl J Med 2000; 342:1334. [PMID: 10793167]

Pleural Effusion

- **Essentials of Diagnosis**
  - Many asymptomatic; pleuritic chest pain, dyspnea in some
  - Decreased breath sounds and percussive dullness; bronchial breathing above effusion
  - Layering on decubitus chest x-rays; ultrasonography occasionally required for confirmation
  - Exudative effusion commonly due to malignancy, infection, auto-immune disease, pulmonary embolism, asbestosis
  - Transudative effusion caused by congestive heart failure, cirrhosis with ascites, nephrotic syndrome, hypothyroidism
  - Exudative effusions have at least one of the following: (1) pleural fluid protein to serum protein ratio > 0.5; (2) pleural fluid LDH to serum LDH ratio > 0.6; or (3) pleural fluid LDH > two-thirds the upper limit of normal serum LDH
  - Markedly reduced glucose in empyema, rheumatoid effusion

- **Differential Diagnosis**
  - Atelectasis
  - Lobar consolidation
  - Chronic pleural thickening
  - Subdiaphragmatic process

- **Treatment**
  - Diagnostic thoracentesis for evaluating cause, with pleural fluid glucose, protein, red and white cells counts, LDH, and relevant cultures
  - Therapy guided by suspected cause
  - Pleural biopsy indicated in selected cases for diagnostic purposes (eg, tuberculosis, mesothelioma)
  - Bleomycin, tetracycline, and talc are the most effective sclerosing agents for malignant pleural effusion

- **Pearl**

Amesotheliocytosis in an exudative pleural effusion implies tuberculosis until proved otherwise.

Reference

Light RW: Pleural effusions. Med Clin North Am 1977;61:1339. [PMID: 21999]

Spontaneous Pneumothorax

- ■ Essentials of Diagnosis

  - Primary spontaneous pneumothorax occurs in the absence of underlying disease; secondary pneumothorax complicates pre-existing pulmonary disease (eg, asthma, COPD)
  - Primary spontaneous pneumothorax occurs in tall, thin boys and young men who smoke
  - Abrupt onset of ipsilateral chest pain (sometimes referred to shoulder or arm) and dyspnea
  - Decreased breath sounds over involved hemithorax, which may be bronchial but distant in 100% pneumothorax; hyperresonance, tachycardia, hypotension, and mediastinal shift toward contra-lateral side if tension is present
  - Chest x-ray diagnostic with retraction of lung from parietal pleura, often best seen by end-expiratory film

- ■ Differential Diagnosis

  - Myocardial infarction
  - Pulmonary emboli
  - Pneumonia with empyema
  - Pericarditis

- ■ Treatment

  - Assessment for cause, eg, pneumocystis pneumonia, lung cancer, COPD
  - Immediate decompression by needle thoracostomy if tension sus-pected
  - Spontaneous pneumothoraces of less than 15% followed by ser-ial radiographs and observation in the hospital; pneumothoraces greater than 15% treated by aspiration of air through small cathe-ter or by tube thoracostomy depending on clinical setting
  - Secondary pneumothoraces (eg, due to COPD, cystic fibrosis) usually require chest tube
  - Discontinue smoking
  - Risk of recurrence is high (up to 50% in those with primary spon-taneous pneumothorax)
  - Therapy for recurrent pneumothorax includes surgical pleuro-desis or stapling of the ruptured blebs

- ■ Pearl

  Pneumothorax during menstruation (catamenial pneumothorax) sug-gests endometriosis.

Reference

Sahn SA et al: Spontaneous pneumothorax. N Engl J Med 2000;342:868. [PMID: 10727592]

Bronchiolitis Obliterans With Organizing Pneumonia (BOOP)

2

- ■ Essentials of Diagnosis
  - Bronchiolitis obliterans in adults—also called cryptogenic organizing pneumonia—may follow infections (eg, mycoplasma, viral infection), may be due to toxic fume inhalation or associated with connective tissue disease or organ transplantation, may complicate local lung lesions, or may be idiopathic
  - Usually characterized by abrupt onset of flu-like symptoms, including dry cough, dyspnea, fever, and weight loss
  - Dry crackles and wheezing by auscultation; clubbing rare
  - Restrictive abnormalities with pulmonary function studies; hypoxemia
  - Chest radiograph typically shows patchy alveolar infiltrates bilaterally
  - Open or thoracoscopic lung biopsy necessary for precise diagnosis

- ■ Differential Diagnosis
  - Idiopathic pulmonary fibrosis
  - AIDS-related lung infections
  - Congestive heart failure
  - Mycobacterial or fungal infection
  - Severe pneumonia due to bacteria, fungi, or tuberculosis

- ■ Treatment
  - Corticosteroids effective in two-thirds of cases
  - Relapse common after short (< 6 months) steroid courses

- ■ Pearl

One of the "new" diseases; consider this when there is untimely resolution of an infiltrate in what you thought was a community-acquired pneumonia.

Reference

Epler GR: Bronchiolitis obliterans organizing pneumonia. Arch Intern Med 2001;161:158. [PMID: 11176728]

Solitary Pulmonary Nodule

2

- ■ **Essentials of Diagnosis**
  - • A round or oval circumscribed lesion less than 5 cm in diameter surrounded by normal lung tissue
  - • Twenty-five percent of cases of bronchogenic carcinoma present as such; the 5-year survival rate so detected is 50%
  - • Factors favoring benign lesion: age under 35 years, asymptomatic status, size under 2 cm, diffuse calcification, smooth margins, and satellite lesions
  - • Factors suggesting malignancy: age over 45 years, symptoms, size greater than 2 cm, lack of calcification, indistinct margins, smoking history
  - • Skin tests, serologies, cytology rarely helpful
  - • Comparison with old chest radiographs essential; follow-up with serial radiographs or CT scans often helpful; CT scan may reveal benign-appearing calcifications
  - • Positron emission tomography (PET) scans are a newly emerging diagnostic modality

- ■ **Differential Diagnosis**
  - • Benign causes: granuloma (eg, tuberculosis or fungal infection), arteriovenous malformation, pseudotumor, fat pad, hamartoma
  - • Malignant causes: primary, metastatic malignancy

- ■ **Treatment**
  - • Options include fine-needle aspiration (FNA), surgical resection, or radiographic follow-up over 2 years; negative FNA does not exclude malignancy due to high false-negative rate, unless a specific benign diagnosis is made
  - • Thoracic CT scan (with thin cuts through nodule) to look for benign-appearing calcifications and evaluate mediastinum for lymphadenopathy
  - • With high-risk clinical or radiographic features, surgical resection is recommended
  - • In low-risk or intermediate-risk cases, close radiographic follow-up may be justified

- ■ **Pearl**

In calcified pulmonary nodules, the first digit of the patient's Social Security number (always present on VA studies) suggests the specific infectious cause.

Reference

Ost D et al: Evaluation and management of the solitary pulmonary nodule. Am J Respir Crit Care Med 2000;162(3 Part 1):782. [PMID: 10988081]

Asthma

2

■ Essentials of Diagnosis

- Episodic wheezing, colds; chronic dyspnea or tightness in the chest; can present as cough
- Some attacks triggered by cold air or exercise
- Prolonged expiratory time, wheezing; if severe, pulsus paradoxus and cyanosis
- Peripheral eosinophilia common; mucus casts, eosinophils, and Charcot-Leyden crystals in sputum
- Obstructive pattern by spirometry supports diagnosis, though may be normal between attacks
- With methacholine challenge, absence of bronchial hyperreactivity makes diagnosis unlikely

■ Differential Diagnosis

- Congestive heart failure
- Chronic obstructive pulmonary disease
- Pulmonary embolism
- Foreign body aspiration
- Pulmonary infection (eg, strongyloidiasis, aspergillosis)
- Churg-Strauss syndrome

■ Treatment

- Avoidance of known precipitants, inhaled corticosteroids in persistent asthma, inhaled bronchodilators for symptoms
- In patients not well controlled on inhaled corticosteroids, long-acting inhaled beta-agonist (eg, salmeterol)
- Treatment of exacerbations: oxygen, inhaled bronchodilators (β_2 agonists or anticholinergics), systemic corticosteroids
- Leukotriene modifiers (eg, montelukast) may provide an option for long-term therapy in mild to moderate disease
- For difficult-to-control asthma, consider exacerbating factors such as gastroesophageal reflux disease and chronic sinusitis

■ Pearl

All that wheezes is not asthma, especially over age 45.

Reference

National Asthma Education and Prevention Program: Expert Panel Report 2: Guidelines for the diagnosis and management of asthma. National Institutes of Health, Publication No. 97-4051, Bethesda, MD, 1997.
http://www.nhlbi.nih.gov/guidelines/asthma/asthgdln.htm

Chronic Cough

- **Essentials of Diagnosis**

  - One of the most common reasons for seeking medical attention
  - Defined as a cough persisting for at least 4 weeks
  - Chest auscultation for wheezing, nasal and oral examination for signs of postnasal drip (eg, cobblestone appearance or erythema of mucosa)
  - Chest x-ray to exclude specific parenchymal lung diseases
  - Consider spirometry before and after bronchodilator, methacholine challenge, sinus CT scan, and 24-hour esophageal pH monitoring
  - Bronchoscopy in selected cases

- **Differential Diagnosis**
  - Angiotensin-converting enzyme-induced cough
  - Postnasal drip
  - Sinusitis
  - Asthma
  - Gastroesophageal reflux
  - Postinfectious cough—can last 4–6 weeks
  - Bronchiectasis
  - Chronic obstructive pulmonary disease
  - Congestive heart failure
  - Interstitial lung disease
  - Sarcoidosis
  - Bronchogenic carcinoma

- **Treatment**
  - Smoking cessation
  - Treat underlying condition if present
  - Trial of inhaled beta-agonist (eg, albuterol)
  - For postnasal drip: antihistamines (H_1-antagonists or may add nasal ipratropium bromide)
  - For suspected gastroesophageal reflux disease, proton pump inhibitors (eg, omeprazole)

- **Pearl**

In undiagnosed chronic cough, think of ACE inhibitors and asthma; these are far more common than appreciated.

Reference

Philp EB: Chronic cough. Am Fam Physician 1997;56:1395. [PMID: 9337762]

Chronic Obstructive Pulmonary Disease (COPD)

2

- ■ **Essentials of Diagnosis**
  - Primarily consisting of emphysema and chronic bronchitis; most patients have components of both
  - Acute or chronic dyspnea (emphysema) or chronic productive cough nearly always in a heavy smoker
  - Tachypnea, barrel chest, distant breath sounds, wheezes or rhonchi, cyanosis; clubbing unusual
  - Hypoxemia and hypercapnia more pronounced with chronic bronchitis than with emphysema
  - Hyperexpansion with decreased markings by chest radiography; variable findings of bullae, thin cardiac shadow
  - Airflow obstruction by spirometry; normal diffusing capacity ($D_L CO$) in bronchitis, reduced in emphysema
  - Ventilation and perfusion well-matched in remaining lung in emphysema, not in chronic bronchitis

- ■ **Differential Diagnosis**
  - Asthma
  - Bronchiectasis
  - α_1-Antiprotease deficiency
  - Congestive heart failure
  - Recurrent pulmonary emboli

- ■ **Treatment**
  - Cessation of cigarette smoking is most important intervention
  - Clinical trial of inhaled anticholinergic agent, eg, ipratropium bromide
  - Pneumococcal vaccination; yearly influenza vaccination
  - Supplemental oxygen for hypoxic patients ($PaO_2 < 55$ mm Hg) reduces mortality
  - For acute exacerbations, treat as acute asthma and identify underlying precipitant; if patient has low baseline peak flow rates, antibiotics may be beneficial
  - Lung reduction surgery in selected patients with emphysema

- ■ **Pearl**

The blue bloater pushes the pink puffer's wheelchair (patients with bronchitis have better exercise tolerance than those with emphysema).

Reference

Barnes PJ: Chronic obstructive pulmonary disease. N Engl J Med 2000;343:269. [PMID: (UI: 10911010]

Cystic Fibrosis

- **Essentials of Diagnosis**

  - A generalized autosomal recessive disorder of the exocrine glands
  - Cough, dyspnea, recurrent pulmonary infections often due to pseudomonas; symptoms of malabsorption, infertility
  - Increased thoracic diameter, distant breath sounds, rhonchi, clubbing, nasal polyps
  - Hypoxemia; obstructive or mixed pattern by spirometry; decreased diffusing capacity
  - Sweat chloride > 60 meq/L
  - Genetic testing for gene mutation can confirm diagnosis even if sweat test is negative

- **Differential Diagnosis**

  - Asthma
  - Bronchiectasis
  - Congenital emphysema (α_1-antiprotease deficiency)
  - Pancreatic insufficiency
  - Other causes of malabsorption

- **Treatment**

  - Comprehensive multidisciplinary therapy required, including genetic and occupational counseling
  - Inhaled bronchodilators and chest physiotherapy
  - Antibiotics for recurrent airway infections guided by cultures and sensitivities (high rate of resistant *Pseudomonas aeruginosa* and *Staphylococcus aureus* infections seen)
  - Pneumococcal vaccination; yearly influenza vaccinations
  - Recombinant human deoxyribonuclease given by aerosol has modest benefit
  - Chest physiotherapy with a variety of devices may be beneficial
  - Lung transplantation is the definitive treatment in selected patients

- **Pearl**

Consider cystic fibrosis in young adults with recurrent pulmonary infections; formes frustes are more common than once thought.

Reference

Rubin BK: Emerging therapies for cystic fibrosis lung disease. Chest 1999; 115:1120. [PMID: 10208218]

Foreign Body Aspiration

2

- ■ Essentials of Diagnosis
  - • Sudden onset of cough, wheeze, and dyspnea
  - • Localized wheezing, hyperresonance, and diminished breath sounds
  - • Localized air trapping or atelectasis on end-expiratory chest radiograph

- ■ Differential Diagnosis
  - • Asthma with mucus plugging
  - • Bronchiolitis
  - • Pyogenic upper airway process (eg. Ludwig's angina, soft tissue abscess, epiglottitis)
  - • Laryngospasm associated with anaphylaxis
  - • Bronchial compression from mass lesion
  - • Substernal goiter
  - • Tracheal cystadenoma

- ■ Treatment
  - • Bronchoscopic or surgical removal of foreign body, often by rigid bronchoscopy
  - • Emergency attention to airway—may require endotracheal intubation

- ■ Pearl

An adult complaining of croup has a substernal goiter until proved otherwise.

Reference

Reilly JS et al: Prevention and management of aerodigestive foreign body injuries in childhood. Pediatr Clin North Am 1996;43:1403. [PMID: 8973519]

Allergic Bronchopulmonary Aspergillosis

- **Essentials of Diagnosis**
  - Caused by an allergy to antigens of aspergillus species that colonize the tracheobronchial tree
  - Recurrent dyspnea, unmasked by corticosteroid withdrawal, with history of asthma; cough productive of brownish plugs of sputum
  - Physical examination as in asthma
  - Peripheral eosinophilia, elevated serum IgE level, precipitating antibody to aspergillus antigen present; positive skin hypersensitivity to aspergillus antigen
  - Infiltrate (often fleeting) and central bronchiectasis by chest radiography

- **Differential Diagnosis**
  - Asthma
  - Bronchiectasis
  - Invasive aspergillosis
  - Churg-Strauss syndrome
  - Löffler's syndrome
  - Chronic obstructive pulmonary disease

- **Treatment**
  - Oral corticosteroids often required for several months
  - Inhaled bronchodilators as for attacks of asthma
  - Treatment with itraconazole (for 16 weeks) improves disease control
  - Complications include hemoptysis, severe bronchiectasis, and pulmonary fibrosis

- **Pearl**

One of the three ways aspergillus causes disease—all different pathophysiologically.

Reference

Stevens DA et al: A randomized trial of itraconazole in allergic bronchopulmonary aspergillosis. N Engl J Med 2000;342:756. [PMID: 10717010]

Bronchiectasis

2

- **Essentials of Diagnosis**
  - A congenital or acquired disorder affecting the large bronchi causing permanent abnormal dilation and destruction of bronchial walls; may be a consequence of untreated pneumonia
  - Chronic cough with copious purulent three-layered sputum, hemoptysis; weight loss, recurrent pneumonias
  - Coarse, moist crackles; clubbing
  - Hypoxemia; obstructive pattern by spirometry
  - Chest x-rays variable, may show multiple cystic lesions at bases in advanced cases
  - High-resolution CT scan is essential for diagnosis in many cases
  - Often associated with underlying systemic disorder (eg, cystic fibrosis, hypogammaglobulinemia, IgA deficiency, common variable immunodeficiency, primary ciliary dyskinesia), chronic pulmonary infection (eg, tuberculosis, lung abscess), and HIV infection

- **Differential Diagnosis**
  - Chronic obstructive pulmonary disease
  - Tuberculosis
  - Chronic lung abscess
  - Pneumonia due to any cause

- **Treatment**
  - Smoking cessation
  - Antibiotics selected by sputum culture and sensitivities
  - Chest physiotherapy
  - Inhaled bronchodilators
  - Surgical resection in selected patients with unresponsive localized disease or massive hemoptysis
  - Complications include cor pulmonale, amyloidosis, and secondary visceral abscesses (eg, brain abscess)

- **Pearl**

Paragonimiasis is the most common cause worldwide, as bronchiectasis is the world's most common cause of hemoptysis.

Reference

Cohen M et al: Bronchiectasis in systemic diseases. Chest 1999;116:1063. [PMID: 10531174]

Acute Tracheobronchitis

- **Essentials of Diagnosis**
  - Poorly defined but common condition characterized by inflammation of the trachea and bronchi
  - Due to infectious agents (bacteria or viruses) or irritants (eg, dust and smoke)
  - Cough is most common symptom; purulent sputum production and malaise common
  - Variable rhonchi and wheezing; fever is often absent but may be prominent in cases caused by *Haemophilus influenzae*
  - Chest x-ray normal
  - Increased incidence in smokers

- **Differential Diagnosis**
  - Asthma
  - Pneumonia
  - Inhaled foreign body
  - Inhalation pneumonitis
  - Viral croup

- **Treatment**
  - Symptomatic therapy with inhaled bronchodilators, cough suppressants
  - Antibiotics are not recommended in all patients because they shorten the disease course by less than 1 day
  - Patients encouraged to stop smoking

- **Pearl**

Sputum culture does not help in this disorder.

Reference

Gonzales R et al: Uncomplicated acute bronchitis. Ann Intern Med 2000;133: 981. [PMID: 119400]

Acute Bacterial Pneumonia

2

- ■ Essentials of Diagnosis
  - Fever, chills, cough with purulent sputum production; early pleuritic pain, often severe, suggests pneumococcal etiology
  - Tachycardia, tachypnea; bronchial breath sounds with percussive dullness and egophony over involved lung; findings may be more pronounced after hydration
  - Leukocytosis with left shift; low white count (< 5000/μL) associated with poor outcome
  - Patchy or lobar infiltrate by chest x-ray
  - Diagnostic Gram stain or culture of sputum, blood, or pleural fluid
  - Causes include *Streptococcus pneumoniae, Haemophilus influenzae,* gram-negative rods, *Staphylococcus aureus,* legionella
  - In ventilator-associated pneumonia, an invasive diagnostic strategy including bronchoscopy may reduce mortality

- ■ Differential Diagnosis
  - Lung abscess
  - Pulmonary embolism
  - Myocardial infarction
  - Atypical or viral pneumonia
  - Bronchiolitis obliterans with organizing pneumonia (BOOP)

- ■ Treatment
  - Empiric antibiotics for common organisms after obtaining cultures
  - Hospitalize selected patients (severe hypoxemia, more than one lobe involved, poor host resistance factors, presence of coexisting illness, leukopenia or marked leukocytosis, hypotension)
  - Pneumococcal vaccine can prevent or lessen the severity of pneumococcal infections in up to 90% of patients

- ■ Pearl

When gram-positive diplococci thrive in neutrophils, think staphylococci, not pneumococci.

Reference

Bartlett JG et al: Community-acquired pneumonia in adults: guidelines for management. The Infectious Diseases Society of America. Clin Infect Dis 1998; 26:811. [PMID: 9564457]

Atypical Pneumonia

- **Essentials of Diagnosis**

  - Cough with scant sputum, fever, malaise, headache; gastrointestinal symptoms variable
  - Physical examination of lungs may be unimpressive
  - Mild leukocytosis; cold agglutinins sometimes positive but not diagnostic
  - Patchy, nonlobar infiltrate by chest x-ray often surprisingly extensive
  - Pathogens include mycoplasma, chlamydia, viral agents
  - Typical and atypical pneumonia not always distinguishable by clinical or radiographic features

- **Differential Diagnosis**

  - Bacterial pneumonia
  - Pulmonary embolism
  - Congestive heart failure
  - Bronchiolitis obliterans with organizing pneumonia (BOOP)
  - Idiopathic pulmonary fibrosis
  - Hypersensitivity pneumonitis

- **Treatment**

  - Empiric antibiotic treatment with doxycycline, erythromycin, or newer macrolide (eg, azithromycin) or fluoroquinolone (eg, levofloxacin)
  - Hospitalize as for bacterial pneumonia

- **Pearl**

In psittacosis, the history of parrot exposure may be difficult to obtain because of illegal importation of the bird.

Reference

Bartlett JG et al: Community-acquired pneumonia in adults: guidelines for management. The Infectious Diseases Society of America. Clin Infect Dis 1998;26:811. [PMID: 9564457]

Anaerobic Pneumonia & Lung Abscess

2

- **Essentials of Diagnosis**
  - Cough producing foul-smelling sputum; hemoptysis; fever, weight loss, malaise
  - Patients with periodontal disease, history of impaired deglutition (eg, neurologic or esophageal disorder or altered consciousness) are predisposed
  - Bronchial breath sounds with dullness and egophony over involved lung
  - Leukocytosis; hypoxemia
  - Chest x-ray density, often with central lucency or air-fluid level
  - Sputum cultures reveal only mouth flora

- **Differential Diagnosis**
  - Tuberculosis
  - Bronchogenic carcinoma
  - Pulmonary mycoses
  - Bronchiectasis
  - Cavitary bacterial pneumonia
  - Pulmonary vasculitis (eg, Wegener's granulomatosis)

- **Treatment**
  - Clindamycin or high-dose penicillin (treatment for 6 or more weeks)
  - Surgery in selected cases (massive abscess; massive or persistent hemoptysis)
  - Supplemental oxygen as needed
  - Bronchoscopic exclusion of carcinoma or foreign body aspiration in patients with atypical features, especially edentulous patients

- **Pearl**

A lung abscess in an edentulous patient is lung cancer until proved otherwise.

Reference

Bartlett, JG et al: Community-acquired pneumonia in adults: guidelines for management. The Infectious Diseases Society of America. Clin Infect Dis 1998; 26:811. [PMID: 9564457]

Pulmonary Tuberculosis

- **Essentials of Diagnosis**
  - Lassitude, weight loss, fever, cough, night sweats, hemoptysis; may be asymptomatic, however
  - Cachexia in many; posttussive apical rales occasionally present
  - Apical or subapical infiltrates with cavities classic in reactivation tuberculosis; pleural effusion in primary tuberculosis, likewise mid-lung infiltration, but any radiographic abnormality is possible
  - Positive skin test to intradermal purified protein derivative (PPD) in most
  - *Mycobacterium tuberculosis* by culture of sputum, pleural fluid, gastric washing, or pleural biopsy; pleural fluid culture usually sterile, however
  - Increasing antibiotic-resistant strains
  - Granuloma on pleural biopsy in patients with effusions; mesothelial cells usually absent from fluid

- **Differential Diagnosis**
  - Bronchogenic carcinoma
  - Bacterial pneumonia or lung abscess
  - Fungal infection
  - Sarcoidosis
  - Pneumoconiosis
  - Pleural effusion of asbestosis
  - Other mycobacterial infections

- **Treatment**
  - Combination antituberculous therapy for 6–9 months; all regimens include isoniazid, but rifampin, ethambutol, pyrazinamide, streptomycin all have activity
  - All cases of suspected *M tuberculosis* infection reported to local health departments
  - Hospitalization should be considered for those incapable of self-care or likely to expose susceptible individuals

- **Pearl**

With respect to pulmonary tuberculosis and HIV infection—if it looks like tuberculosis it isn't, and if it doesn't it is.

Reference

Diagnostic Standards and Classification of Tuberculosis in Adults and Children. This official statement of the American Thoracic Society and the Centers for Disease Control and Prevention was adopted by the ATS Board of Directors, July 1999. This statement was endorsed by the Council of the Infectious Disease Society of America, September 1999. Am J Respir Crit Care Med 2000;161(4 Part 1):1376. [PMID: 10764337]

2

Idiopathic Pulmonary Fibrosis (Usual Interstitial Pneumonia)

- **Essentials of Diagnosis**
  - Insidious onset of dyspnea and dry cough in patients usually in their sixth or seventh decades
  - Inspiratory crackles by auscultation; clubbing
  - Hypoxemia, especially exertional; antinuclear antibody and rheumatoid factor often positive but nonspecific
  - Diffuse interstitial infiltration by chest x-ray, which may progress to honeycombing pattern
  - Restrictive pattern with decreased total lung capacity and diffusing capacity (D_LCO)
  - High-resolution thoracic CT scan helpful
  - Thoracoscopic and open lung biopsy are best methods for definitive diagnosis; cellular pattern on bronchoalveolar lavage also helpful

- **Differential Diagnosis**
  - Bronchiolitis obliterans organizing pneumonia (BOOP)
  - Interstitial lung disease due to infection
  - Drug-induced fibrosis (eg, bleomycin, nitrofurantoin)
  - Sarcoidosis
  - Pneumoconiosis
  - Asbestosis
  - Hypersensitivity pneumonitis

- **Treatment**
  - Supportive therapy, including supplemental oxygen
  - High-dose oral corticosteroids ineffective
  - Adjunctive cytotoxic therapy in selected patients may improve outcome
  - Early referral to lung transplantation center is critical for good candidates; gamma interferon is a promising new therapy

- **Pearl**

Progression from desquamative interstitial pneumonia to usual interstitial pneumonia does not occur; the former is a nonspecific alveolar response to smoking.

Reference

American Thoracic Society. Idiopathic pulmonary fibrosis: diagnosis and treatment. International consensus statement. American Thoracic Society (ATS), and the European Respiratory Society (ERS). Am J Respir Crit Care Med 2000;161(2 Part 1):646. [PMID: 10673212]

Sarcoidosis

■ Essentials of Diagnosis

- A disease of unknown cause with an increased incidence in North American blacks and Northern European whites
- Malaise, fever, dyspnea of insidious onset; symptoms referable to eyes, skin, nervous system, liver, or heart also common; often presents asymptomatically
- Iritis, erythema nodosum, parotid enlargement, lymphadenopathy, hepatosplenomegaly
- Hypercalcemia (5%) less common than hypercalciuria (20%)
- Pulmonary function testing may show evidence of obstruction, but restriction with decreased $D_{L}CO$ is more common
- Symmetric hilar and right paratracheal adenopathy, interstitial infiltrates, or both seen on chest x-ray
- Tissue reveals noncaseating granuloma; transbronchial biopsy gives high yield, even without parenchymal disease on chest film
- Increased angiotensin-converting enzyme levels are neither sensitive nor specific; cutaneous anergy in 70%

■ Differential Diagnosis

- Tuberculosis
- Lymphoma, including lymphocytic interstitial pneumonitis
- Histoplasmosis or coccidioidomycosis
- Idiopathic pulmonary fibrosis
- Pneumoconiosis
- Berylliosis

■ Treatment

- Oral systemic corticosteroid therapy indicated for symptomatic pulmonary disease, cardiac involvement, iritis unresponsive to local therapy, hypercalcemia, central nervous system involvement, arthritis, skin disease
- Asymptomatic patients with normal pulmonary function may not require corticosteroids—they should receive close clinical follow-up

■ Pearl

The only disease in medicine in which steroids reverse anergy.

Reference

Statement on sarcoidosis. Am J Respir Crit Care Med 1999;160:736. [PMID: 10430755]

Pulmonary Thromboembolism

2

- **Essentials of Diagnosis**
  - Seen in immobilized patients, congestive failure, malignancies, and after pelvic trauma or surgery
  - Abrupt onset of dyspnea and anxiety, with or without pleuritic chest pain, cough with hemoptysis; syncope rare, but suggestive of extensive disease
  - Tachycardia, tachypnea, most common; loud P_2 with right-sided S_3 characteristic but unusual; findings of peripheral venous thrombosis often absent
  - Acute respiratory alkalosis and hypoxemia
  - Characteristic perfusion defect on ventilation-perfusion scan, confirmed by pulmonary angiography in selected patients
  - Lower extremity ultrasound will demonstrate deep venous thrombosis in about half of cases
  - Spiral CT scan is newly emerging diagnostic technique with unclear utility

- **Differential Diagnosis**
  - Pneumonia
  - Myocardial infarction
  - Atelectasis
  - Any cause of acute respiratory distress (eg, pneumothorax, aspiration, pulmonary edema, or asthma) or pleural effusion
  - Early sepsis
  - Dressler's syndrome

- **Treatment**
  - Anticoagulation: acutely with heparin for several days, instituting warfarin concurrently and continuing for a minimum of 3 months
  - Thrombolytic therapy initially in selected patients with hemodynamic compromise, but no effect on mortality
  - Intravenous filter placement in inferior vena cava for selected patients not candidates for or unresponsive to anticoagulation

- **Pearl**

Ten percent of pulmonary emboli originate from upper extremity veins.

Reference

Rathbun SW et al: Sensitivity and specificity of helical computed tomography in the diagnosis of pulmonary embolism: a systematic review. Ann Intern Med 2000;132:227. [PMID: 10651604]

Primary Pulmonary Hypertension

- **Essentials of Diagnosis**

  - A rare disorder seen primarily in young and middle-aged women
  - Defined as pulmonary hypertension and elevated peripheral vascular resistance in the absence of lung or heart disease
  - Progressive dyspnea, malaise, chest pain, exertional syncope
  - Tachycardia, right ventricular lift, increased P_2, systolic ejection click, right-sided S_3; may have evidence of right-sided heart failure (peripheral edema, hepatomegaly, ascites)
  - Right ventricular strain or hypertrophy by electrocardiography
  - Large central pulmonary arteries by chest x-ray, with oligemia distally
  - Characteristic plexogenic arteriopathy on pathologic examination

- **Differential Diagnosis**

  - Mitral stenosis
  - Sleep apnea
  - Chronic pulmonary embolism
  - Autoimmune disease
  - Ischemic heart disease
  - Congenital heart disease
  - Cirrhosis of the liver with portal hypertension
  - Pulmonary veno-occlusive disease

- **Treatment**

  - Continuous intravenous prostacyclin infusion improves survival
  - Empiric anticoagulation may confer survival benefit
  - Other vasodilator agents of unpredictable and uncertain efficacy
  - Bilateral lung or heart-lung transplantation important options; all eligible patients should be referred to a transplant center for evaluation

- **Pearl**

All murmurs of mitral stenosis may be missing in that condition, leading to an inaccurate diagnosis of primary pulmonary hypertension.

Reference

Gaine SP et al: Primary pulmonary hypertension. Lancet 1998;352:719. [PMID: 9729004]

Silicosis

- **Essentials of Diagnosis**
  - A typical pneumoconiosis: a chronic fibrotic lung disease caused by the inhalation of various dusts
  - History of extensive prolonged exposure to dust containing silicon dioxide (eg, foundry work, sandblasting, hard rock mining)
  - Progressive dyspnea, often over months to years
  - Dry inspiratory crackles by auscultation
  - Characteristic changes on chest radiograph with bilateral fibrosis and nodules (upper greater than lower lobes), hilar lymphadenopathy with "eggshell" calcification
  - Pulmonary function studies yield mixed obstructive and restrictive pattern

- **Differential Diagnosis**
  - Other inhalation pneumoconioses (eg, asbestosis)
  - Tuberculosis (often complicates silicosis)
  - Sarcoidosis
  - Histoplasmosis
  - Coccidioidomycosis
  - Idiopathic pulmonary fibrosis

- **Treatment**
  - Supportive care; chronic oxygen if sustained hypoxemia present
  - Chemoprophylaxis with isoniazid necessary for all silicotic patients with positive tuberculin reactivity (given the markedly increased incidence of tuberculosis in silicosis)

- **Pearl**

One of the associations with tuberculosis which is paradoxical; many clinically similar processes do not share this association.

Reference

Mossman BT et al: Mechanisms in the pathogenesis of asbestosis and silicosis. Am J Respir Crit Care Med 1998;157(5 Part 1):1666. [PMID: 9603153]

Asbestosis

- **Essentials of Diagnosis**

  - History of exposure to dust containing asbestos particles (eg, from work in mining, insulation, construction, shipbuilding)
  - Progressive dyspnea, rarely pleuritic chest pain
  - Dry inspiratory crackles common; clubbing and cyanosis occasionally seen
  - Interstitial fibrosis, later coalescing into nodules, is characteristic (lower field greater than upper field); pleural thickening, plaques, and diaphragmatic calcification common but unrelated to parenchymal disease; in some, exudative pleural effusion develops before parenchymal disease
  - High-resolution CT scan often confirmatory
  - Pulmonary function testing shows a restrictive defect with a diminished $D_L CO$ often the earliest abnormality

- **Differential Diagnosis**

  - Other inhalation pneumoconioses (eg, silicosis)
  - Fungal disease
  - Sarcoidosis
  - Idiopathic pulmonary fibrosis
  - Mesothelioma

- **Treatment**

  - Supportive care; chronic oxygen supplementation for sustained hypoxemia
  - Legal counseling regarding compensation for occupational exposure

- **Pearl**

Remember that the highest exposures on ships or boats come from sweeping the floor on submarines, not working on the structure of the vessel.

Reference

Wagner GR: Asbestosis and silicosis. Lancet 1997;349:1311. [PMID: 9142077]

Pulmonary Alveolar Proteinosis

- **Essentials of Diagnosis**
  - May be idiopathic or secondary (ie, post lung infection, immuno-compromised host)
  - Progressive dyspnea and low-grade fever
  - Physical examination often normal
  - Hypoxemia; bilateral alveolar infiltrates suggestive of pulmonary edema on chest radiography
  - Characteristic intra-alveolar phospholipid accumulation without fibrosis at open lung biopsy
  - Superinfection with nocardia or fungi may occur

- **Differential Diagnosis**
  - Congestive heart failure
  - Acute pneumonia
  - Bronchiolitis obliterans with organizing pneumonia (BOOP)

- **Treatment**
  - Periodic whole lung lavage reduces exertional dyspnea
  - Natural history variable with occasional spontaneous remissions seen

- **Pearl**

If the lab tells you they see faintly acid-fast organisms on a screen of the sputum in a patient with new-onset "pulmonary edema," here is your diagnosis.

Reference

Wang BM et al: Diagnosing pulmonary alveolar proteinosis. A review and an update. Chest 1997;111:460. [PMID: 9041997]

Chronic Eosinophilic Pneumonia

- **Essentials of Diagnosis**
  - Fever, dry cough, wheezing, dyspnea, and weight loss—all variable from transient to severe and progressive
  - Wheezing, dry crackles occasionally appreciated by auscultation
  - Peripheral blood eosinophilia present in most cases
  - Peripheral pulmonary infiltrates on radiographs in many cases (ie, "the radiologic negative" of pulmonary edema) shown to be eosinophilic by bronchoalveolar lavage or open lung biopsy

- **Differential Diagnosis**
  - Acute infectious pneumonia
  - Asthma
  - Idiopathic pulmonary fibrosis
  - Bronchiolitis obliterans with organizing pneumonia (BOOP)
  - Allergic bronchopulmonary aspergillosis
  - Churg-Strauss syndrome
  - Other eosinophilic pulmonary syndromes (eg, drug or parasite-related)

- **Treatment**
  - Corticosteroid therapy often results in dramatic improvement in idiopathic cases; recurrence is common
  - Most patients require corticosteroid therapy for a year or more (sometimes indefinitely)

- **Pearl**

Always pause and consider strongyloidiasis before giving steroids to a patient with pulmonary disease and eosinophilia.

Reference

Allen JN et al: Eosinophilic lung diseases. Am J Respir Crit Care Med 1994;150(5 Part 1):1423. [PMID: 7952571]

Hypersensitivity Pneumonitis

2

- **Essentials of Diagnosis**
  - Work and environmental history suggesting link between activities and symptoms
  - Acute form: 4–12 hours after exposure, onset of cough, dyspnea, fever, chills, myalgias; tachypnea, tachycardia, inspiratory crackles; leukocytosis with lymphopenia and neutrophilia; eosinophilia unusual
  - Subacute or chronic form: exertional dyspnea, cough, fatigue, anorexia, weight loss; basilar crackles
  - Caused by exposure to microbial agents (eg, thermophilic actinomyces in farmer's lung, aspergillus), animal proteins (eg, bird fancier's lung) with resultant IgG complement deposition, and chemical sensitizers (eg, isocyanates, trimetallic anhydride)
  - IgG precipitating antibodies are not sensitive or specific—markers of antigen exposure, not disease
  - Pulmonary function tests reveal restrictive pattern and decreased $D_L CO$
  - High-resolution thoracic CT scan reveals fine reticulonodular pattern or diffuse ground-glass appearance
  - Bronchoalveolar lavage reveals marked lymphocytosis
  - Transbronchial or thoracoscopic lung biopsy can confirm diagnosis in unclear cases

- **Differential Diagnosis**
  - Sarcoidosis
  - Asthma
  - Atypical pneumonia
  - Collagen-vascular disease, eg, systemic lupus erythematosus
  - Idiopathic pulmonary fibrosis
  - Lymphoma

- **Treatment**
  - Identification and removal of exposure is essential
  - Consider systemic corticosteroids in subacute or chronic forms

- **Pearl**

Bagassosis and sequoiosis are two examples: a history of exposure to sugar cane or fallen lumber, respectively, makes the diagnosis.

Reference

Kaltreider HB. Hypersensitivity pneumonitis. West J Med 1993;159:570. [PMID: 8279154]

Sleep-Related Breathing Disorders (Sleep Apnea)

- **Essentials of Diagnosis**

  - Excessive daytime somnolence or fatigue, morning headache, weight gain, erectile dysfunction; bed partner may report restless sleep and loud snoring
  - Obesity, systemic hypertension common; signs of pulmonary hypertension or cor pulmonale may develop over time in a few
  - Erythrocytosis common
  - Sleep study—either formal polysomnography or a screening study—reveals periods of apnea
  - Most cases are of mixed central or obstructive origin; pure central sleep apnea is rare

- **Differential Diagnosis**

  - Alcohol or sedative abuse
  - Narcolepsy
  - Depression
  - Seizure disorder
  - Chronic obstructive pulmonary disease
  - Hypothyroidism

- **Treatment**

  - Weight loss and avoidance of sedatives or hypnotic medications mandatory
  - Nocturnal nasal continuous positive airway pressure (CPAP) and supplemental oxygen frequently abolish obstructive apnea
  - Protriptyline effective in minority of patients
  - Surgical approaches (uvulopalatopharyngoplasty, nasal septoplasty, tracheostomy) reserved for selected cases

- **Pearl**

When a plethoric clinic patient nods off during the history, it's sleep apnea until proved otherwise; if the historian does, it's a post-call resident.

Reference

Piccirillo JF et al: Obstructive sleep apnea. JAMA 2000;284:1492. [PMID: (UI: 11000621]

3

Gastrointestinal Diseases

Gastroesophageal Reflux Disease

- **Essentials of Diagnosis**
  - Substernal burning (pyrosis) or pressure, aggravated by recumbency and relieved with sitting; waterbrash, dysphagia; nocturnal regurgitation, cough, or wheezing common
  - Esophageal reflux or hiatal hernia may be found by fluoroscopy at barium study; iron deficiency anemia secondary to occult blood loss may be encountered
  - Manometry reveals incompetent lower esophageal sphincter; endoscopy with biopsy may be necessary for diagnosis
  - Esophageal pH monitoring helpful in excluding disease when symptoms are present during monitoring
  - Conditions associated with diminished lower esophageal sphincter tone include obesity, pregnancy, hiatal hernia, nasogastric tube, recurrent emesis, and Raynaud's phenomenon

- **Differential Diagnosis**
  - Peptic ulcer disease
  - Cholecystitis
  - Angina pectoris
  - Achalasia
  - Esophageal spasm

- **Treatment**
  - Weight loss if indicated, avoidance of late-night meals or snacks, elevation of head of bed
  - Avoid substances reducing lower esophageal sphincter tone (chocolate, caffeine, tobacco, alcohol, fried or fatty foods)
  - Antacids, high-dose H_2 blockers, or proton pump inhibitors (eg, omeprazole)
  - Gastrointestinal motility stimulants (eg, bethanechol, metoclopramide) in selected patients
  - Surgical fundoplication via abdominal (Hill, Nissen) or thoracic (Belsey) approach for rare cases refractory to medical management

- **Pearl**

Eradication of Helicobacter pylori may actually worsen GERD by increasing gastric acid secretion.

Reference

Katzka DA: Digestive system disorders: gastroesophageal reflux disease. West J Med 2000;173:48.

Diffuse Esophageal Spasm

- **Essentials of Diagnosis**
  - Dysphagia, substernal pain, hypersalivation, reflux of recently ingested food
  - May be precipitated by ingestion of hot or cold foods
  - Endoscopic, radiographic, and manometric demonstration of non-propulsive hyperperistalsis; lower esophageal sphincter relaxes normally
  - "Nutcracker esophagus" variant with prolonged, high pressure (> 175 mm Hg) propulsive contractions

- **Differential Diagnosis**
  - Angina pectoris
  - Esophageal or mediastinal tumors
  - Aperistalsis
  - Achalasia
  - Psychoneurosis

- **Treatment**
  - Nitrates often effective
  - Esophageal myotomy for refractory patients with severe disease

- **Pearl**

Like all esophageal motor disorders, consider myocardial ischemia as responsible until proved otherwise.

Reference

Patti MG et al: Evaluation and treatment of primary esophageal motility disorders. West J Med 1997;166:263.

Achalasia

■ **Essentials of Diagnosis**

- Progressive dysphagia, odynophagia, and regurgitation of undigested food
- Barium swallow demonstrates a dilated upper esophagus with a narrowed cardioesophageal junction ("bird's beak" esophagus); chest x-ray may reveal a retrocardiac air-fluid level
- Lack of primary peristalsis by manometry or cineradiography and incomplete lower esophageal sphincter relaxation with swallowing

■ **Differential Diagnosis**

- Diffuse esophageal spasm
- Aperistalsis
- Benign lower esophageal stricture
- Esophageal or mediastinal tumors (esophageal carcinoma may complicate achalasia, however)
- Scleroderma of esophagus

■ **Treatment**

- Nifedipine, 10–20 mg sublingually 30 minutes before meals
- Botulinum toxin injection endoscopically in patients who are not good surgical candidates
- Pneumatic esophageal dilation
- Surgical extramucosal myotomy (esophagocardiomyotomy) in refractory cases
- Consider yearly esophagoscopy to evaluate for carcinoma

■ **Pearl**

In patients with retrocardiac air-fluid levels on chest x-ray, consider this diagnosis—it's not always a lung abscess.

Reference

Bassotti G et al: Review article: pharmacological options in achalasia. Aliment Pharmacol Therap 1999;13:1391.

Esophageal Web

- **Essentials of Diagnosis**
  - Dysphagia
  - Plummer-Vinson syndrome if associated with iron deficiency anemia, glossitis, and spooning of nails; may be higher incidence of hypopharyngeal carcinoma
  - Barium swallow (lateral view often required), esophagoscopy diagnostic (but often misses cervical esophageal webs)

- **Differential Diagnosis**
  - Achalasia
  - Esophageal diverticulum
  - Aperistalsis
  - Esophageal or mediastinal tumor
  - Esophageal stricture

- **Treatment**
  - Treat the iron deficiency after finding its cause—the web may resolve spontaneously
  - Esophagoscopy with disruption of webs adequate in most cases
  - Bougienage required on occasion

- **Pearl**

Webs do not cause iron deficiency; the iron deficiency comes first, and the web is a connective tissue effect of low iron.

Reference

Chung S et al: Gastrointestinal: upper oesophageal web. J Gastroenterol Hepatology 1999;14:611.

Benign Stricture of Esophagus

- ### Essentials of Diagnosis
  - Dysphagia for solids more than liquids; odynophagia
  - Smooth narrowing of lumen radiographically; esophagoscopy and biopsy or cytology mandatory to exclude malignancy
  - Onset months to years following esophageal insult, including gastroesophageal reflux, indwelling nasogastric tube, corrosive ingestion, infectious esophagitis, or endoscopic injury

- ### Differential Diagnosis
  - Achalasia
  - Esophageal or mediastinal tumor
  - Esophageal web
  - Schatzki's ring
  - Left atrial enlargement
  - Pericardial effusion

- ### Treatment
  - Monthly bougienage dilation is definitive therapy for most patients
  - Surgical therapy required rarely

- ### Pearl

When reflux is the cause, be wary of adenocarcinoma developing within columnar metaplasia induced by the acid (see next page).

Reference

Johanson JF: Epidemiology of esophageal and supraesophageal reflux injuries. Am J Med 2000;108(Suppl 4a):99S.

Barrett's Esophagus

- **Essentials of Diagnosis**
  - Dysphagia, heartburn, regurgitation in supine position
  - Upper endoscopy with biopsy reveals columnar epithelium replacing squamous epithelium
  - May be complicated by esophageal stricture or, in area of columnar epithelium, ulceration
  - Esophageal adenocarcinoma may develop in up to 10% of patients

- **Differential Diagnosis**
  - Achalasia
  - Esophageal or mediastinal tumor
  - Esophageal web
  - Benign stricture
  - Left atrial enlargement or pericardial effusion

- **Treatment**
  - Acid suppression (pH > 4) with proton pump inhibitors
  - Surgical fundoplication in selected patients
  - Endoscopic laser or photodynamic therapy in selected patients with dysplasia who are not surgical candidates
  - Surveillance esophagoscopy with biopsy at 1- or 2-year intervals

- **Pearl**

When brisk upper gastrointestinal bleeding occurs in a patient with Barrett's esophagus, suspect cardioesophageal fistula.

Reference

Bremner CG et al: Barrett's esophagus. Surg Clin North Am 1997;77:1115.

Mallory-Weiss Syndrome
(Mucosal Laceration of the Gastroesophageal Junction)

- ■ Essentials of Diagnosis
  - Because many patients are hypovolemic, portal pressure is low and bleeding not impressive
  - Hematemesis of bright red blood, often following prolonged or forceful vomiting or retching; majority lack this history
  - More impressive in alcoholics with brisk bleeding because of associated esophageal varices
  - Endoscopic demonstration of vertical mucosal tear at cardio-esophageal junction or proximal stomach
  - Hiatal hernia often associated

- ■ Differential Diagnosis
  - Peptic ulcer
  - Esophageal varices
  - Gastritis
  - Reflux, infectious, or pill esophagitis

- ■ Treatment
  - Usually none required; spontaneous resolution of bleeding unless concomitant varices present
  - Endoscopic hemostatic intervention with epinephrine injection or thermal coaptation for active bleeding; rarely, balloon tamponade, embolization, or surgery is required for uncontrolled bleeding

- ■ Pearl

Hyperemesis of pregnancy is the most common cause, but bleeding is seldom reported by the patient since it is trivial due to absence of factors noted in alcoholics.

Reference

Bharucha AE et al: Clinical and endoscopic risk factors in the Mallory-Weiss syndrome. Am J Gastroenterol 1997;92:805.

Emetogenic Esophageal Perforation (Boerhaave's Syndrome)

- ■ Essentials of Diagnosis
  - History of alcoholic binge drinking, excessive and rapid food intake, or both
  - Violent vomiting or retching followed by sudden pain in chest or abdomen, odynophagia, dyspnea
  - Fever, shock, profound systemic toxicity, subcutaneous emphysema, mediastinal crunching sounds, rigid abdomen, tachypnea
  - Leukocytosis, salivary hyperamylasemia
  - Chest x-ray shows mediastinal widening, mediastinal emphysema, pleural effusion (often delayed)
  - Demonstration of rupture of lower esophagus by esophagogram with water-soluble opaque media or CT scan; no role for endoscopy

- ■ Differential Diagnosis
  - Myocardial infarction, pericarditis
  - Pulmonary embolism, pulmonary abscess
  - Aortic dissection
  - Ruptured viscus
  - Acute pancreatitis
  - Shock due to other causes
  - Caustic ingestion, pill esophagitis
  - Instrumental esophageal perforation

- ■ Treatment
  - Aggressive supportive measures with broad-spectrum antibiotics covering mouth organisms, nasogastric tube suctioning, and total parenteral nutrition
  - Surgical consultation with repair

- ■ Pearl

One of the few causes in medicine of hydrophobia.

Reference

Achem, SR: Boerhaave's syndrome. Dig Dis 1999;17:256.

Foreign Bodies in the Esophagus

- **Essentials of Diagnosis**
  - Most common in children, edentulous older patients, and the severely mentally impaired
  - Occurs at physiologic areas of narrowing (upper esophageal sphincter, the level of the aortic arch, or the diaphragmatic hiatus)
  - Other predisposing factors favoring impaction include Zenker's diverticulum, webs, achalasia, peptic strictures, or malignancy
  - Recent ingestion of food or foreign material (coins most commonly in children), but the history may be missing
  - Vague discomfort in chest or neck, dysphagia, inability to handle secretions, odynophagia, hypersalivation, and stridor or dyspnea in children
  - Radiographic or endoscopic evidence of esophageal obstruction by foreign body

- **Differential Diagnosis**
  - Esophageal stricture
  - Esophageal or mediastinal tumor
  - Angina pectoris

- **Treatment**
  - Endoscopic removal with airway protection as needed and the use of an overtube if sharp objects are present
  - Emergent endoscopy should be used for sharp objects, disk batteries (secondary to risk of perforation due to their caustic nature), or evidence of the inability to handle secretions
  - Endoscopy is successful in over 90% of cases
  - Observation and delayed endoscopy may be considered if the patient is without symptoms and radiologic studies are negative

- **Pearl**

Treatment is ordinarily straightforward; diagnosis may not be.

Reference

Stack LB et al: Foreign bodies in the gastrointestinal tract. Emerg Med Clin North Am 1996;493.

Gastritis

■ **Essentials of Diagnosis**

- May be acute (erosive) or indolent (atrophic)
- Symptoms often vague and include nausea, vomiting, anorexia, nondescript upper abdominal distress; significant hemorrhage may occur with or without symptoms
- Mild epigastric tenderness to palpation; in some, physical signs absent
- Iron deficiency anemia not unusual
- Endoscopy with gastric biopsy for definitive diagnosis
- Multiple associations include stress (burns, sepsis, critical illness), drugs (NSAIDs, salicylates), atrophic states (aging, pernicious anemia), previous surgery (gastrectomy, Billroth II), *Helicobacter pylori* infection, acute or chronic alcoholism

■ **Differential Diagnosis**

- Peptic ulcer
- Hiatal hernia
- Malignancy of stomach or pancreas
- Cholecystitis
- Ischemic cardiac disease

■ **Treatment**

- Avoidance of alcohol, caffeine, salicylates, tobacco, and NSAIDs
- Investigate for presence of *Helicobacter pylori*; eradicate if present
- Proton pump inhibitors in patients receiving oral feedings, H_2 inhibitors, or sucralfate
- Prevention in high-risk patients (eg, intensive care setting) using these same agents

■ **Pearl**

Ninety-five percent of gastroenterologists and a high proportion of other health care workers carry H pylori.

Reference

Tytgat GN: Ulcers and gastritis. Endoscopy 2000;32:108.

Duodenal Ulcer

- **Essentials of Diagnosis**
  - Epigastric pain 45–60 minutes following meals or nocturnal pain, both relieved by food or antacids, sometimes by vomiting; symptoms chronic and periodic; radiation to back common
  - Iron deficiency anemia, positive fecal occult blood; amylase elevated with posterior penetration
  - Ulcer crater or deformity of duodenal bulb demonstrated radiographically or endoscopically
  - Caused by *Helicobacter pylori* in 70% of cases, NSAIDs in 20–30%, Zollinger-Ellison syndrome in less than 1%; *H pylori* infection may be diagnosed serologically
  - Complications include hemorrhage, intractable pain, perforation, and obstruction

- **Differential Diagnosis**
  - Reflux esophagitis
  - Gastritis
  - Pancreatitis
  - Cholecystitis
  - Other peptic disease, eg, Zollinger-Ellison syndrome or gastric ulcer

- **Treatment**
  - Eradicate *H pylori* when present
  - Avoid tobacco, alcohol, xanthines, and ulcerogenic drugs, especially NSAIDs
  - H_2 blockers, proton pump inhibitors, and sucralfate
  - Surgery—now far less common—may be needed for ulcers refractory to medical management (rare) or for the management of complications (eg, perforation, uncontrolled bleeding); supraselective vagotomy preferred unless patient unstable or is obstructed

- **Pearl**

Once an ulcer, always an ulcer. Patients with first episodes have a higher incidence of recurrence throughout life.

Reference

Wilcox CM: Relationship between nonsteroidal anti-inflammatory drug use, *Helicobacter pylori,* and gastroduodenal mucosal injury. Gastroenterology 1997;113(6 Suppl):S85.

Zollinger-Ellison Syndrome (Gastrinoma)

- ■ Essentials of Diagnosis
  - Severe, recurrent, intractable peptic ulcer disease, often associated with concomitant esophagitis; ulcers may be in atypical locations, like jejunum, but most in usual sites
  - Eighty percent of cases are sporadic; the rest are associated with multiple endocrine neoplasia type 1 (MEN 1)
  - Serum gastrin > 150 pg/mL (often much higher) in the setting of a low gastric pH; elevated serum chromogranin A
  - Diarrhea common, caused by inactivation of pancreatic enzymes; relieved by nasogastric tube suctioning immediately
  - Gastrinomas may arise in pancreas, duodenum, or lymph nodes; over 50% are malignant but not usually aggressive
  - Localization techniques include somatostatin receptor scintigraphy, thin-cut CT, MRI, endoscopic ultrasound, or intraoperative localization

- ■ Differential Diagnosis
  - Peptic ulcer disease of other cause
  - Esophagitis
  - Gastritis
  - Pancreatitis
  - Cholecystitis
  - Diarrhea or malabsorption from other causes

- ■ Treatment
  - High-dose proton pump inhibitor (with goal of < 10 meq/h of gastric acid secretion)
  - Exploratory laparotomy for patients without preoperative evidence of unresectable metastatic disease
  - Chemotherapy ineffective; interferon, octreotide, and hepatic artery embolization, for metastatic disease
  - Resection for localized disease
  - Family counseling
  - MEN 1-associated gastrinoma appears to have a lower incidence of hepatic metastases and a better long-term prognosis

- ■ Pearl

In Zollinger-Ellison syndrome, isolated gastric ulcer is never encountered.

Reference

Qureshi W et al: Zollinger-Ellison syndrome. Improved treatment options for this complex disorder. Postgrad Med 1998;104:155.

Gastric Ulcer

- **Essentials of Diagnosis**
  - Epigastric pain unpredictably relieved by food or antacids; weight loss, anorexia, vomiting
  - Iron deficiency anemia, fecal occult blood positive
  - Ulcer demonstrated by barium study or endoscopy
  - Caused by *Helicobacter pylori* (in 70% of cases), NSAIDs, gastric malignancy, Zollinger-Ellison syndrome
  - Endoscopic biopsy or documentation of complete healing necessary to exclude malignancy
  - Complications include hemorrhage, perforation, and obstruction

- **Differential Diagnosis**
  - Other peptic ulcer disease
  - Gastric carcinoma
  - Cholecystitis
  - Esophagitis
  - Gastritis
  - Irritable or functional bowel disease

- **Treatment**
  - Eradicate *H pylori* when present
  - Avoid tobacco, alcohol, xanthines, and ulcerogenic drugs, especially NSAIDs
  - Proton pump inhibitors, sucralfate, H_2 receptor antagonists
  - Surgery may be needed for ulcers refractory to medical management (rare) or for the management of complications (eg, perforation, uncontrolled bleeding)

- **Pearl**

Gastric ulcers lose weight; duodenal ulcers gain it.

Reference

Barkin J: The relation between *Helicobacter pylori* and nonsteroidal anti-inflammatory drugs. Am J Med 1998;105(5A):22S.

Crohn's Disease

- **Essentials of Diagnosis**
  - Insidious onset, with intermittent bouts of diarrhea, low-grade fever, right lower quadrant pain; peripheral arthritis, spondylitis; rash less common but may be presenting symptom
  - Complications include fistula formation, perianal disease with abscess, right lower quadrant mass and tenderness
  - Anemia, leukocytosis, positive fecal occult blood
  - Radiographic findings of thickened, stenotic bowel with ulceration, stricturing, or fistulas; characteristic skip areas
  - Histologic demonstration of submucosal inflammation with fibrosis and granulomatous lesions

- **Differential Diagnosis**
  - Ulcerative colitis
  - Appendicitis
  - Diverticulitis
  - Intestinal tuberculosis
  - Mesenteric adenitis
  - Lymphoma, other tumors of small intestine
  - Miscellaneous arthropathies and skin diseases

- **Treatment**
  - Low-residue, lactose-free diet, antidiarrheals, antispasmodics, vitamin B_{12} and calcium supplementation as needed
  - Sulfasalazine or mesalamine for colonic disease
  - Corticosteroids or mercaptopurine for acute flares or extraintestinal complications
  - Infliximab for refractory or fistulous disease
  - Surgery for refractory obstruction, fistula, or abscess

- **Pearl**

Ileocecal disease is present in 40–50%, isolated small bowel disease in 30–40%, and isolated colonic disease in 20%.

Reference

Rampton DS: Management of Crohn's disease. BMJ 1999;319:1480.

Celiac & Tropical Sprue

■ **Essentials of Diagnosis**

- Caused by gluten in diet (celiac sprue)
- Bulky, pale, frothy, greasy stools (steatorrhea); abdominal distention, flatulence, weight loss, and evidence of fat-soluble vitamin deficiencies
- Hypochromic or megaloblastic anemia; abnormal D-xylose absorption; increased fecal fat on quantitative studies
- Deficiency pattern on small bowel radiographic studies; villous atrophy on small bowel biopsy

■ **Differential Diagnosis**

- Crohn's disease
- Functional blind loop (especially jejunal diverticulosis)
- Intestinal tuberculosis (may be associated with celiac sprue)
- Intestinal lymphoma (may also complicate celiac sprue)
- Whipple's disease
- Pancreatic insufficiency

■ **Treatment**

- For tropical sprue: folic acid, vitamin B_{12} replacement if necessary, tetracycline or trimethoprim-sulfamethoxazole for 1–6 months
- For celiac sprue: strict elimination of gluten from diet (ie, wheat, rye, barley, and oat products); vitamin supplementation (especially vitamin B_{12}) and steroids in selected patients

■ **Pearl**

Flat gut occurs where it comes into contact with gluten; if gluten is introduced past the upper small bowel by nasogastric tube, the gut will be spared.

Reference

Ryan B et al: Refractory celiac disease. Gastroenterology 2000;119:243.

Disaccharidase (Lactase) Deficiency

- ■ Essentials of Diagnosis
  - Congenital in Asians and blacks, in whom it is nearly ubiquitous; can also be acquired temporarily after gastroenteritis of other causes
  - Symptoms vary from abdominal bloating, distention, cramps, and flatulence to explosive diarrhea in response to disaccharide ingestion
  - Stool pH < 5.5; reducing substances present in stool
  - Flat glucose response to disaccharide loading, abnormal hydrogen breath test, or resolution of symptoms on lactose-free diet suggests the diagnosis

- ■ Differential Diagnosis
  - Chronic mucosal malabsorptive disorders
  - Irritable bowel syndrome
  - Inflammatory bowel disease
  - Pancreatic insufficiency
  - Giardiasis

- ■ Treatment
  - Restriction of dietary lactose; usually happens by experience in blacks from early life
  - Lactase enzyme supplementation
  - Maintenance of adequate nutritional and calcium intake

- ■ Pearl

Consider this in undiagnosed diarrhea; the patient may not be aware of ingesting lactose.

Reference

Shaw AD et al: Lactose intolerance: problems in diagnosis and treatment. J Clin Gastroenterol 1999;28:208.

Whipple's Disease

■ **Essentials of Diagnosis**

- Caused by infection with the bacillus *Tropheryma whippelii*
- Rare in women and blacks
- Insidious onset of fever, abdominal pain, malabsorption, arthralgias, weight loss, symptoms of steatorrhea, polyarthritis
- Lymphadenopathy, arthritis, macular skin rash, various neurologic findings
- Anemia, hypoalbuminemia, hypocarotenemia
- Small bowel mucosal biopsy reveals characteristic foamy mononuclear cells filled with periodic acid-Schiff (PAS) staining material; electron microscopy shows bacilli in multiple affected organs

■ **Differential Diagnosis**

- Celiac or tropical sprue
- Crohn's disease
- Ulcerative colitis
- Intestinal lymphoma
- Rheumatoid arthritis or HLA-B27 spondyloarthropathy
- Hyperthyroidism
- HIV infection

■ **Treatment**

- Penicillin and streptomycin (ceftriaxone and streptomycin for central nervous system disease) for 10–14 days followed by trimethoprim-sulfamethoxazole (cefixime or doxycycline in sulfonamide-allergic patients)
- Treatment for at least 1 year

■ **Pearl**

Oculomasticatory myorhythmia (continuous rhythmic motion of the eye muscles with mastication) or ocular-facial-skeletal myorhythmia is Whipple's disease and nothing else.

Reference

Ramaiah C et al: Whipple's disease. Gastroenterol Clin North Am 1998;27:683.

Intestinal Tuberculosis

- ■ Essentials of Diagnosis
  - Chronic abdominal pain, anorexia, bloating; weight loss, fever, diarrhea, new-onset ascites in many
  - Mild right lower quadrant tenderness; fistula-in-ano sometimes seen
  - Barium study may reveal mucosal ulcerations or scarring and fibrosis with narrowing of the small or large intestine
  - In peritonitis, ascitic fluid has high protein and mononuclear pleocytosis; peritoneal biopsy with granulomas
  - Complications include intestinal obstruction, hemorrhage, fistula formation, and bacterial overgrowth with malabsorption

- ■ Differential Diagnosis
  - Carcinoma of the colon or small bowel
  - Inflammatory bowel disease
  - Ameboma
  - Intestinal lymphoma or amyloidosis
  - Ovarian or peritoneal carcinomatosis
  - *Mycobacterium avium-intracellulare* infection

- ■ Treatment
  - Standard therapy for tuberculosis

- ■ Pearl

Historically, many patients underwent exploratory laparotomy for suspected small bowel obstruction; improvement inevitably ensued without specific therapy.

Reference

Kapoor VK: Abdominal tuberculosis. Postgrad Med J 1998;74:459.

Irritable Bowel Syndrome

- **Essentials of Diagnosis**
  - Chronic functional disorder characterized by abdominal pain, alteration in bowel habits, constipation and diarrhea (often alternating), dyspepsia, anxiety or depression
  - Variable abdominal tenderness
  - Sigmoidoscopy may reveal spasm or mucous hypersecretion; other studies normal

- **Differential Diagnosis**
  - Inflammatory bowel disease
  - Ischemic colitis
  - Diverticular disease
  - Peptic ulcer disease
  - Pancreatitis

- **Treatment**
  - Reassurance and explanation
  - High-fiber diet with or without fiber supplements; restricting dairy products may be helpful
  - Antispasmodic agents (eg, dicyclomine, hyoscyamine, propantheline), antidiarrheal or anticonstipation agents
  - Amitriptyline, serotonin selective reuptake inhibitors, and behavioral modification with relaxation techniques helpful for some patients

- **Pearl**

Irritable bowel syndrome is the most common diagnosis resulting in office visits to a gastroenterologist; it ranks highly with primary care providers, too.

Reference

Schmulson MW et al: Diagnostic approach to the patient with irritable bowel syndrome. Am J Med 1999;107(5A):20S.

Ulcerative Colitis

- **Essentials of Diagnosis**
  - Role of personality debated; half are normal
  - Low-volume diarrhea, often bloody; tenesmus and cramping lower abdominal pain; associated with fever, weight loss, rash
  - Mild abdominal tenderness, mucocutaneous lesions, erythema nodosum or pyoderma gangrenosum
  - Anemia, accelerated sedimentation rate, hypoproteinemia, absent stool pathogens
  - Ragged mucosa with loss of haustral markings on barium enema; colon involved contiguously from rectum, seldom if ever sparing it
  - Crypt abscesses on rectal mucosal biopsy
  - Increased incidence of adenocarcinoma with young age at onset, long-standing active disease, pancolitis

- **Differential Diagnosis**
  - Bacterial, amebic, or ischemic colitis
  - Diverticular disease
  - Adenocarcinoma of the colon
  - Benign colonic stricture
  - Pseudomembranous colitis
  - Granulomatous colitis or Crohn's disease
  - Antibiotic-associated diarrhea
  - Radiation colitis or collagenous colitis

- **Treatment**
  - Topical mesalamine or corticosteroids by enema or suppository
  - Fiber supplements, lactose-free diet
  - Sulfasalazine, mesalamine, or olsalazine for chronic therapy
  - Mesalamine, corticosteroids, or cyclosporine for acute flares; obtain amebic serologies before systemic steroids
  - Fish oil, ciprofloxacin, nicotine may be of benefit in refractory disease
  - Colectomy for toxic megacolon unresponsive to medical therapy, severe extracolonic manifestations, colonic malignancy or dysplasia, or (in selected patients with long-standing disease) for cancer prophylaxis
  - Yearly colonoscopy

- **Pearl**

Four hepatobiliary complications: pericholangitis, chronic active hepatitis, sclerosing cholangitis, cholangiocarcinoma.

Reference

Ghosh S et al: Ulcerative colitis. BMJ 2000;320:1119.

Polyps of the Colon & Rectum

- **Essentials of Diagnosis**
  - Discrete mass lesions arising from colonic epithelium and protruding into the intestinal lumen; polyps may be pedunculated or sessile
  - Most patients asymptomatic; can be associated with chronic occult blood loss
  - Family history may be present
  - Diagnosed by sigmoidoscopy, colonoscopy, or barium enema
  - Removing polyps decreases the incidence of adenocarcinoma

- **Differential Diagnosis**
  - Adenocarcinoma
  - Radiographic artifact

- **Treatment**
  - Surgical or endoscopic polypectomy in all cases with histologic review
  - Colectomy for familial polyposis or Gardner's syndrome
  - Surveillance colonoscopy every 3–5 years

- **Pearl**

The incidence curves of adenomatous polyps and carcinoma by age are superimposable.

Reference

Kronborg O: Colon polyps and cancer. Endoscopy 2000;32:124.

Anal Fissure
(Fissura-in-Ano, Anal Ulcer)

- ■ Essentials of Diagnosis
  - • Linear disruption of the anal epithelium
  - • Rectal pain with defecation; bleeding and constipation
  - • Acute anal tenderness to digital examination
  - • Ulceration and stenosis of anal canal, hypertrophic anal papilla, external skin tag on anoscopy

- ■ Differential Diagnosis
  - • Rectal syphilis, tuberculosis, herpes, chlamydial infections
  - • Crohn's disease
  - • Acute monocytic leukemia
  - • Malignant epithelioma leukemia

- ■ Treatment
  - • High-fiber diet, psyllium, bran, stool softeners, sitz baths, hydro-cortisone suppositories
  - • Topical nitrate therapy or botulinum toxin injection
  - • Lateral internal sphincterotomy if no improvement with medical therapy

- ■ Pearl

Unexplained cases call for white count with differential.

Reference

Janicke DM et al: Anorectal disorders. Emerg Med Clin North Am 1996;14:757.

Acute Pancreatitis

- **Essentials of Diagnosis**
  - Background of alcohol binge or gallstones
  - Abrupt onset of epigastric pain, often with radiation to the back; nausea, vomiting, low-grade fever, and dehydration
  - Abdominal tenderness, distention
  - Leukocytosis, elevated serum and urine amylase; hypocalcemia and hemoconcentration in severe cases; hypertriglyceridemia (> 1000 mg/dL) may be causative, likewise hypercalcemia
  - Radiographic "sentinel loop" may be seen on plain films of the abdomen, signifying localized ileus
  - CT for patients highly symptomatic or for suspected abscesses

- **Differential Diagnosis**
  - Acute cholecystitis or cholangitis
  - Penetrating or perforating duodenal ulcer
  - Mesenteric infarction
  - Gastritis
  - Nephrolithiasis
  - Abdominal aortic aneurysm
  - Small bowel obstruction

- **Treatment**
  - Nasogastric suction for nausea or ileus, prompt intravenous fluid and electrolyte replacement, analgesics, and antiemetics
  - Antibiotics (imipenem) for documented infection or evidence of necrotizing pancreatitis on CT; discontinue drugs capable of causing the disease, eg, thiazides, corticosteroids
  - Aggressive surgical debridement for sterile pancreatic necrosis without clinical improvement with conservative measures or for infected pancreatic necrosis
  - Early endoscopic retrograde cholangiopancreatography with sphincterotomy for pancreatitis with associated jaundice and cholangitis resulting from choledocholithiasis

- **Pearl**

In "idiopathic" pancreatitis, obtain more history from someone other than the patient. You can be sure alcohol is in the picture.

Reference

Janicke DM et al: Anorectal disorders. Emerg Med Clin North Am 1996;14:757.

Chronic Pancreatitis

- **Essentials of Diagnosis**
  - Persistent or recurrent abdominal pain
  - Pancreatic calcification by radiographic study
  - Pancreatic insufficiency with malabsorption and diabetes in one-third of patients
  - Occurs in patients with alcoholism (most common), hereditary pancreatitis, or untreated hyperparathyroidism; or after abdominal trauma
  - Diagnostic studies include endoscopic retrograde cholangiopancreatography (beading of pancreatic duct with ectatic side branches), endoscopic ultrasound (stippling or stranding of parenchyma with ductal dilation or thickening), magnetic resonance cholangiopancreatography, and an abnormal secretin pancreatic stimulation test

- **Differential Diagnosis**
  - Diabetes mellitus
  - Malabsorption due to other causes
  - Intractable duodenal ulcer
  - Carcinoma of the pancreas
  - Gallstones
  - Irritable bowel syndrome

- **Treatment**
  - Low-fat diet, pancreatic enzyme supplements, avoidance of alcohol
  - Pain management includes opioids and amitriptyline
  - Endoscopic sphincterotomy and pancreatic duct stenting as well as endoscopic ultrasound-guided celiac block for pain management have yielded disappointing results
  - Treatment of hyperlipidemia if present
  - Intravenous fluid and electrolyte replacement for acute exacerbations
  - Surgical therapy to restore free flow of bile or to treat intractable pain

- **Pearl**

Alcohol and trauma are the causes of chronic relapsing pancreatitis. As always, the history will tell the story.

Reference

Apte MV et al: Chronic pancreatitis: complications and management. J Clin Gastroenterol 1999;29:225.

Clostridium difficile (Pseudomembranous) Colitis

- **Essentials of Diagnosis**
  - Profuse watery, green, foul-smelling, or bloody diarrhea
  - Cramping abdominal pain
  - Fecal leukocytes present in over half of patients
  - Fevers, marked abdominal tenderness, leukocytosis, hypovolemia, dehydration, and hypoalbuminemia are common
  - History of antibiotic use (especially penicillin family antibiotics and clindamycin)
  - Many cases may be asymptomatic or associated with minimal symptoms
  - Diagnosis confirmed by positive stool antigen test or via sigmoidoscopy or colonoscopy.

- **Differential Diagnosis**
  - Antibiotic-associated diarrhea (without *C difficile* or pseudomembranous colitis)
  - Other bacterial diarrheas
  - Inflammatory bowel disease
  - Parasitic (amebiasis) and viral (cytomegalovirus) causes of diarrhea and colitis

- **Treatment**
  - Discontinue offending antibiotic therapy
  - Replacement of fluid and electrolyte losses
  - Oral metronidazole, with vancomycin reserved for metronidazole-resistant cases or critically ill patients; treatment is for 10–14 days
  - Surgical therapy is needed rarely (1–3%) for severe cases with megacolon or impending perforation
  - Avoid opioids and antidiarrheal agents

- **Pearl**

The cause of the highest benign white count in all of medicine save pertussis.

Reference

Taege AJ et al: *Clostridium difficile* diarrhea and colitis: a clinical overview. Cleve Clin J Med 1999;66:503.

Acute Colonic Pseudo-Obstruction (Ogilvie's Syndrome)

3

- ■ Essentials of Diagnosis
  - Often seen in elderly hospitalized patients
  - Associated with a history of trauma, fractures, cardiac disease, infection, or the use of opioids, antidepressants, and anticholinergics
  - Often detected as a distended, tympanitic abdomen with abdominal x-ray revealing gross colonic dilation (cecum > 10 cm), scant air-fluid levels, a gradual transition to collapsed bowel, and air and stool present in the rectum
  - May mimic true obstruction, and obstruction should be evaluated with radiologic studies using diatrizoate (Hypaque) enema
  - Fevers, marked abdominal tenderness, leukocytosis, and acidosis may be present in advanced cases with impending perforation

- ■ Differential Diagnosis
  - Mechanical obstruction
  - Toxic megacolon
  - Chronic intestinal pseudo-obstruction

- ■ Treatment
  - Cessation of oral intake, nasogastric and rectal suctioning, intravenous fluids
  - Correction of electrolyte abnormalities (Ca^{2+}, Mg^{2+}, K^+)
  - Discontinue offending medications and treat underlying infections
  - Frequent enemas (tap water) and patient repositioning may be of benefit
  - Neostigmine (2 mg intravenously) in appropriately selected patients
  - Colonoscopic decompression for patients failing neostigmine or in whom neostigmine therapy is contraindicated
  - Surgical consultation (for tube cecostomy) for patients with peritoneal signs or impending perforation

- ■ Pearl

Many patients with this disorder have surprisingly unimpressive examinations. Sequential abdominal films in high-risk ICU patients are prudent irrespective of symptoms.

Reference

Di Lorenzo C: Pseudo-obstruction: current approaches. Gastroenterology 1999; 116:980.

4

Hepatobiliary Disorders

Acute Viral Hepatitis

- **Essentials of Diagnosis**
  - Anorexia, nausea, vomiting, malaise, symptoms of flu-like syndrome, arthralgias, and aversion to smoking
  - Jaundice, fever, chills; enlarged, tender liver
  - Normal to low white cell count; abnormal liver function studies (ALT > AST); serologic tests for hepatitis A (IgM antibody), hepatitis B (HBsAg), or hepatitis C (antibody) may be positive
  - Liver biopsy shows characteristic hepatocellular necrosis and mononuclear infiltrates
  - Hepatitis A: oral-fecal transmission, short incubation period; good prognosis, but rare cases of fulminant hepatic failure
  - Hepatitis B and hepatitis C: parenteral transmission, longer incubation period, progression to chronic disease more likely

- **Differential Diagnosis**
  - Alcoholic hepatitis
  - Leptospirosis
  - Secondary syphilis
  - Q fever
  - Choledocholithiasis
  - Carcinoma of the pancreas
  - Cholestatic jaundice secondary to drugs
  - Acetaminophen toxicity
  - Hepatic vein thrombosis

- **Treatment**
  - Supportive care
  - Avoidance of hepatotoxins: alcohol, acetaminophen

- **Pearl**

Hepatitis A is the only viral hepatitis causing spiking fevers.

Reference

Sjögren MH: Serologic diagnosis of viral hepatitis. Med Clin North Am 1996; 80:929. [PMID: 8804369]

Chronic Viral Hepatitis

- ■ Essentials of Diagnosis
  - Fatigue, right upper quadrant discomfort, arthralgias, depression, nausea, anorexia
  - In advanced cases (cirrhosis): jaundice, variceal bleeding, encephalopathy, ascites, spontaneous bacterial peritonitis, and hepatocellular carcinoma
  - Persistent elevation in ALT (> 6 months)
  - In hepatitis B, positive hepatitis B DNA with HBeAg present
  - In hepatitis C, positive hepatitis C RNA

- ■ Differential Diagnosis
  - Alcoholic cirrhosis
  - Metabolic liver disorders, eg, Wilson's disease, hemochromatosis
  - Autoimmune hepatitis
  - Cholestatic jaundice secondary to drugs

- ■ Treatment
  - Avoidance of alcohol, acetaminophen
  - Interferon alfa or lamivudine for patients with chronic active hepatitis B and interferon alfa and ribavirin for symptomatic patients with hepatitis C
  - Liver transplantation for advanced disease

- ■ Pearl

Hepatitis C is the most common reason for liver transplantation.

Reference

Berenguer M et al: Hepatitis. Advances in antiviral therapy for hepatitis. Lancet 1998;352(Suppl 4):SIV15. [PMID: 9873162]

Autoimmune Hepatitis

- **Essentials of Diagnosis**
  - Insidious onset; usually affects young women
  - Fatigue, anorexia, arthralgias; dark urine; light stools in some
  - Jaundice, spider angiomas, hepatomegaly, acne, hirsutism
  - Abnormal liver function tests, most notably increased amino-transferases, polyclonal gammopathy
  - Associated with arthritis, thyroiditis, nephritis, Coombs-positive hemolytic anemia
  - ANA or anti-smooth muscle antibody-positive
  - Patients may develop cirrhosis, predicted by biopsy features of chronic active hepatitis

- **Differential Diagnosis**
  - Chronic viral hepatitis
  - Sclerosing cholangitis
  - Primary biliary cirrhosis
  - Wilson's disease
  - Hemochromatosis

- **Treatment**
  - General supportive measures (including exercise, calcium, and hormonal therapy to prevent osteoporosis)
  - Prednisone with or without azathioprine
  - Liver transplantation for decompensated cirrhosis

- **Pearl**

Spider angiomas never occur below the waist.

Reference

Czaja AJ: The variant forms of autoimmune hepatitis. Ann Intern Med 1996; 125:588. [PMID: 8815758]

Alcoholic Hepatitis

- **Essentials of Diagnosis**
  - Onset usually after years of alcohol intake; anorexia, nausea, abdominal pain
  - Fever, jaundice, tender hepatomegaly, ascites, encephalopathy
  - Macrocytic anemia, leukocytosis with left shift, thrombocytopenia, abnormal liver function tests (AST > ALT, increased bilirubin, prolonged prothrombin time), hypergammaglobulinemia; AST rarely exceeds 300 units/L despite severity of illness
  - Liver biopsy confirms diagnosis

- **Differential Diagnosis**
  - Cholecystitis, cholelithiasis
  - Cirrhosis due to other causes
  - Non-alcoholic fatty liver
  - Viral hepatitis
  - Drug-induced hepatitis

- **Treatment**
  - General supportive measures, withdrawal of alcohol, avoidance of hepatotoxins (especially acetaminophen)
  - Methylprednisolone (32 mg/d for 4 weeks) may be beneficial in severe disease when discriminant function (4.6 [PT − control] + bilirubin [mg/dL]) is > 32

- **Pearl**

Acute alcoholic hepatitis can be indistinguishable from acute chole-cystitis with or without cholangitis. This is the most useful application of abdominal ultrasound.

Reference

Hill DB et al: Alcoholic liver disease. Treatment strategies for the potentially reversible stages. Postgrad Med 1998;103:261. [PMID: 9553600]

Cirrhosis

- ■ **Essentials of Diagnosis**
    - The outcome of many types of hepatitis—viral, toxic, immune, and metabolic
    - Insidious onset of malaise, weight loss, increasing abdominal girth, erectile dysfunction in men
    - Jaundice, spider angiomas, palpable firm hepatomegaly, palmar erythema, Dupuytren's contractures, gynecomastia, ascites, edema, encephalopathy with asterixis
    - Macrocytic anemia, thrombocytopenia, abnormal liver function (increased prothrombin time, hypoalbuminemia)
    - Biopsy diagnostic with micro- or macronodular fibrosis
    - Complications include esophageal or gastric varices, gastrointestinal bleeding, spontaneous bacterial peritonitis, encephalopathy, hepatorenal syndrome

- ■ **Differential Diagnosis**
    - Congestive heart failure
    - Constrictive pericarditis
    - Hemochromatosis
    - Primary biliary cirrhosis
    - Wilson's disease
    - Schistosomiasis
    - Nephrotic syndrome
    - Hypothyroidism

- ■ **Treatment**
    - Supportive care, abstinence from alcohol, vitamin supplementation
    - Beta-blockers in patients with established varices
    - Diuretics or large-volume paracenteses for ascites and edema
    - Antibiotic treatment and, debatably, prophylaxis for spontaneous bacterial peritonitis
    - Lactulose for encephalopathy
    - Transjugular intrahepatic portosystemic shunt for bleeding esophageal varices or refractory ascites
    - Liver transplantation in selected cases

- ■ **Pearl**

Hepatitis A never causes cirrhosis.

Reference

Menon KV et al: Managing the complications of cirrhosis. Mayo Clin Proc 2000;75:501. [PMID: 10807079]

Primary Biliary Cirrhosis

- **Essentials of Diagnosis**
  - Usually affects women aged 40–60 with the insidious onset of pruritus, jaundice, and hepatomegaly
  - Hepatomegaly in 70% with splenomegaly in 35%
  - Malabsorption, xanthomatous neuropathy, osteomalacia, and portal hypertension may be complications
  - Increased alkaline phosphatase, cholesterol, bilirubin; positive antimitochondrial antibody in 95%

- **Differential Diagnosis**
  - Chronic biliary tract obstruction, ie, cholelithiasis-related stricture
  - Bile duct carcinoma
  - Inflammatory bowel disease complicated by cholestatic liver disease
  - Sarcoidosis
  - Sclerosing cholangitis
  - Drug-induced cholestasis

- **Treatment**
  - Cholestyramine, colestipol, or rifampin for pruritus
  - Calcium and supplementation with vitamins A, D, E, and K
  - Ursodeoxycholic acid, colchicine, or methotrexate may be helpful
  - Liver transplant for refractory cirrhosis

- **Pearl**

The perfect disease for cure by transplantation: no virus, no malignancy in explant.

Reference

Neuberger J: Primary biliary cirrhosis. Lancet 1997;350:875. [PMID: 9310614]

Hepatic Vein Obstruction (Budd-Chiari Syndrome)

- **Essentials of Diagnosis**
  - Spectrum of disorders characterized by occlusion of the hepatic veins from a variety of causes
  - Acute or chronic onset of tender, painful hepatic enlargement, jaundice, splenomegaly, and ascites
  - Liver scintigraphy may show a prominent caudate lobe since its venous drainage may not be occluded; liver biopsy reveals characteristic central lobular congestion
  - Doppler ultrasound or venography demonstrates occlusion of the hepatic veins
  - Associations include caval webs, polycythemia, right-sided heart failure, malignancy, "bush teas" (pyrrolizidine alkaloids), paroxysmal nocturnal hemoglobinuria, birth control pills, pregnancy, hypercoagulable states

- **Differential Diagnosis**
  - Cirrhosis
  - Constrictive pericarditis
  - Restrictive or dilated cardiomyopathy
  - Metastatic disease involving the liver
  - Granulomatous liver disease

- **Treatment**
  - Treatment of complications, eg, ascites, encephalopathy
  - Lifelong anticoagulation or treatment of underlying disease
  - Portacaval, mesocaval, or mesoatrial shunt may be required
  - Transvenous intravascular portosystemic shunt may be considered in noncirrhotic patients
  - Liver transplantation for severe hepatocellular dysfunction

- **Pearl**

"Idiopathic" Budd-Chiari syndrome has been shown to be caused in many cases by subclinical myeloproliferative diseases.

Reference

Mahmoud A et al: New approaches to the Budd-Chiari syndrome. J Gastroenterol Hepatol 1996;11:1121. [PMID: 9034920]

Pyogenic Hepatic Abscess

- ### Essentials of Diagnosis
  - Right-sided or midabdominal pain, anorexia, nausea; weight loss, pleuritic chest pain, cough
  - Fever, jaundice, right upper quadrant tenderness, weight loss, pleuritic chest pain, cough
  - Leukocytosis with left shift; nonspecific abnormalities of liver function studies
  - Most common organisms are *Escherichia coli, Proteus vulgaris, Enterobacter aerogenes,* and anaerobic species
  - Elevated right hemidiaphragm by radiography; ultrasound, CT scan, or liver scan demonstrates intrahepatic defect
  - Predisposing factors: malignancy, recent endoscopy or surgery, diabetes, Crohn's disease, diverticulitis, appendicitis, recent trauma

- ### Differential Diagnosis
  - Amebic hepatic abscess
  - Acute hepatitis
  - Right lower lobe pneumonia
  - Cholelithiasis, cholecystitis
  - Appendicitis

- ### Treatment
  - Antibiotics with coverage of gram-negative organisms and anaerobes
  - Needle or surgical drainage for cases refractory to medical management

- ### Pearl

The classic triad of fever, jaundice, and hepatomegaly is found in less than 10% of cases.

Reference

Ch Yu S et al: Pyogenic liver abscess: treatment with needle aspiration. Clin Radiol 1997;52:912. [PMID: 9413964]

Amebic Hepatic Abscess

- ■ **Essentials of Diagnosis**
  - Right-sided abdominal pain, right pleuritic chest pain; preceding or concurrent diarrheal illness in minority
  - History of travel to endemic region
  - Fever, tender palpable liver ("punch" tenderness), localized intercostal tenderness
  - Anemia, leukocytosis with left shift, nonspecific liver test abnormalities
  - Positive serologic tests for *Entamoeba histolytica* in over 95% of patients, though may be initially nondiagnostic
  - Increased right hemidiaphragm by radiography; ultrasound, CT scan, or liver scan demonstrates location and number of lesions

- ■ **Differential Diagnosis**
  - Pyogenic abscess
  - Acute hepatitis
  - Right lower lobe pneumonia
  - Cholelithiasis, cholecystitis
  - Appendicitis

- ■ **Treatment**
  - Metronidazole drug of choice; repeated courses occasionally necessary
  - Percutaneous needle aspiration for toxic patient
  - Oral course of luminal amebicides (iodoquinol, paromomycin sulfate) following acute therapy to eradicate intestinal cyst phase

- ■ **Pearl**

Amebic liver abscess presents with amebic colitis in only 10% of cases. Aspiration of abscess reveals odorless yellow to dark brown "anchovy paste" material.

Reference

Fujihara T et al: Amebic liver abscess. J Gastroenterol 1996;31:659. [PMID: 8887031]

Cholelithiasis (Gallstones)

- ■ Essentials of Diagnosis
  - • Frequently asymptomatic but may be associated with recurrent bouts of right-sided or midepigastric pain and nausea or vomiting after eating
  - • Ultrasound, CT scan, and plain films demonstrate stones within the gallbladder
  - • Increased incidence with female gender, chronic hemolysis, obesity, Native American origin, inflammatory bowel disease, diabetes mellitus, pregnancy, hypercholesterolemia

- ■ Differential Diagnosis
  - • Acute cholecystitis
  - • Acute pancreatitis
  - • Peptic ulcer disease
  - • Acute appendicitis
  - • Acute hepatitis
  - • Right lower lobe pneumonia
  - • Myocardial infarction
  - • Radicular pain in T6–T10 dermatome

- ■ Treatment
  - • Laparoscopic or open cholecystectomy for symptomatic patients only
  - • Bile salts (cheno- and ursodeoxycholic acid) may cause dissolution of cholesterol stones
  - • Lithotripsy with concomitant bile salts administration may be successful

- ■ Pearl

In a patient with right upper quadrant densities on a plain film of the abdomen associated with hyperchromia and microcytosis, consider hereditary spherocytosis with premature cholelithiasis due to lifelong hemolysis.

Reference

Agrawal S et al: Gallstones, from gallbladder to gut. Management options for diverse complications. Postgrad Med 2000;108:143. [PMID: 11004941]

Choledocholithiasis

■ Essentials of Diagnosis

- Often a history of biliary tract disease; episodic attacks of right abdominal or epigastric pain that may radiate to the right scapula or shoulder; occasionally painless jaundice
- Pain, fever, and jaundice (Charcot's triad); associated with nausea, vomiting, hypothermia, shock, and leukocytosis with a left shift
- Elevated serum amylase and liver function tests, especially bilirubin and alkaline phosphatase
- Abdominal imaging studies may reveal gallstones
- Ultrasound or CT scan shows dilated biliary tree
- Endoscopic retrograde cholangiopancreatography (ERCP) or magnetic resonance cholangiopancreatography (MRCP) localizes the degree and location of obstruction

■ Differential Diagnosis

- Carcinoma of the pancreas, ampulla of Vater, or common duct
- Acute hepatitis
- Biliary stricture
- Drug-induced cholestatic jaundice
- Pancreatitis
- Other septic syndromes

■ Treatment

- Intravenous broad-spectrum antibiotics
- Endoscopic papillotomy and stone extraction followed by laparoscopic or open cholecystectomy
- A T tube may be placed in the common duct to decompress it for at least 7–8 postoperative days

■ Pearl

Although choledocholithiasis is often asymptomatic, onset of septic shock may occur within hours. The sun should never set on this diagnosis.

Reference

Soetikno RM et al: Endoscopic management of choledocholithiasis. J Clin Gastroenterol 1998;27:296. [PMID: 9855257]

Sclerosing Cholangitis

- **Essentials of Diagnosis**
  - Progressively obstructive jaundice, pruritus, malaise, anorexia, and indigestion, most common in young men aged 20–40 years
  - Two-thirds of cases have associated ulcerative colitis
  - Positive antineutrophil cytoplasmic antibody found in 70%; elevated total bilirubin and alkaline phosphatase common
  - Endoscopic retrograde cholangiopancreatography (ERCP) demonstrates thick or narrowed biliary ductal system
  - Absence of previous biliary stones, biliary surgery, congenital abnormalities, biliary cirrhosis, and cholangiocarcinoma necessary to make the diagnosis

- **Differential Diagnosis**
  - Choledocholithiasis
  - Drug-induced cholestasis
  - Carcinoma of pancreas or biliary tree
  - Hepatitis due to any cause
  - *Clonorchis sinensis* infection

- **Treatment**
  - At present, no specific medical therapy has been shown to have a major impact on the prevention of complications or survival
  - Ursodeoxycholic acid may improve liver function tests but does not alter natural history
  - Stenting or balloon dilation of localized strictures by ERCP
  - Liver transplantation for decompensated disease

- **Pearl**

Most sclerosing cholangitis is seen in ulcerative colitis, but most ulcerative colitis is not complicated by sclerosing cholangitis.

Reference

Angulo P et al: Primary sclerosing cholangitis. Hepatology 1999;30:325. [PMID: 10385674]

Variceal Bleeding

- **Essentials of Diagnosis**
  - Sudden, painless large-volume episode of hematemesis with melena or hematochezia typical
  - Antecedent history of liver disease and stigmas of liver disease or portal hypertension on physical examination
  - A hepatic portal venous pressure gradient of ≥12 mm Hg is generally necessary for variceal bleeding
  - Fifty percent of patients with alcoholic cirrhosis will present with esophageal varices within 2 years of diagnosis
  - A 30–50% risk of death with each episode

- **Differential Diagnosis**
  - Mallory-Weiss tear
  - Alcoholic gastritis
  - Peptic ulcer disease
  - Esophagitis
  - Bleeding from portal hypertensive gastropathy

- **Treatment**
  - Appropriate resuscitation (intravenous resuscitation, correction of coagulopathy, blood transfusions, airway protection, antibiotic therapy for spontaneous bacterial peritonitis prophylaxis)
  - Intravenous octreotide (100 μg bolus, 50 μg/h drip)
  - Urgent endoscopic evaluation and treatment with band ligation or sclerotherapy; less successful in gastric varices
  - Balloon tamponade (Minnesota-Sengstaken-Blakemore) as a temporizing measure or for endoscopic failures
  - Transjugular intrahepatic portosystemic shunt (TIPS) or shunt surgery for refractory cases of esophageal or gastric varices
  - Liver transplantation for appropriate candidates with recurrent bleeding episodes
  - Prophylaxis of recurrent bleeding with endoscopic (band ligation) and pharmacologic therapy (propranolol, nadolol)

- **Pearl**

In a patient with any possible lifetime exposure, eg, a person born in Puerto Rico with no other liver disease, consider schistosomiasis— even if there has been no visit to the endemic area for over 20 years.

Reference

Luketic VA et al: Esophageal varices. I. Clinical presentation, medical therapy, and endoscopic therapy. Gastroenterol Clin North Am 2000;29:337. [PMID: 10836186]

Ascites

- ■ Essentials of Diagnosis
  - Usually associated with liver disease; but heart or kidney disease should also be sought
  - Evidence of shifting dullness, bulging flanks
  - Paracentesis for new-onset ascites or symptoms suggestive of spontaneous bacterial peritonitis
  - Fluid sent for cell count, albumin, total protein; glucose, amylase, LDH, bacterial stains, cytology examination, and triglycerides in some
  - Serum–ascites albumin gradient ≥ 1.1 g/dL is virtually diagnostic of portal hypertension
  - > 250 neutrophils/μL with a percentage greater than 50% characteristic of infection

- ■ Differential Diagnosis
  - Chronic liver disease (80–85% of all cases)
  - Malignancy-related (10%)
  - Cardiac failure (3%)
  - Tuberculosis
  - Dialysis-related
  - Pancreatic
  - Lymphatic tear (chylous)

- ■ Treatment

  Treat as follows for ascites due to portal hypertension:
  - Sodium restriction (< 2g/d)
  - Fluid restriction if serum sodium < 120 mmol/L
  - Diuretics: usually spironolactone and furosemide
  - Large-volume paracentesis (4–6 L) for tense or refractory ascites with albumin replacement (6–10 g/L)
  - Transjugular intrahepatic portosystemic shunt (TIPS) or surgical shunting in refractory cases
  - Patients with spontaneous bacterial peritonitis treated for 5 days with a third-generation cephalosporin (eg, cefotaxime)
  - Spontaneous bacterial peritonitis prophylaxis (with norfloxacin or trimethoprim-sulfisoxazole) for patients with spontaneous bacterial peritonitis, gastrointestinal hemorrhage, or low-protein ascites (< 1.5 g/dL)

- ■ Pearl

Once spontaneous bacterial peritonitis occurs, liver transplant may be the only intervention that prolongs life.

Reference

Menon KV et al: Managing the complications of cirrhosis. Mayo Clin Proc 2000;75:501. [PMID: 10807079]

Hepatic Encephalopathy

- **Essentials of Diagnosis**
  - Neurologic and psychiatric abnormalities resulting from liver dysfunction due to acute liver failure, cirrhosis, or major non-cirrhotic portosystemic shunting
  - Diagnosis requires history and physical examination suggestive of liver disease or portosystemic shunting
  - Clinical manifestations range from mild confusion, personality changes, and sleep disturbances (stage I) to coma (stage IV)
  - Asterixis, hyperreflexia, muscular rigidity, extensor plantar response, parkinsonian features, immobile facies, slow and monotonous speech
  - Often triggered by gastrointestinal bleeding, infection, lactulose noncompliance, dietary protein overload, hypokalemia

- **Differential Diagnosis**
  - Systemic or central nervous system sepsis
  - Hypoxia or hypercapnia
  - Acidosis
  - Uremia
  - Medication
  - Postictal confusion
  - Wernicke-Korsakoff syndrome
  - Acute liver failure (cerebral edema or hypoglycemia)
  - Delirium tremens
  - Hyponatremia

- **Treatment**
  - Identify and treat precipitating factors listed above
  - Lactulose, 30–60 mL by mouth or nasogastric tube every 2 hours until bowel movements occur; titrate to maintain two or three loose stools per day
  - Flumazenil of temporary benefit
  - Dietary protein restriction (< 70 g/d but > 40 g/d)
  - Liver transplantation for chronic hepatic encephalopathy

- **Pearl**

In a stable cirrhotic with encephalopathy and none of the above precipitants, hepatocellular carcinoma is the most likely explanation.

Reference

Butterworth RF: Complications of cirrhosis III. Hepatic encephalopathy. J Hepatol 2000;32(1 Suppl):171. [PMID: 10728803]

Hepatocellular Carcinoma

- **Essentials of Diagnosis**
  - One of the world's most common visceral tumors
  - Hepatitis B, hepatitis C, alcoholic cirrhosis, hemochromatosis among the important risk factors
  - Symptoms may not help, as they are similar to those of underlying liver disease
  - Even a palpable mass can be confusing because of regenerating nodules
  - Edema due to inferior vena cava invasion
  - Elevated—sometimes markedly—alpha-fetoprotein in some but not all; characteristic arterial phase helical CT scan

- **Differential Diagnosis**
  - Metastatic primary of other source
  - Regenerating nodule

- **Treatment**
  - Surgical resection if uninvolved liver not cirrhotic (as in virus carriers) and only one lobe involved
  - Transplant in highly selected patients

- **Pearl**

A normal hematocrit in cirrhosis suggests this diagnosis; the tumor may manufacture erythropoietin, and most cirrhotics are anemic.

Reference

Bergsland EK et al: Hepatocellular carcinoma. Curr Opin Oncol 2000;12:357. [PMID: 10888422]

5

Hematologic Diseases

Iron Deficiency Anemia

- ■ Essentials of Diagnosis
  - Lassitude; in children under age 2, poor muscle tone, delayed motor development
  - Pallor, cheilosis, and koilonychia
  - Hypochromic microcytic red cells late in disease; indices normal early
  - Serum iron low, total iron-binding capacity increased; absent marrow iron; serum ferritin < 15 ng/mL classically, but concomitant illness may elevate it
  - Newer tests include increased serum soluble transferrin receptor and transferrin receptor:log ferritin ratio
  - Occult blood loss invariably causative in adults; malabsorption or dietary insufficiency rarely if ever causes deficiency

- ■ Differential Diagnosis
  - Anemia of chronic disease
  - Thalassemia
  - Sideroblastic anemias, including lead intoxication

- ■ Treatment
  - Oral ferrous sulfate or ferrous gluconate three times daily for 6–12 months
  - Parenteral iron dextran for selected patients with severe, clinically significant iron deficiency with continuing chronic blood loss
  - Evaluation for occult blood loss

- ■ Pearl

Remember iron deficiency as a treatable cause of obesity; ice cream craving is one of many associated picas.

Reference

Frewin R et al: ABC of clinical haematology. Iron deficiency anaemia. BMJ; 1997;314:360. [PMID: 9040336]

Anemia of Chronic Disease

- **Essentials of Diagnosis**
  - Known chronic disease, particularly inflammatory; symptoms and signs usually those of responsible disease
  - Modest anemia (Hct ≥ 25%); red cells normal morphologically but may be slightly microcytic
  - Low serum iron with normal or low total iron-binding capacity, normal or high serum ferritin, normal or increased bone marrow iron stores, low soluble transferrin receptor and soluble transferrin receptor:log ferritin ratio

- **Differential Diagnosis**
  - Iron deficiency anemia
  - Sideroblastic anemia
  - Thalassemia

- **Treatment**
  - None usually necessary
  - Red blood cell transfusions for symptomatic anemia, recombinant erythropoietin (epoetin alfa) in patients with associated renal disease

- **Pearl**

In anemia of chronic disease, the hemoglobin and hematocrit should not fall below 60% of baseline; if lower, some other cause of anemia is present.

Reference

Spivak JL: The blood in systemic disorders. Lancet 2000;355:1707. [PMID: 10905258]

Disseminated Intravascular Coagulation

- ■ Essentials of Diagnosis
  - • Evidence of abnormal bleeding or clotting, usually in a critically ill patient
  - • Occurs as a result of activation and consumption of clotting and antithrombotic factors due to severe stressors such as sepsis, burns, massive hemorrhage
  - • May occur in chronic, indolent form, usually associated with malignancy
  - • Anemia, thrombocytopenia, elevated prothrombin time and, later, partial thromboplastin time, low fibrinogen, elevated fibrin degradation products and fibrin D-dimers

- ■ Differential Diagnosis
  - • Severe liver disease
  - • Thrombotic thrombocytopenic purpura
  - • Vitamin K deficiency
  - • Other microangiopathic hemolytic anemias (eg, prosthetic heart valve)
  - • Sepsis-induced thrombocytopenia or anemia
  - • Heparin-induced thrombocytopenia

- ■ Treatment
  - • Treat underlying disorder
  - • Replacement of consumed blood factors with fresh frozen plasma, cryoprecipitate, and potentially antithrombin III
  - • Heparin in selected cases, particularly acute promyelocytic leukemia
  - • Antifibrinolytic therapy (aminocaproic acid or tranexamic acid) for refractory bleeding, but only in presence of heparin therapy

- ■ Pearl

Remember that platelets and fibrinogen may be normal in chronic DIC.

Reference

Levi M et al: Disseminated intravascular coagulation. N Engl J Med 1999; 341:586. [PMID: 10451465]

Thrombotic Thrombocytopenic Purpura (TTP)

- ■ Essentials of Diagnosis
  - • Petechial rash, mucosal bleeding, fever, altered mental status, renal failure; many cases in HIV infection
  - • Laboratory reports are notable for anemia, dramatically elevated LDH, normal prothrombin and partial thromboplastin times, fibrin degradation products, and thrombocytopenia
  - • Most cases probably related to acquired inhibitor of von Willebrand factor-cleaving protease; may also be secondary to drugs, chemotherapy, or cancer
  - • Demonstrating presence or decreased activity of vWF-cleaving protease inhibitor may be diagnostic, but tests not commonly available

- ■ Differential Diagnosis
  - • Disseminated intravascular coagulation
  - • Preeclampsia-eclampsia
  - • Other microangiopathic hemolytic anemias
  - • Hemolytic-uremic syndrome

- ■ Treatment
  - • Immediate plasmapheresis
  - • Fresh-frozen plasma infusions help if plasmapheresis not readily available
  - • Splenectomy and immunosuppressive or cytotoxic medications for refractory cases

- ■ Pearl

A previously rare disease which doubled in incidence during the AIDS epidemic.

Reference

George JN: How I treat patients with thrombotic thrombocytopenic purpura-hemolytic uremic syndrome. Blood 2000;96:1223. [PMID: 10942361]

Hemolytic-Uremic Syndrome

- **Essentials of Diagnosis**
  - Petechial rash, hypertension, acute-to-subacute renal failure
  - Often preceded by gastroenteritis or exposure to offending medication
  - Frequently associated with antecedent campylobacter infection (may be very mild to occult)
  - Laboratory reports notable for thrombocytopenia, anemia, renal failure, elevated LDH, normal prothrombin time and partial thromboplastin time as well as fibrin and fibrinogen degeneration products

- **Differential Diagnosis**
  - Disseminated intravascular coagulation
  - Thrombotic thrombocytopenic purpura
  - Pre-eclampsia–eclampsia
  - Other microangiopathic hemolytic anemias

- **Treatment**
  - In children, disease is most often self-limited and managed with supportive care
  - In adults, stop potentially offending drugs
  - Plasmapheresis for refractory cases

- **Pearl**

Many childhood cases are precipitated by E coli O157:H7 infection.

Reference

van Gorp EC et al: Review: infectious diseases and coagulation disorders. J Infect Dis 1999;180:176. [PMID: 10353876]

Autoimmune Hemolytic Anemia

- **Essentials of Diagnosis**
  - Acquired anemia caused by IgG autoantibody
  - Fatigue, malaise in many; occasional abdominal or back pain
  - Pallor, jaundice, but palpable spleen uncommon
  - Persistent anemia with microspherocytes and reticulocytosis; elevated indirect bilirubin and serum LDH
  - Positive Coombs (direct antiglobulin) test
  - Various drugs, underlying autoimmune or lymphoproliferative disorder may be causative

- **Differential Diagnosis**
  - Hemoglobinopathy
  - Hereditary spherocytosis
  - Nonspherocytic hemolytic anemia
  - Sideroblastic anemia
  - Cold agglutinin disease
  - Megaloblastic anemia

- **Treatment**
  - High-dosage steroids
  - Intravenous immune globulin, or plasmapheresis in severe cases
  - Cross-match difficult because of autoantibodies, so least incompatible blood used
  - Splenectomy for refractory or recurrent cases
  - More intensive immunosuppressive regimens available for refractory cases after splenectomy

- **Pearl**

When therapeutic splenectomy is being contemplated, give prophylactic pneumococcal vaccine.

Reference

Smith LA: Autoimmune hemolytic anemias: characteristics and classification. Clin Lab Sci 1999;12:110. [PMID: 10387488]

Drug-Induced Hemolytic Anemia

- ■ Essentials of Diagnosis
  - Immune hemolytic anemia due to host antibody recognition of drug and red blood cell membrane
  - Acute to subacute onset; elevated LDH, hyperbilirubinemia, reticulocytosis
  - Rarely, fulminant presentation with laboratory abnormalities as noted plus hemoglobinemia-hemoglobinuria, renal failure, and hemodynamic instability
  - Positive Coombs test with patient's blood; study using reagent red blood cells positive only in presence of offending drug

- ■ Differential Diagnosis
  - Autoimmune hemolytic anemia
  - Microangiopathic hemolytic anemia (eg, disseminated intravascular coagulation, thrombotic thrombocytopenic purpura)
  - Delayed transfusion-related hemolysis
  - Blood loss

- ■ Treatment
  - Discontinue offending drug
  - Plasmapheresis for severe cases, especially if drug has long serum half-life
  - Intravenous immune globulin, steroids potentially of benefit

- ■ Pearl

An annoying prospect in an internal medicine patient: since many drugs can cause it and since typical patients are taking many drugs, the only way to be sure is to peel off the drugs one by one until improvement is noted.

Reference

Wright MS: Drug-induced hemolytic anemias: increasing complications to therapeutic interventions. Clin Lab Sci 1999;12:115. [PMID: 10387489]

Hemolytic Transfusion Reaction

■ Essentials of Diagnosis

- Chills and fever during blood transfusion
- Back, chest pain; dark urine
- Associated with vascular collapse, renal failure, and disseminated intravascular coagulation
- Hemolysis, hemoglobinuria, and severe anemia

■ Differential Diagnosis

- Leukoagglutination reaction
- IgA deficiency with anaphylactic transfusion reaction
- Myocardial infarction
- Acute abdomen due to other causes
- Pyelonephritis
- Bacteremia due to contaminated blood product

■ Treatment

- Stop transfusion immediately
- Hydration and intravenous mannitol to prevent renal failure

■ Pearl

Any adverse clinical event during transfusion should be considered and evaluated as a hemolytic reaction.

Reference

Sloop GD et al: Complications of blood transfusion. How to recognize and respond to noninfectious reactions. Postgrad Med 1995;98:159. [PMID: 7603944]

Hereditary Spherocytosis

- **Essentials of Diagnosis**
  - Chronic hemolytic anemia of variable severity, often with exacerbations during coincident illnesses
  - Malaise, abdominal discomfort in symptomatic patients
  - Jaundice, splenomegaly in severely affected patients
  - Variable anemia with spherocytosis and reticulocytosis; elevated MCHC; increased osmotic fragility test and increased red cell fragility as measured with ektacytometry (ie, measurement of the shear stress a red blood cell can withstand before lysing)
  - Negative Coombs test
  - Family history of anemia, jaundice, splenectomy

- **Differential Diagnosis**
  - Autoimmune hemolytic anemia
  - Hemoglobin C disease
  - Iron deficiency anemia
  - Alcoholism
  - Burns

- **Treatment**
  - Oral folic acid supplementation
  - Pneumococcal vaccination if splenectomy contemplated
  - Splenectomy for symptomatic patients

- **Pearl**

The only condition in medicine causing a hyperchromic, microcytic anemia.

Reference

Tse WT et al: Red blood cell membrane disorders. Br J Haematol 1999;104:2. [PMID: 10027705]

5

Paroxysmal Nocturnal Hemoglobinuria

- **Essentials of Diagnosis**
  - Episodic red-brown urine, especially on first morning specimen
  - Variable anemia with or without leukopenia, thrombocytopenia; reticulocytosis; positive urine hemosiderin, elevated serum LDH
  - Flow cytometry of red cells negative for CD55 or CD59, positive sucrose hemolysis test or Ham's test
  - Iron deficiency often concurrent
  - Intra-abdominal venous thrombosis in some patients

- **Differential Diagnosis**
  - Hemolytic anemias
  - Myelodysplasia
  - Pancytopenia due to other causes

- **Treatment**
  - Prednisone for moderate to severe cases
  - Oral iron replacement if iron-deficient
  - Allogeneic bone marrow transplantation for severe cases
  - Long-term anticoagulation for thrombotic events

- **Pearl**

One of the few hemolytic anemias associated with iron deficiency; most hemolysis occurs extravascularly with conservation of iron.

Reference

Nishimura J et al: Paroxysmal nocturnal hemoglobinuria: An acquired genetic disease. Am J Hematol 1999;62:175. [PMID: 10539884]

Thalassemia Major

- **Essentials of Diagnosis**
  - Severe anemia from infancy; positive family history
  - Massive splenomegaly
  - Hypochromic, microcytic red cells with severe poikilocytosis, target cells, acanthocytes, and basophilic stippling on smear
  - Mentzer's index (MCV/RBC) < 13
  - Greatly elevated hemoglobin F level

- **Differential Diagnosis**
  - Other hemoglobinopathies
  - Congenital nonspherocytic hemolytic anemia

- **Treatment**
  - Regular red blood cell transfusions
  - Oral folic acid supplementation
  - Splenectomy for secondary hemolysis due to hypersplenism
  - Deferoxamine to avoid iron overload
  - Allogeneic bone marrow transplantation in selected cases

- **Pearl**

With low-MCV anemia in a patient of Mediterranean origin, thalassemia is the presumptive diagnosis until proved otherwise.

Reference

Rund D et al: New trends in the treatment of beta-thalassemia. Crit Rev Oncol Hematol 2000;33:105. [PMID: 10737372]

Beta-Thalassemia Minor

- ■ Essentials of Diagnosis
  - Symptoms variable depending on degree of anemia; no specific physical findings
  - Mild and persistent anemia, hypochromia with microcytosis and target cells; red blood cell count normal or elevated
  - Similar findings in one of patient's parents
  - Patient often of Mediterranean, African, or southern Chinese ancestry
  - Elevated hemoglobin A_2 and hemoglobin F
  - Mentzer's index (MCV/RBC) < 13

- ■ Differential Diagnosis
  - Iron deficiency anemia
  - Other hemoglobinopathies, especially hemoglobin C disorders
  - Sideroblastic anemia
  - Alpha-thalassemia
  - Anemia of chronic disease

- ■ Treatment
  - Oral folic acid supplementation
  - Avoidance of medicinal iron or oxidative agents
  - Red blood cell transfusions during pregnancy or stress (intercurrent illness) if hemoglobin falls below 9 g/dL

- ■ Pearl

The hemoglobinopathies exhibit central red cell targeting; liver disease targeting tends to be eccentric.

Reference

Olivieri NF: The beta-thalassemias. N Engl J Med 1999;341:99. [PMID: 10395635]

Alpha-Thalassemia Trait

- **Essentials of Diagnosis**
  - Commonly comes to attention because of CBC done for other reasons
  - Increased frequency in persons of African, Mediterranean, or southern Chinese ancestry
  - Microcytosis out of proportion to anemia; occasional target cells and acanthocytes on smear but far less so than beta; normal iron studies
  - Mentzer's index (MCV/RBC) < 13
  - No increase in hemoglobin A_2 or hemoglobin F
  - Diagnosis of exclusion in patient with modest anemia (definitive diagnosis depends on hemoglobin gene mapping)

- **Differential Diagnosis**
  - Iron deficiency anemia
  - Other hemoglobinopathies
  - Sideroblastic anemia
  - Beta-thalassemia minor

- **Treatment**
  - Oral folic acid supplementation
  - Avoidance of medicinal iron or oxidative agents
  - Red blood cell transfusions during pregnancy or stress (intercurrent illness) if hemoglobin falls below 9 g/dL

- **Pearl**

Microcytosis without anemia or hyperchromia is with few exceptions alpha-thalassemia.

Reference

Bowie LJ et al: Alpha thalassemia and its impact on other clinical conditions. Clin Lab Med 1997;17:97. [PMID: 9138902]

Sickle Cell Anemia

■ Essentials of Diagnosis

- Caused by substitution of valine for glutamine in the sixth position on the beta chain
- Recurrent episodes of fever with pain in arms, legs, or abdomen starting in early childhood
- Splenomegaly in early childhood *only;* jaundice, pallor; adults are functionally asplenic
- Anemia and elevated reticulocyte count with irreversibly sickled cells on peripheral smear; elevated indirect bilirubin, LDH; positive sickling test; hemoglobin S and F on electrophoresis
- Complications include salmonella osteomyelitis, remarkably high incidence of encapsulated infections, and ischemic complications in any sluggish or hypoxic part of the circulation (eg, medullary interstitium of kidney)
- Five types of crises: pain, aplastic, megaloblastic, sequestration, hemolytic
- Positive family history and lifelong history of hemolytic anemia

■ Differential Diagnosis

- Other hemoglobinopathies
- Acute rheumatic fever
- Osteomyelitis
- Acute abdomen due to any cause
- If hematuria present, renal stone or tumor

■ Treatment

- Chronic oral folic acid supplementation
- Hydration and analgesics
- Hydroxyurea for patients with frequent crises
- Partial exchange transfusions for intractable vaso-occlusive crises, acute chest syndrome, stroke or transient ischemic attack, priapism
- Transfusion for hemolytic or aplastic crises and during third trimester of pregnancy
- Pneumonia vaccination
- Genetic counseling

■ Pearl

In regard to sickle cell anemia: anything disease can do, so may trait.

Reference

Serjeant GR: Sickle-cell disease. Lancet 1997;350:725. [PMID: 92911916]

Hemoglobin SC Disease

- **Essentials of Diagnosis**
  - Recurrent attacks of abdominal, joint, or bone pain
  - Splenomegaly, retinopathy (similar to diabetes)
  - Mild anemia, reticulocytosis, and few sickle cells on smear but many targets; 50% hemoglobin C, 50% hemoglobin S on electrophoresis
  - In situ thrombi of pulmonary artery and venous sinus of brain may simulate pulmonary emboli, may cause stroke

- **Differential Diagnosis**
  - Sickle cell anemia
  - Sickle thalassemia
  - Hemoglobin C disease
  - Cirrhosis
  - Pulmonary embolism
  - Beta thalassemia

- **Treatment**
  - No specific therapy for most patients
  - Otherwise treat as for SS hemoglobin

- **Pearl**

Unique among hemoglobinopathies, thrombotic complications are most severe during pregnancy.

Reference

Moll S et al: Hemoglobin SC disease. Am J Hematol 1997;54:313. [PMID: 9092687]

Hemoglobin S–Thalassemia Disease

- ■ Essentials of Diagnosis
  - • Recurrent attacks of abdominal, joint, or bone pain
  - • Splenomegaly
  - • Mild to moderate anemia with low MCV; reticulocytosis; few sickle cells on smear with many target cells; increased hemoglobin A_2 by electrophoresis distinguishes from sickle cell disease, hemoglobin C

- ■ Differential Diagnosis
  - • Sickle cell anemia
  - • Hemoglobin C disease
  - • Hemoglobin SC disease
  - • Cirrhosis

- ■ Treatment
  - • Chronic oral folic acid supplementation
  - • Acute therapy as in sickle cell anemia

- ■ Pearl

Like other sickle hemoglobin positives, complications tend to be less severe than in SC disease.

Reference

Clarke GM et al: Laboratory investigation of hemoglobinopathies and thalassemias: review and update. Clin Chem 2000;46(8 Part 2):1284. [PMID: 10926923]

Sideroblastic Anemia

- **Essentials of Diagnosis**
  - Dimorphic (ie, normal and hypochromic) red blood cell population on smear
  - Hematocrit may reach 20%
  - Most often result of clonal stem cell disorder, though rarely may be drugs, lead, or alcohol; may be a megaloblastic component
  - Elevated serum iron with high percentage saturation; marrow is diagnostic with abnormal ringed sideroblasts (iron deposits encircling red blood cell precursor nuclei)
  - Minority progress to acute leukemia

- **Differential Diagnosis**
  - Iron deficiency anemia
  - Post-transfusion state
  - Anemia of chronic disease
  - Thalassemia

- **Treatment**
  - Remove offending toxin if present
  - Chelation therapy for lead toxicity
  - Pyridoxine 200 mg/d occasionally helpful
  - Does not respond to erythropoietin (epoetin alfa)

- **Pearl**

In the anemic alcoholic patient who is not bleeding, sideroblastic anemia may be the diagnosis; reticulocytosis 3 days after discontinuation of ethanol is characteristic, at which time the serum iron falls abruptly.

Reference

Sheth S et al: Genetic disorders affecting proteins of iron metabolism: clinical implications. Annu Rev Med 2000;51:443. [PMID: 10774476]

Vitamin B_{12} Deficiency

- **Essentials of Diagnosis**
  - Dyspnea on exertion, nonspecific gastrointestinal symptoms
  - Constant symmetric numbness and tingling of the feet; later, poor balance and dementia manifest
  - Pallor, mild jaundice, decreased vibratory and position sense
  - Pancytopenia with oval macrocytes and hypersegmented neutrophils, increased MCV, megaloblastic bone marrow; low serum vitamin B_{12}; positive Schilling test
  - Neurologic manifestations occur without anemia in rare cases, including dementia
  - Hematologic response to pharmacologic doses of folic acid
  - History of total gastrectomy, bowel resection, bacterial overgrowth, fish tapeworm, Crohn's disease, or autoimmune endocrinopathies (eg, diabetes mellitus, hypothyroidism)

- **Differential Diagnosis**
  - Folic acid deficiency
  - Myelodysplastic syndromes
  - Occasional hemolytic anemias with megaloblastic red cell precursors in marrow
  - Infiltrative granulomatous or malignant processes causing pancytopenia
  - Hypersplenism
  - Paroxysmal nocturnal hemoglobinuria
  - Acute leukemia

- **Treatment**
  - Vitamin B_{12} 100 μg intramuscularly daily during first week, then weekly for 1 month
  - Lifelong B_{12} 100 μg intramuscularly every month thereafter
  - Hypokalemia may complicate early therapy

- **Pearl**

An arrest in reticulocytosis shortly after institution of therapy means concealed iron deficiency until proved otherwise.

Reference

Hoffbrand AV et al: Nutritional anemias. Semin Hematol 1999;36(4 Suppl 7):13. [PMID: 10595751]

Folic Acid Deficiency

- ■ **Essentials of Diagnosis**
  - Nonspecific gastrointestinal symptoms, fatigue, dyspnea without neurologic complaints in a patient with malnutrition, often related to alcoholism
  - Pallor, mild jaundice
  - Pancytopenia, but counts not as low as in vitamin B_{12} deficiency; oval macrocytosis and hypersegmented neutrophils; megaloblastic marrow; normal vitamin B_{12} levels
  - Red blood cell folate < 150 ng/mL diagnostic

- ■ **Differential Diagnosis**
  - Vitamin B_{12} deficiency
  - Myelodysplastic syndromes
  - Infiltrative granulomatous or neoplastic bone marrow process
  - Hypersplenism
  - Paroxysmal nocturnal hemoglobinuria
  - Acute leukemia

- ■ **Treatment**
  - Exclude vitamin B_{12} deficiency prior to therapy
  - Oral folic acid supplementation

- ■ **Pearl**

In countries such as England where vegetables may be overcooked, folate deficiency may occur in otherwise adequately nourished persons.

Reference

Snow CF: Laboratory diagnosis of vitamin B_{12} and folate deficiency: a guide for the primary care physician. Arch Intern Med 1999;159:1289. [PMID: 103865055]

Pure Red Cell Aplasia

■ **Essentials of Diagnosis**

- Autoimmune disease in which IgG antibody attacks erythroid precursors
- Lassitude, malaise; nonspecific examination except for pallor
- Severe anemia with normal red blood cell morphology; myeloid and platelet lines unaffected; low or absent reticulocyte count
- Reduced or absent erythroid precursors in normocellular marrow
- Rare associations with systemic lupus erythematosus, chronic lymphocytic leukemia, non-Hodgkin's lymphoma and thymoma

■ **Differential Diagnosis**

- Aplastic anemia
- Myelodysplastic syndromes
- Drug-induced red cell aplasia
- Parvovirus B19 infection

■ **Treatment**

- Evaluate for underlying disease
- Immunosuppressive therapy with prednisone, cyclophosphamide, antithymocyte globulin
- High-dose intravenous immune globulin in selected patients
- Thymectomy in patients with thymoma may be beneficial

■ **Pearl**

In patients who have red cell aplasia and arthritis without other features of systemic lupus erythematosus, parvovirus B19 infection is an underappreciated diagnosis.

Reference

Erslev AJ et al: Pure red-cell aplasia: a review. Blood Rev 1996;10:20. [PMID: 8861276]

Agranulocytosis

- ### Essentials of Diagnosis
  - Malaise of abrupt onset, chills, fever, sore throat
  - Mucosal ulceration
  - History of drug ingestion common (eg, trimethoprim-sulfameth-oxazole, ganciclovir, propylthiouracil)
  - Profound granulocytopenia with relative lymphocytosis

- ### Differential Diagnosis
  - Aplastic anemia
  - Myelodysplasia
  - Systemic lupus erythematosus (SLE)
  - Viral infection (HIV, CMV, hepatitis)
  - Acute leukemia
  - Felty's syndrome

- ### Treatment
  - Stop offending drugs
  - Broad-spectrum antibiotics for fever
  - Trial of filgrastim (granulocyte cell-stimulating factor) for severe neutropenia
  - Allogeneic bone marrow transplant for appropriate refractory patients

- ### Pearl
Sequential neutrophil counts are valueless in at-risk patients; a normal neutrophil count today may be agranulocytosis tomorrow.

Reference
Mylonakis E et al: Resolution of drug-induced agranulocytosis. Geriatrics 2000; 55:89. [PMID: 10711310]

Aplastic Anemia

- **Essentials of Diagnosis**
  - Lassitude, fatigue, malaise, other nonspecific symptoms
  - Pallor, purpura, mucosal bleeding, petechiae, signs of infection
  - Pancytopenia with normal cellular morphology; hypocellular bone marrow with fatty infiltration
  - Occasional history of exposure to an offending drug or radiation

- **Differential Diagnosis**
  - Bone marrow infiltrative process (tumor, some infections, granulomatous diseases)
  - Myelofibrosis
  - Acute leukemia
  - Hypersplenism
  - Viral infections including HIV, hepatitis
  - SLE

- **Treatment**
  - Allogeneic bone marrow transplantation for patients under age 30
  - Intensive immunosuppression with antithymocyte globulin, cyclosporine if transplant not feasible
  - Oral androgens may be of benefit
  - If SLE associated, plasmapheresis and corticosteroids effective
  - Avoid transfusions if possible in patients who may be transplant candidates; otherwise, red blood cells and platelet transfusions, filgrastim (granulocyte cell-stimulating factor) or sargramostim (granulocyte-macrophage cell-stimulating factor) as necessary

- **Pearl**

The risk of aplastic anemia from chloramphenicol is one in 40,000 courses; chloramphenicol is underused because of this overexaggerated risk.

Reference

Ball SE: The modern management of severe aplastic anaemia. Br J Haematol 2000;110:41. [PMID: 10930978]

Acute Leukemia

- **Essentials of Diagnosis**
  - Crisp onset of fever, weakness, malaise, bleeding, bone or joint pain, infection
  - Pallor, fever, petechiae; lymphadenopathy, generally unimpressive; splenomegaly unusual
  - Leukocytosis or cytopenia of any or all three cell lines; immature, abnormal white cells in bone marrow, often in peripheral blood
  - Abnormal cells are either lymphoblasts (ALL) or myeloblasts (AML); Auer rods indicate the latter
  - Seven types of morphology depending on cell of origin in patients with AML

- **Differential Diagnosis**
  - Aplastic anemia
  - Idiopathic thrombocytopenia purpura
  - Infectious mononucleosis
  - Hodgkin's or non-Hodgkin's lymphoma
  - Pertussis
  - Metastatic malignancy to bone marrow
  - Miliary tuberculosis
  - Paroxysmal nocturnal hemoglobinuria

- **Treatment**
  - Aggressive combination chemotherapy with specific drugs dictated by cell type
  - Conventional-dose chemotherapy curative in minority of adults with acute leukemia; allogeneic and autologous bone marrow transplantation considered for appropriate patients

- **Pearl**

Remember that pain in expansile bone marrow can simulate mechanical back pain with bilateral leg radiation.

Reference

Löwenberg B et al: Acute myeloid leukemia. N Engl J Med 1999;341:1051. [PMID: 10502596]

Chronic Myelogenous Leukemia

- ■ **Essentials of Diagnosis**
  - Symptoms variable; often diagnosed by examination or blood count done for unrelated reasons
  - Splenomegaly in all cases; sternal tenderness in some
  - Leukocytosis, typically striking; immature white cells in peripheral blood and bone marrow; thrombocytosis, eosinophilia, basophilia common
  - Diagnosis relies on demonstration of Philadelphia chromosome t(9:22) by conventional cytogenetics, PCR of peripheral blood or bone marrow, or fluorescent in situ hybridization
  - Low leukocyte alkaline phosphatase level, markedly elevated serum vitamin B_{12} due to high B_{12} binding transcobalamins
  - Results in acute leukemia in 3–5 years

- ■ **Differential Diagnosis**
  - Leukemoid reactions associated with infection, inflammation, or cancer
  - Other myeloproliferative disorders

- ■ **Treatment**
  - Tyrosine kinase inhibitor (STI571; imitanib mesylate [Gleevec]) targeting specific molecular defect in CML cells is now first-line therapy in many centers
  - Combination of cytarabine (Ara-C) and interferon leads to cytogenetic complete remissions in small minority of patients
  - Allogeneic bone marrow transplantation remains useful therapy for appropriate candidates

- ■ **Pearl**

Pseudohypoglycemia and pseudohyperkalemia are in vitro artifacts resulting from continuing white cell metabolism of glucose and release of potassium into serum after clotting. They should be considered before inappropriate therapy is initiated.

Reference

Druker BJ et al: Efficacy and safety of a specific inhibitor of the BCR-ABL tyrosine kinase in chronic myeloid leukemia. N Engl J Med 2001;344:1031. [PMID: 11287972]

Polycythemia Vera

- **Essentials of Diagnosis**
  - Acquired myeloproliferative disorder with overproduction of all three hematopoietic cell lines; dominated by erythrocytosis
  - Pruritus (especially following a hot shower), tinnitus, blurred vision in some
  - Venous thromboses, often in uncommon sites (eg, splenic or portal vein thromboses); plethora, splenomegaly
  - Erythrocytosis; leukocytosis with eosinophilia and basophilia, thrombocytosis common; elevated total red blood cell mass, normal P_{O_2}
  - Increased serum vitamin B_{12}, leukocyte alkaline phosphatase levels usually elevated; hyperuricemia
  - Increased incidence of leukemia late in course; higher incidence of peptic ulcer

- **Differential Diagnosis**
  - Hypoxemia (pulmonary or cardiac disease, high altitude)
  - Carboxyhemoglobin (tobacco use)
  - Certain hemoglobinopathies characterized by tight O_2 binding
  - Erythropoietin-secreting tumors
  - Cystic renal disease
  - Spurious erythrocytosis with decreased plasma volume and high normal red cell mass (Gaisböck's syndrome)
  - Other myeloproliferative disorders

- **Treatment**
  - Phlebotomy to Hct < 45%
  - Myelosuppressive therapy with radiophosphorus (^{32}P) or alkylating agents only for patients with high phlebotomy requirements, intractable pruritus, or marked thrombocytosis
  - Avoidance of medicinal iron; low-iron diet
  - Aspirin 325 mg/d if at high risk for arterial thrombosis or history of clotting
  - Deep venous thrombosis prophylaxis for any surgical procedure or prolonged period of immobilization

- **Pearl**

Do not give iron to a patient with anemia from a bleeding ulcer and a palpable spleen—the hemorrhage may be concealing this disease.

Reference

Tefferi A et al: A clinical update in polycythemia vera and essential thrombocythemia. Am J Med 2000;109:141. [PMID: 10967156]

Essential Thrombocytosis

- **Essentials of Diagnosis**
  - Sustained elevated platelet count without other cause
  - Painful burning of palms and soles (erythromelalgia) promptly and completely relieved with low-dose aspirin
  - Arterial > venous thromboses
  - Low likelihood of progression to fibrotic "spent" stage or acute leukemia
  - May have mild elevations in white count and hematocrit; basophilia, eosinophilia, hypervitaminosis B_{12}

- **Differential Diagnosis**
  - Other myeloproliferative disorders (especially polycythemia vera)
  - Chronic infection or autoimmune disease, visceral malignancy (reactive thrombocytosis)
  - Iron deficiency

- **Treatment**
  - Platelet-lowering therapy for those with high risk of clotting (history of prior clotting, older patients, established arterial vascular disease)
  - Anagrilide and hydroxyurea most commonly used agents

- **Pearl**

It is the qualitative (not quantitative) platelet defect that results in clotting; reactive thrombocytosis is not a hypercoagulable state.

Reference

Tefferi A et al: A clinical update in polycythemia vera and essential thrombocythemia. Am J Med 2000;109:141. [PMID: 10967156]

Myelofibrosis

- **Essentials of Diagnosis**
  - Fatigue, abdominal discomfort, bleeding, bone pain
  - Massive splenomegaly, variable hepatomegaly
  - Anemia, leukocytosis or leukopenia; leukoerythroblastic peripheral smear with marked poikilocytosis, giant platelets, left-shifted myeloid series
  - Dry tap on bone marrow aspiration

- **Differential Diagnosis**
  - Chronic myelocytic leukemia
  - Other myeloproliferative disorders
  - Hemolytic anemias
  - Lymphoma
  - Metastatic cancer involving bone marrow
  - Hairy cell leukemia

- **Treatment**
  - Red blood cell transfusion support
  - Androgenic steroids may decrease transfusion requirements
  - Splenectomy for painful splenomegaly, severe thrombocytopenia, or extraordinary red blood cell requirements
  - Interferon alfa or erythropoietin (epoetin alfa)—or both—may be of benefit in selected patients

- **Pearl**

With hilar adenopathy, transverse myelitis, or any mass lesion complicating myelofibrosis, extramedullary hematopoiesis may be responsible.

Reference

Tefferi A: Myelofibrosis with myeloid metaplasia. N Engl J Med 2000;342: 1255. [PMID: 10781623]

Myelodysplastic Syndromes

- **Essentials of Diagnosis**

  - Clonal hematopoietic disorder characterized by ineffective hematopoiesis leading to peripheral cytopenias and variable presence of blasts
  - Progression as follows: refractory anemia → refractory anemia with ringed sideroblasts → refractory anemia with excess blasts (RAEB) → RAEB in transition → chronic myelomonocytic leukemia
  - Evolution to acute leukemia may take up to 15 years
  - Morphologic dysplasia frequently seen in cells of myeloid-lineage (eg, Pelger-Huët anomaly, hypogranular-hypolobulated neutrophils, giant platelets)
  - Previous chemotherapy (eg, procarbazine, melphalan) predisposes

- **Differential Diagnosis**

  - Acute myeloblastic leukemia
  - Anemia of chronic disease
  - Alcohol-induced sideroblastic anemia
  - Other causes of specific cytopenias
  - Other causes of macrocytic anemias

- **Treatment**

  - Supportive care with red cell or platelet transfusions
  - Erythropoietin (epoietin alfa) and filgrastim (G-CSF) may benefit selected patients
  - Poor results with low-dose chemotherapy; azacitidine may be most effective single agent
  - Allogeneic bone marrow transplantation for appropriate patients

- **Pearl**

Consider myelodysplastic syndrome in older patients with hematocrits less than 60% of lifetime high and no other obvious cause.

Reference

Heaney ML et al: Myelodysplasia. N Engl J Med 1999;340:1649. [PMID: 10341278]

Chronic Lymphocytic Leukemia

- **Essentials of Diagnosis**
  - Fatigue in some; most asymptomatic; often discovered incidentally
  - Pallor, lymphadenopathy, splenomegaly common also
  - Sustained lymphocytosis > 5000/μL or higher, with some counts up to 1,000,000/μL; morphologically mature cells in most cases
  - Coombs-positive hemolytic anemia, immune thrombocytopenia, hypogammaglobulinemia late in course
  - Anemia, thrombocytopenia, bulky lymphadenopathy associated with poorer prognosis
  - Flow cytometry separates CLL from reactive lymphocytosis
  - May transform into high-grade lymphoid neoplasm (Richter transformation)

- **Differential Diagnosis**
  - Infectious mononucleosis
  - Pertussis
  - Lymphoma in leukemic stage
  - Mantle cell lymphoma
  - Hairy cell leukemia

- **Treatment**
  - Given the chronic, frequently indolent nature of the disease, chemotherapy is reserved for symptomatic patients or for young patients with advanced disease
  - Conventional chemotherapy unlikely to be curative; much interest, however, in combinations of chemotherapy and immunotherapy
  - Steroids, immunoglobulin may help associated immune cytopenias

- **Pearl**

Smudged lymphocytic nuclei result from crushing of fragile cells during preparation of blood smear.

Reference

Mead GM: ABC of clinical haematology. Malignant lymphomas and chronic lymphocytic leukaemia. BMJ 1997;314:1103. [PMID: 9133896]

Hairy Cell Leukemia

- ■ Essentials of Diagnosis
  - • Fatigue, abdominal pain, but often asymptomatic; susceptibility to bacterial infections
  - • Pallor, prominent splenomegaly, rare lymphadenopathy
  - • Pancytopenia, "hairy cell" morphology of leukocytes in periphery and marrow at high magnification
  - • "Dry tap" on bone marrow aspiration; diagnosis confirmed by flow cytometry; tartrate-resistant acid phosphatase (TRAP) stain also positive

- ■ Differential Diagnosis
  - • Myelofibrosis
  - • Chronic lymphocytic leukemia
  - • Waldenström's macroglobulinemia
  - • Non-Hodgkin's lymphoma
  - • Aplastic anemia
  - • Acute leukemia
  - • Infiltration of marrow by tumor or granuloma
  - • Paroxysmal nocturnal hemoglobinuria

- ■ Treatment
  - • Azacitidine gives durable remissions in > 80% of patients
  - • Splenectomy for severe cytopenias or chemotherapy-resistant disease

- ■ Pearl

Involved cells coexpress CD11c and CD22 on immunophenotyping.

Reference

Pettitt AR et al: Hairy-cell leukaemia: biology and management. BMJ 1999; 106:2. [PMID: 10444156]

Multiple Myeloma

- ### Essentials of Diagnosis
  - Weakness, weight loss, recurrent infection, bone (especially back) pain, often resulting in pathologic fractures
  - Pallor, bony tenderness; spleen is not enlarged
  - Anemia; accelerated sedimentation rate; elevated serum calcium, renal insufficiency; normal alkaline phosphatase; narrowed anion gap in most
  - Nephrotic syndrome (with associated amyloidosis causing albuminuria or by light chains in urine)
  - Elevated serum globulin with monoclonal spike on protein electrophoresis
  - Immature plasma cells infiltrating bone marrow; diagnostic only when > 30% or in sheets
  - Lytic bone lesions with negative bone scan

- ### Differential Diagnosis
  - Metastatic cancer
  - Lymphoma with monoclonal spike
  - Hyperparathyroidism
  - Waldenström's macroglobulinemia
  - Benign monoclonal gammopathy
  - Primary amyloidosis

- ### Treatment
  - Pamidronate for patients with extensive bone disease or hypercalcemia
  - Autologous bone marrow transplant now standard for disease palliation, though unlikely to be curative
  - Combination chemotherapy with alkylating agents (eg, melphalan), steroids, and vincristine used frequently pretransplant, or for patients not able to undergo transplantation.
  - Radiation therapy for local bone pain or pathologic fractures
  - Thalidomide effective for those with advanced or relapsed or refractory disease

- ### Pearl

The counterintuitive three noes of myeloma: no fever, no increased alkaline phosphatase, no splenomegaly.

Reference

George ED et al: Multiple myeloma: recognition and management. Am Fam Physician 1999;59:1885. [PMID: 10208707]

Waldenström's Macroglobulinemia

- **Essentials of Diagnosis**
  - Fatigue, symptoms of hyperviscosity (altered mental status, bleeding, or thrombosis)
  - Variable hepatosplenomegaly and lymphadenopathy; boxcar retinal vein engorgement
  - Anemia with rouleau formation; monoclonal IgM paraprotein; increased serum viscosity; narrowed anion gap
  - Plasmacytoid infiltrate in marrow
  - Absence of bone lesions

- **Differential Diagnosis**
  - Benign monoclonal gammopathy
  - Chronic lymphocytic leukemia with M spike
  - Multiple myeloma
  - Lymphoma

- **Treatment**
  - Plasmapheresis for severe hyperviscosity (stupor or coma)
  - Chemotherapy including chlorambucil, cyclophosphamide, fludarabine, cladribine
  - Monoclonal antibody therapy (rituximab) may be effective

- **Pearl**

There are rouleaux and then there are rouleaux; some can be found on any blood smear, but they are abundant in Waldenström's macroglobulinemia and myeloma.

Reference

Owen RG et al: Waldenström's macroglobulinaemia: laboratory diagnosis and treatment. Hematol Oncol 2000;18:41. [PMID: (UI: 10960874]

Non-Hodgkin's Lymphoma

- ■ Essentials of Diagnosis
  - Many symptom-free and come to attention because of lymphadenopathy
  - Fever, night sweats, weight loss in many
  - Common in HIV infection, where isolated central nervous system lymphoma and other extranodal involvement are typical
  - Behaves as though origin is multicentric
  - Variable hepatosplenomegaly; rubbery enlargement of lymph nodes
  - Lymphatic and extranodal masses on imaging; elevated LDH in many, bone marrow positive in one-third
  - Lymph node or involved extranodal tissue biopsies diagnostic; most useful clinical classification (based on nodal architecture) is low-, medium-, and high-grade

- ■ Differential Diagnosis
  - Hodgkin's disease
  - Metastatic cancer
  - Infectious mononucleosis
  - Cat-scratch disease
  - Pseudolymphoma caused by phenytoin
  - Sarcoidosis
  - Primary HIV infection

- ■ Treatment
  - Staging with CT scans of the chest, abdomen, and pelvis; gallium or PET scan (for aggressive disease); bone marrow biopsy and lumbar puncture in selected cases
  - Treatment individualized depending on histology and prognostic factors: age, stage, serum LDH, extranodal disease, performance status
  - With indolent disease, local radiation therapy; chemotherapy for symptomatic, more aggressive advanced disease; monoclonal antibody therapy useful in relapses.
  - Autologous bone marrow transplantation effective in relapsed aggressive lymphoma and perhaps for high-risk primary lymphoma.

- ■ Pearl

A single intracranial lesion in an AIDS patient is lymphoma, multiple lesions toxoplasmosis until proved otherwise.

Reference

DeVita VT Jr et al: The lymphomas. Semin Hematol 1999;36(4 Suppl 7):84. [PMID: 10595757]

Hodgkin's Disease

- **Essentials of Diagnosis**
  - In most cases the disorder starts in one node group and spreads in an orderly, contiguous fashion
  - Regionally enlarged, rubbery, painless lymphadenopathy (often cervical); hepatosplenomegaly variable
  - Reed-Sternberg cells (or variants) in lymph node or bone marrow biopsy diagnostic
  - Patients considered stage A if no constitutional symptoms are present and stage B if they have fevers, night sweats, or significant weight loss
  - Younger patients have supradiaphragmatic disease with favorable histology; older individuals tend toward more aggressive pathology, infradiaphragmatic involvement

- **Differential Diagnosis**
  - Non-Hodgkin's lymphoma
  - Lymphadenitis secondary to infections (tuberculosis and cat-scratch disease)
  - Pseudolymphoma caused by phenytoin
  - Lymphomatoid granulomatosis
  - Sarcoidosis
  - HIV disease
  - SLE

- **Treatment**
  - Staging (I–IV) with chest x-ray, CT scans of chest, abdomen, and pelvis, gallium or PET scan, and bone marrow biopsy; laparotomy (if results would alter therapy) now infrequently necessary
  - Radiation therapy for localized disease or short course of combination chemotherapy with less extensive radiation
  - Combination chemotherapy for disseminated disease with or without radiation to bulky areas of disease

- **Pearl**

When a patient develops pain in a lymph node soon after drinking alcohol, think Hodgkin's.

Reference

Eghbali H et al: Current treatment of Hodgkin's disease. Crit Rev Oncol Hematol 2000;35:49. [PMID: 10863151]

Idiopathic Thrombocytopenic Purpura

- **Essentials of Diagnosis**
  - Mucosal bleeding, easy bruising and bleeding
  - Petechiae, ecchymoses; splenomegaly rare
  - Severe thrombocytopenia, prolonged bleeding time; elevated platelet-associated IgG in 95%, though nonspecific; bone marrow with normal to increased megakaryocytes
  - May be associated with autoimmune diseases (eg, SLE), HIV infection, lymphoproliferative disorders, or with Coombs-positive hemolytic anemia (Evans's syndrome)

- **Differential Diagnosis**
  - Acute leukemia
  - Myelodysplastic syndrome
  - TTP
  - Disseminated intravascular coagulation
  - Chronic lymphocytic leukemia
  - Aplastic anemia
  - Alcohol abuse
  - Drug toxicity (eg, quinidine, digoxin)
  - AIDS
  - SLE

- **Treatment**
  - Prednisone, intravenous immune globulin, or anti Rh-D immune globulin (WinRho) in Rh-positive patients all have high rates of success acutely
  - Splenectomy if no response to initial therapy, for relapsed disease, or for patients requiring high doses of steroids to maintain an acceptable platelet count
  - Danazol, vincristine, vinblastine, azathioprine, or cyclophosphamide for refractory cases; plasma immunoadsorption may also be successful in some refractory cases
  - Reserve platelet transfusion for life-threatening hemorrhages; bleeding sometimes stops even as the platelet count rises slightly if at all

- **Pearl**

The order of platelet bleeding as the count falls: first skin, then mucous membrane, finally viscera. Thus, absence of cutaneous petechiae means a low likelihood of intracranial hemorrhage.

Reference

George JN et al: Idiopathic thrombocytopenic purpura: diagnosis and management. Am J Med Sci 1998;316:87. [PMID: 9704662]

Von Willebrand's Disease

- **Essentials of Diagnosis**
  - History of lifelong excessive bruising and mucosal bleeding; excessive bleeding during previous surgery, dental extraction, or childbirth
  - Usually prolonged bleeding time, especially after aspirin, but platelet count normal
  - Variable abnormalities in factor VIII level, von Willebrand factor, or ristocetin cofactor activity
  - Prolonged partial thromboplastin time when factor VIII levels decreased

- **Differential Diagnosis**
  - Qualitative platelet disorders
  - Waldenström's macroglobulinemia
  - Aspirin ingestion
  - Hemophilias
  - Dysfibrinogenemia

- **Treatment**
  - Avoid aspirin
  - vWF and factor VIII concentrates for severe bleeding or for surgical procedures in most cases
  - Desmopressin acetate in type I disease may be sufficient to raise vWF and factor VIII to acceptable levels
  - Tranexamic acid for bleeding not responsive to other interventions

- **Pearl**

Remember von Willebrand's disease in patients who have a past surgical history of erratic bleeding patterns; aspirin may have been given in the bleeding instances, other analgesics when hemostasis was more easily achieved.

Reference

Aledort LM: von Willebrand disease: from the bedside to therapy. Thromb Haemost 1997;78:562. [PMID: 9198216]

Hemophilia A & B

- **Essentials of Diagnosis**
  - Lifelong history of space bleeding in a male
  - Slow, prolonged bleeding after minor injury or surgery; spontaneous hemarthroses common
  - Prolonged partial thromboplastin time corrected by mixing patient's plasma with a normal specimen
  - Low factor VIII coagulant activity (hemophilia A) or factor IX coagulant activity (hemophilia B)

- **Differential Diagnosis**
  - Von Willebrand's disease
  - Disseminated intravascular coagulation
  - Afibrinogenemia and dysfibrinogenemia
  - Heparin administration
  - Acquired factor deficiencies or inhibitors (eg, paraproteins with anti-VIII or anti-IX activity)

- **Treatment**
  - Avoidance of aspirin
  - Factor replacement for any bleeding with factor VIII concentrates (hemophilia A) or factor IX complex (hemophilia B) or during invasive procedures
  - Increased factor dosing, steroids, or immunosuppressants if factor inhibitor develops
  - Desmopressin acetate before surgical procedures for hemophilia A may benefit selected patients

- **Pearl**

Christmas disease (factor IX deficiency) is the index patient's name, not the holiday.

Reference

Mannucci PM et al: The hemophilias: progress and problems. Semin Hematol 1999;36(4 Suppl 7):104. [PMID: 10595759]

6

Rheumatologic & Autoimmune Disorders

Degenerative Joint Disease (Osteoarthritis)

- **Essentials of Diagnosis**
  - Progressive degeneration of articular cartilage and hypertrophy of bone at the articular margin
  - Affects almost all joints, especially weight-bearing and frequently used joints; hips, knees, shoulders, and first carpometacarpal joint most common
  - May be primary (idiopathic) or secondary to trauma, metabolic abnormality, or other articular disease
  - Primary degenerative joint disease most commonly affects the terminal interphalangeal joints (Heberden's nodes), hips, and first carpometacarpal joints
  - Morning stiffness brief; articular inflammation minimal
  - Radiographs reveal narrowing of the joint spaces, osteophytes, increased density of subchondral bone, subchondral cysts

- **Differential Diagnosis**
  - Rheumatoid arthritis
  - Seronegative spondyloarthropathies
  - Crystal-induced arthritides
  - Hyperparathyroidism
  - Multiple myeloma
  - Hemochromatosis

- **Treatment**
  - Weight reduction
  - Exercises to strengthen muscles around affected joints
  - Aspirin, other NSAIDs (eg, ibuprofen, 600 mg three times daily) or COX-2 inhibitors
  - Glucosamine and chondroitin sulfate appear to be effective
  - Intra-articular corticosteroid injection (eg, triamcinolone, 10–40 mg) in selected cases
  - Surgery for severely affected joints, especially hip

- **Pearl**

The first metatarsophalangeal joint harbors the most subclinical degenerative disease and thus is the most common nidus for gout.

Reference

Manek NJ et al: Osteoarthritis: current concepts in diagnosis and management. Am Fam Physician 2000;61:1795. [PMID: 10750883]

Gout

- **Essentials of Diagnosis**
    - Spectrum of disease, including recurrent arthritic attacks, tophi, interstitial nephropathy, and uric acid nephrolithiasis
    - First attack typically nocturnal and usually monarticular; may be polyarticular with repeated attacks
    - Affects first metatarsophalangeal joint (podagra), mid foot, ankle, knees, wrist, elbow—hips and shoulders spared
    - Hyperuricemia may be primary (caused by overproduction [10%] or underexcretion [90%] of uric acid) or secondary to diuretic use, cytotoxic drugs (especially cyclosporine), myeloproliferative disorders, multiple myeloma, hemoglobinopathies, chronic renal disease, hypothyroidism
    - After long periods of untreated hyperuricemia, tophi (monosodium urate deposits with an associated foreign body reaction) develop in subcutaneous tissues, bone, cartilage, joints, and other tissues
    - Identification of weakly negatively birefringent, needle-like sodium urate crystals in joint fluid or tophi is diagnostic

- **Differential Diagnosis**
    - Cellulitis
    - Septic arthritis
    - Pseudogout
    - Rheumatoid arthritis
    - Calcium oxalate deposition disease
    - Chronic lead intoxication (saturnine gout)

- **Treatment**
    - Treat the acute arthritis first and the hyperuricemia later, if at all
    - For acute attacks: dramatic therapeutic response to NSAIDs (eg, indomethacin, 50 mg three times daily), colchicine, intra-articular or systemic corticosteroids
    - For chronic prophylaxis in patients with frequent acute attacks, tophaceous deposits, or renal damage: allopurinol and probenecid (uricosuric agent) with concomitant colchicine
    - Avoid thiazides and loop diuretics

- **Pearl**

Long-standing "rheumatoid arthritis" sparing the shoulders and hips is most likely gout.

Reference

Pascual E: Gout update: from lab to the clinic and back. Curr Opin Rheumatol 2000;12:213. [PMID: 10803751]

Chondrocalcinosis & Pseudogout
(Calcium Pyrophosphate Dihydrate Deposition Disease)

- **Essentials of Diagnosis**
  - Chondrocalcinosis a central feature
  - Subacute, recurrent, and (rarely) chronic arthritis, usually involving large joints (especially knees, shoulders, and wrists) and almost always accompanied by chondrocalcinosis of the affected joints
  - May be hereditary, idiopathic, or associated with metabolic disorders, including hemochromatosis, hypoparathyroidism, osteoarthritis, ochronosis, diabetes mellitus, hypothyroidism, Wilson's disease, and gout
  - Identification of calcium pyrophosphate rhomboidal crystals (strong positive birefringence) in the joint fluid is diagnostic
  - Radiographs may reveal chondrocalcinosis or signs of degenerative joint disease at the following sites: knee (medial meniscus), fibrocartilaginous portion of the symphysis pubica, and articular disk of the wrist

- **Differential Diagnosis**
  - Gout
  - Calcium phosphate disease (hydroxyapatite arthropathy)
  - Calcium oxalate deposition disease
  - Degenerative joint disease
  - Rheumatoid arthritis

- **Treatment**
  - Treat underlying disease if present
  - Aspirin, other NSAIDs (eg, indomethacin, 50 mg three times daily)
  - Intra-articular injection of corticosteroids (eg, triamcinolone, 10–40 mg)
  - Colchicine, 0.6 mg twice daily, occasionally useful for prophylaxis

- **Pearl**

Pseudogout and gout may coexist in the same joint at the same time.

Reference

Fam AG: What is new about crystals other than monosodium urate? Curr Opin Rheumatol 2000;12:228. [PMID: 10803754]

Rheumatoid Arthritis

- ■ Essentials of Diagnosis
  - Symmetric polyarthritis of peripheral joints with pain, tenderness, and swelling; morning stiffness common
  - Chronic, persistent synovitis with formation of pannus that erodes cartilage, bone, ligaments, and tendons
  - Joint deformities may develop; ulnar deviation common
  - IgM rheumatoid factor present in up to 85%; 20% of seropositive patients have subcutaneous nodules
  - Extra-articular manifestations include vasculitis, pleural effusion (low in glucose), scleritis, sicca symptoms, Felty's syndrome; usually in strongly seropositive patients
  - Radiographic findings include juxta-articular and sometimes generalized osteopenia, narrowing of the joint spaces, and bony erosions, particularly of the MCPs and ulnar styloid

- ■ Differential Diagnosis
  - SLE
  - Degenerative joint disease; polymyalgia rheumatica
  - Gout or pseudogout
  - Lyme disease
  - Sjögren's syndrome
  - Inflammatory osteoarthritis

- ■ Treatment
  - Pharmacologic doses of aspirin, other NSAIDs
  - Corticosteroid-sparing agents such as COX-2 inhibitors are as effective as other NSAIDs (eg, ibuprofen, 800 mg three times daily) with less gastrointestinal toxicity
  - Disease-modifying drugs, including methotrexate, sulfasalazine, hydroxychloroquine, azathioprine, and leflunomide (alone or in combination) in patients with moderate disease activity or poor prognostic features
  - Refractory disease and the presence of poor prognostic features may be treated with anti-TNF therapy (infliximab or etanercept)
  - Hydroxychloroquine and minocycline have modest efficacy for mild disease
  - Surgery for severely affected joints

- ■ Pearl

A flare of a single joint in a patient with established rheumatoid arthritis means infection until excluded.

Reference

Fries JF: Current treatment paradigms in rheumatoid arthritis. Rheumatology 2000;39(Suppl 1):30. [PMID: 11001377]

Adult Still's Disease

- **Essentials of Diagnosis**
  - Occurs in adults usually under 35; some cases into the fifties
  - Fevers > 39 °C may antedate arthritis by months; occasional cases entirely nonarticular
  - Polyarthritis or oligoarthritis usually affects the proximal interphalangeal and metacarpophalangeal joints, wrists, knees, hips, and shoulders
  - Characteristic evanescent, salmon-colored maculopapular rash involving the trunk and extremities during fever spikes; may be elicited by mechanical irritation
  - Additional findings commonly seen include hepatosplenomegaly, lymphadenopathy, pleuropericarditis, leukocytosis, thrombocytosis, anemia, and elevations in the erythrocyte sedimentation rate and the C-reactive protein level
  - A positive ANA > 1 : 100 or rheumatoid factor > 1 : 80 excludes the diagnosis

- **Differential Diagnosis**
  - Leukemia or lymphoma
  - Arthritis associated with inflammatory bowel disease or psoriasis
  - Chronic infection (eg, culture-negative endocarditis)
  - Systemic vasculitis
  - SLE
  - Lyme disease
  - Granulomatous diseases (eg, sarcoidosis, Crohn's disease)

- **Treatment**
  - Unless contraindicated, aspirin (1g four times daily) often dramatically lyses fever
  - NSAIDs (eg, ibuprofen, 800 mg three times daily)
  - Corticosteroids, hydroxychloroquine, methotrexate, azathioprine, and other immunosuppressive agents are used as second-line agents

- **Pearl**

One of three diseases in all of medicine with biquotidian fever spikes.

Reference

Sobieska M et al: Still's disease in children and adults: a distinct pattern of acute-phase proteins. Clin Rheumatol 1998;17:258. [PMID: 9694067]

Systemic Lupus Erythematosus

- **Essentials of Diagnosis**
  - Predominantly in young women
  - Multisystem inflammatory autoimmune disorder with periods of exacerbation and remission
  - Four or more of the following 11 criteria must be present: malar ("butterfly") rash, discoid rash, photosensitivity, oral ulcers, arthritis, serositis, renal disease, neurologic disease, hematologic disorders, positive antinuclear antibody (ANA), and immunologic abnormalities (eg, antibody to native double stranded DNA or to Sm, or false-positive serologic test for syphilis)
  - Also associated with fever, myositis, alopecia, myocarditis, pericarditis, vasculitis, lymphadenopathy, conjunctivitis, antiphospholipid antibodies with hypercoagulability and miscarriages, thrombocytopenia, glomerulonephritis (focal, membranoproliferative, or membranous), sicca complex
  - Syndrome may be drug-induced (eg, procainamide, hydralazine), in which case brain and kidney usually spared

- **Differential Diagnosis**
  - Rheumatoid arthritis
  - Vasculitis
  - Sjögren's syndrome
  - Systemic sclerosis
  - Endocarditis
  - Lymphoma
  - Glomerulonephritis due to other cause

- **Treatment**
  - Mild disease (ie, arthralgias with dermatologic findings) often responds to hydroxychloroquine and COX-2 inhibitors or NSAIDs
  - Moderate disease activity (ie, refractory to antimalarials): corticosteroids and azathioprine, methotrexate, or mycophenolate mofetil
  - Corticosteroids and cyclophosphamide for lupus cerebritis and lupus nephritis
  - Withdraw offending agent if drug-induced lupus suspected
  - Avoid sun exposure

- **Pearl**

The classic malar rash of SLE spares the nasolabial folds.

Reference

Strand V: New therapies for systemic lupus erythematosus. Rheum Dis Clin North Am 2000;26:389. [PMID: 10768219]

Systemic Sclerosis (Scleroderma)

- ■ Essentials of Diagnosis
  - Diffuse systemic sclerosis in 20% of patients with generalized fibrotic changes of the skin and internal organ systems
  - Raynaud's phenomenon typical; may be associated with intestinal hypomotility, pulmonary fibrosis, myocarditis, pericarditis, hypertension and renal failure, acral ulceration
  - Limited disease (80% of patients) or CREST syndrome (calcinosis cutis, Raynaud's phenomenon, esophageal hypomotility, sclerodactyly, and telangiectasia): skin tightening limited to the distal extremities and feet, with lower risk of renal disease, later onset of pulmonary hypertension and biliary cirrhosis, and an overall better prognosis
  - ANA frequently useful in systemic sclerosis; anticentromere antibody positive in 1% of patients with diffuse scleroderma and 50% of those with CREST syndrome; antitopoisomerase I (Scl-70) in one-third of patients with diffuse systemic sclerosis and 20% of those with CREST syndrome, and a poor prognostic factor

- ■ Differential Diagnosis
  - Eosinophilic fasciitis
  - Overlap syndromes with scleroderma
  - Graft-versus-host disease
  - Amyloidosis
  - Morphea
  - Raynaud's disease
  - Cryoglobulinemia

- ■ Treatment
  - Angiotensin-converting enzyme blockers to treat hypertensive crisis occasionally seen in patients with systemic sclerosis
  - Corticosteroids not helpful; penicillamine may be
  - Warm clothing, smoking cessation, and extended-release calcium channel blockers for Raynaud's phenomenon; intravenous iloprost may be helpful for digital ulcers
  - H_2 receptor antagonists or omeprazole for esophageal reflux

- ■ Pearl

Malabsorption in systemic sclerosis is due not to intestinal fibrosis but to bacterial overgrowth from hypomotility.

Reference

Clements PJ: Systemic sclerosis (scleroderma) and related disorders: clinical aspects. Baillieres Best Pract Res Clin Rheumatol 2000;14:1. [PMID: 10882211]

Overlap Syndromes (Mixed Connective Tissue Disease & Undifferentiated Connective Tissue Syndrome)

- **Essentials of Diagnosis**
  - Clinical features of more than one disease (SLE, systemic sclerosis, polymyositis, and rheumatoid arthritis)
  - Sicca complex (xerostomia, xerophthalmia, dry cough) and myositis in virtually all patients
  - Presence of a specific antibody to ribonuclear protein
  - Suggested clinical criteria include three of the following: edema of the hands, synovitis, myositis, Raynaud's phenomenon, and acrosclerosis
  - Associated with pulmonary fibrosis, pericarditis, myocarditis, esophageal hypomotility, glomerulonephritis
  - May evolve to one predominant phenotype over time

- **Differential Diagnosis**
  - SLE
  - Systemic sclerosis
  - Polymyositis
  - Sjögren's syndrome
  - Rheumatoid arthritis
  - Eosinophilic fasciitis
  - Graft-versus-host disease

- **Treatment**
  - NSAIDs (eg, ibuprofen, 800 mg three times daily) and COX-2 inhibitors
  - Corticosteroids often first-line agent; response good at modest doses
  - Symptomatic relief of dryness with artificial tears, chewing gum, sialagogues, frequent sips of water
  - Warm clothing, smoking cessation, and extended-relief calcium channel blockers for Raynaud's phenomenon

- **Pearl**

Sicca syndrome is a cause of "refractory" angina; a drop of water with nitroglycerin makes it stable angina.

Reference

Kasukawa R: Mixed connective tissue disease. Intern Med 1999;38:386. [PMID: 10397074]

Polymyositis-Dermatomyositis

- **Essentials of Diagnosis**
  - Bilateral proximal muscle weakness
  - Periorbital edema and a purplish (heliotrope) rash over the upper eyelids in many
  - Violaceous, occasionally scaly papules overlying the dorsal surface of the interphalangeal joints of the hands (Gottron's papules)
  - Serum CK elevated; ANA only uncommonly positive save in overlap syndromes; anti-Jo-1 antibodies in the subset of patients who have associated interstitial lung disease; anti-Mi-2 is more specific for dermatomyositis but is insensitive
  - Muscle biopsy and characteristic electromyographic pattern are diagnostic
  - May be associated with rheumatoid arthritis, SLE, scleroderma, mixed connective tissue disease; increased incidence of malignancy, especially in older patients

- **Differential Diagnosis**
  - Endocrine myopathies (eg, hyperthyroidism)
  - Polymyalgia rheumatica
  - Myasthenia gravis; Eaton-Lambert syndrome
  - Muscular dystrophy
  - Rhabdomyolysis
  - Parasitic myositis
  - Drug-induced myopathies (eg, corticosteroids, alcohol, colchicine, statins, zidovudine, hydroxychloroquine, one batch of L-tryptophan)
  - Adult glycogen storage disease
  - Mitochondrial myopathy

- **Treatment**
  - Corticosteroids
  - Methotrexate or azathioprine spares steroids
  - Intravenous immune globulin for some cases of dermatomyositis
  - Search for malignancy unwarranted unless historical or examination findings indicate it

- **Pearl**

Biopsy at the site of a previous EMG will show inflammation; pick the same muscle on the other side.

Reference

Callen JP: Dermatomyositis. Lancet 2000;355:53. [PMID: 10615903]

Sjögren's Syndrome

- **Essentials of Diagnosis**
  - Destruction of exocrine glands, leading to mucosal and conjunctival dryness
  - Dry mouth (xerostomia) and dry eyes (keratoconjunctivitis sicca), decreased tear production, parotid enlargement, severe dental caries, loss of taste and smell
  - Occasionally associated with glomerulonephritis, renal tubular acidosis, biliary cirrhosis, pancreatitis, neuropsychiatric dysfunction, polyneuropathy, interstitial pneumonitis, thyroiditis, cardiac conduction defects
  - Over 50% have cytoplasmic antibodies, anti-Ro (SS-A), and anti-La (SS-B)
  - Decreased lacrimation measured by Schirmer's filter paper test; biopsy of minor salivary glands of lower lip confirms diagnosis
  - May also be observed in patients with rheumatoid arthritis, SLE, systemic sclerosis, polymyositis, polyarteritis, fibrosis; increased incidence of lymphoma and Waldenström's macroglobulinemia, especially in isolated sicca syndrome

- **Differential Diagnosis**
  - Sicca complex associated with other autoimmune diseases such as sarcoidosis, rheumatoid arthritis, SLE, and systemic sclerosis as noted
  - Anticholinergic medications
  - Chronic irritation from smoking

- **Treatment**
  - Symptomatic relief of dryness with artificial tears, chewing gum, sialagogues
  - Cholinergic drugs such as pilocarpine
  - Meticulous care of teeth and avoidance of sugar-containing candies
  - Corticosteroids or azathioprine; cyclophosphamide for peripheral neuropathy, interstitial pneumonitis, glomerulonephritis, and vasculitis

- **Pearl**

Consider parotid tumors before making the diagnosis of Sjögren's syndrome.

Reference

Fox RI et al: Current issues in the diagnosis and treatment of Sjögren's syndrome. Curr Opin Rheumatol 1999;11:364. [PMID: 10503656]

Polyarteritis Nodosa

- **Essentials of Diagnosis**
  - Fever, hypertension, abdominal pain, arthralgias, myalgias
  - Cotton-wool spots and microaneurysms in fundus; pericarditis, myocarditis, palpable purpura, mononeuritis multiplex, livedo reticularis
  - Acceleration of sedimentation rate in most; serologic evidence of hepatitis B or hepatitis C in 30–50%
  - ANCA positive in most
  - Diagnosis confirmed by biopsy or visceral angiography
  - Renal or pulmonary involvement in variant microscopic poly-arteritis

- **Differential Diagnosis**
  - Wegener's granulomatosis
  - Churg-Strauss vasculitis
  - Hypersensitivity vasculitis
  - Subacute endocarditis
  - Essential mixed cryoglobulinemia
  - Cholesterol atheroembolic disease

- **Treatment**
  - Corticosteroids with cyclophosphamide for systemic vasculitis; azathioprine is used as a maintenance immunosuppressant

- **Pearl**

  Treat polyarteritis nodosa with immunosuppressives at your own risk if endocarditis has not been definitively excluded.

Reference

Savage C et al: ABC of arterial and vascular disease: vasculitis. BMJ 2000; 320:1325. [PMID: 10807632]

Polymyalgia Rheumatica & Giant Cell Arteritis

- **Essentials of Diagnosis**
  - Patients usually over age 50
  - Polymyalgia rheumatica characterized by pain and stiffness, not weakness, of the shoulder and pelvic girdle lasting 1 month or more without evidence of infection or malignancy
  - Associated with fever, little if any joint swelling, sedimentation rate > 40mm/h, and rapid response to prednisone 15 mg/d
  - Giant cell (temporal) arteritis frequently coexists with polymyalgia rheumatica; headache, transient or permanent blindness, jaw claudication, or temporal artery tenderness; lingual Raynaud's phenomenon, scalp necrosis
  - Diagnosis confirmation by 5 cm temporal artery biopsy remains reliable for 1–2 weeks after starting steroids

- **Differential Diagnosis**
  - Multiple myeloma
  - Chronic infection, eg, endocarditis, visceral abscess
  - Neoplasm
  - Rheumatoid arthritis
  - Depression
  - Myxedema
  - Carotid plaque with embolic amaurosis fugax
  - Carotid Takayasu's arteritis

- **Treatment**
  - Prednisone 10–20 mg/d for polymyalgia rheumatica
  - Prednisone 60 mg/d immediately on suspicion of temporal arteritis; treat for at least 4 months depending on response of symptoms—not sedimentation rate
  - Methotrexate or azathioprine spares steroids in some patients with side effects on high doses

- **Pearl**

Instruct patients with polymyalgia rheumatica to keep 60 mg of prednisone with them at all times and to take it and come in if there are any visual symptoms.

Reference

Epperly TD et al: Polymyalgia rheumatica and temporal arthritis. Am Fam Physician 2000;62:789. [PMID: 10969858]

Churg-Strauss Vasculitis
(Allergic Granulomatosis & Angiitis)

- ■ Essentials of Diagnosis
  - • Granulomatous vasculitis of small- and medium-sized arteries
  - • Four of the following have a sensitivity of 85% and specificity of 100% for diagnosis: asthma; allergic rhinitis; transient pulmonary infiltrates; palpable purpura or extravascular eosinophils; mononeuritis multiplex; and eosinophilia

- ■ Differential Diagnosis
  - • Wegener's granulomatosis
  - • Eosinophilic pneumonia
  - • Polyarteritis nodosa (often overlaps)
  - • Hypersensitivity vasculitis

- ■ Treatment
  - • Corticosteroids
  - • Cyclophosphamide in addition probably has better outcome

- ■ Pearl

Leukotriene inhibitors such as montelukast, given for asthma, have been implicated as causing some cases of Churg-Strauss syndrome.

Reference

Eustace JA et al: Disease of the month. The Churg Strauss Syndrome. J Am Soc Nephrol 1999;10:2048. [PMID: 10477159]

Hypersensitivity Vasculitis

- **Essentials of Diagnosis**
  - Leukocytoclastic vasculitis of small blood vessels
  - Palpable purpura of lower extremities the predominant feature
  - Secondary to numerous drugs, neoplasms, connective tissue disorders, congenital complement deficiency, serum sickness, viral or bacterial infection
  - On occasion associated with fever, arthralgias, abdominal pain with or without gastrointestinal bleeding, pulmonary infiltrates, kidney involvement with hematuria

- **Differential Diagnosis**
  - Polyarteritis nodosa
  - Henoch-Schönlein purpura
  - Essential mixed cryoglobulinemia
  - Meningococcemia
  - Gonococcemia

- **Treatment**
  - Treat underlying disease if present
  - Discontinue offending drug
  - Corticosteroids in severe cases

- **Pearl**

The palpable purpura of hypersensitivity vasculitis is dependent and thus may be prominent on the backs of bedfast patients.

Reference

Savage CO et al: ABC of arterial and vascular disease: vasculitis. BMJ 2000; 320:1325. [PMID: 10807632]

Wegener's Granulomatosis

- Essentials of Diagnosis
  - Vasculitis associated with glomerulonephritis and necrotizing granulomas of upper and lower respiratory tracts
  - Slight male predominance with peak incidence in fourth and fifth decades
  - Ninety percent present with upper or lower respiratory tract symptoms, including perforation of nasal septum, chronic sinusitis, otitis media, mastoiditis, cough, dyspnea, hemoptysis
  - Proptosis, scleritis, arthritis, purpura, or neuropathy (mononeuritis multiplex) may also be present
  - cANCA in 90%; sinus, lung, or renal biopsy makes the diagnosis, though the latter is seldom specific, showing focal glomerulonephritis; eosinophilia not a feature
  - Chest film may reveal large nodular densities; urinalysis may show hematuria, red cell casts; CT scans of sinuses often reveal bony erosion
  - Increased risk of bladder cancer and lymphoma

- Differential Diagnosis
  - Polyarteritis nodosa
  - Churg-Strauss vasculitis
  - Goodpasture's syndrome
  - Takayasu's arteritis
  - Microscopic polyarteritis
  - Lymphomatoid granulomatosis
  - Lymphoproliferative disorders (especially angiocentric T cell lymphoma)

- Treatment
  - Corticosteroids
  - Primarily oral cyclophosphamide or methotrexate in addition
  - Trimethoprim-sulfamethoxazole effective in mild disease; given to all patients not allergic to sulfonamides

- Pearl

In 10% of renal biopsies, pathognomonic granulomatous vasculitis is seen in renal arterioles.

Reference

Esper GJ et al: Update on the treatment of Wegener's granulomatosis. Bull the Rheumat Dis 1999;48:1. [PMID: 10721552]

Cryoglobulinemia

- ■ Essentials of Diagnosis
  - • Refers to any globulin precipitable at lower than body temperature
  - • Any elevation of globulin may be associated
  - • Monoclonal gammopathies, reactive hypergammaglobulinemia, cryoprecipitable immune complexes are the main causes; first two have acral cold symptoms because of higher titers of cryo-proteins
  - • Symptoms and signs depend upon type
  - • Low erythrocyte sedimentation rate; correctable by doing 37 °C ESR

- ■ Differential Diagnosis
  - • Multiple myeloma, Waldenström's macroglobulinemia
  - • Chronic inflammatory diseases such as endocarditis, sarcoidosis, rheumatoid arthritis
  - • Essential mixed cryoglobulinemia: palpable purpura and glomeru-lonephritis in patients serologically positive for hepatitis C

- ■ Treatment
  - • Entirely dependent on cause

- ■ Pearl

In a patient with back pain whose blood "clots" per the laboratory despite heparinization of the specimen, the diagnosis is myeloma with a cryoprecipitable M-spike.

Reference

Lamprecht P et al: Cryoglobulinemic vasculitis. Arthritis Rheum 1999;42:2507. [PMID: 10615995]

Takayasu's Arteritis ("Pulseless Disease")

- **Essentials of Diagnosis**
  - Large-vessel vasculitis involving the aortic arch and its major branches
  - A disease of Asian women under 40
  - Associated with myalgias, arthralgias, headaches, angina, claudication, erythema nodosum-like lesions; hypertension, bruits, absent pulses, cerebrovascular insufficiency, aortic insufficiency
  - Angiography reveals narrowing, stenosis, and aneurysms of the aortic arch and its major branches
  - Bruits may be heard over the subclavian arteries or aorta in up to 40% of patients; additionally, there may be a > 10 mm Hg difference in systolic blood pressure in the two arms
  - Rich collateral flow visible in the shoulder, chest, and neck areas

- **Differential Diagnosis**
  - Giant cell arteritis
  - Syphilitic aortitis
  - Severe atherosclerosis

- **Treatment**
  - Corticosteroids
  - Cyclophosphamide or methotrexate added for severe disease
  - Surgical bypass or reconstruction of affected vessels

- **Pearl**

Clinically and pathologically identical to giant cell arteritis except in the strikingly disparate epidemiology.

Reference

Numano F et al: Takayasu arteritis—beyond pulselessness. Intern Med 1999; 38:226. [PMID: 10337931]

Thromboangiitis Obliterans (Buerger's Disease)

- **Essentials of Diagnosis**
  - Inflammatory disease involving small- and medium-sized arteries and veins of the distal upper and lower extremities
  - Occurs primarily in young Jewish men who are heavy cigarette smokers
  - Associated with migratory superficial segmental thrombophlebitis of superficial veins, absent peripheral pulses, claudication, numbness, paresthesias, Raynaud's phenomenon, ulceration and gangrene of fingertips and toes
  - Angiography reveals multiple occluded segments in the small- and medium-sized arteries of the arms and legs

- **Differential Diagnosis**
  - Atherosclerosis
  - Raynaud's disease
  - Livedo reticularis due to other cause
  - Antiphospholipid antibody syndrome
  - Cholesterol atheroembolic disease

- **Treatment**
  - Smoking cessation is essential
  - Warm clothing, nifedipine for Raynaud's phenomenon
  - Surgical sympathectomy of some value
  - Amputation required in some

- **Pearl**

The addiction to nicotine is fierce; patients continue to smoke even with limb prostheses.

Reference

Olin JW: Thromboangiitis obliterans (Buerger's disease). N Engl J Med 2000; 343:864. [PMID: 10995867]

Behçet's Syndrome

- **Essentials of Diagnosis**
  - Usually occurs in young adults from Mediterranean countries or Japan; incidence decreases if patient's descendants emigrate elsewhere
  - Most common: recurrent oral aphthous ulcerations (99%), genital ulcers (80%), ocular lesions in half (uveitis, hypopyon, iritis, keratitis, optic neuritis), and skin lesions (erythema nodosum, superficial thrombophlebitis, cutaneous hypersensitivity, folliculitis)
  - Less common: gastrointestinal erosions, epididymitis, glomerulonephritis, cranial nerve palsies, aseptic meningitis, and focal neurologic lesions
  - Pathergy test—a papule or a pustule forms 24–48 hours after simple trauma such as a needle prick.
  - Diagnosis is clinical
  - HLA-B5 histocompatibility antigen often present

- **Differential Diagnosis**
  - HLA-B27 spondyloarthropathies
  - Oral aphthous ulcers
  - Herpes simplex infection
  - Erythema multiforme
  - SLE
  - HIV infection
  - Infective endocarditis

- **Treatment**
  - Local mydriatics in all patients with eye findings to prevent synechiae from forming
  - Corticosteroids
  - Colchicine (for erythema nodosum and arthralgia)
  - Azathioprine, cyclosporine in some

- **Pearl**

Stroke in a young native Japanese woman is Behçet's syndrome unless proved otherwise.

Reference

Sakane T et al: Behçet's disease. N Engl J Med 1999;341:1284. [PMID: 10528040]

Ankylosing Spondylitis

- ■ Essentials of Diagnosis
  - Gradual onset of backache in adults under age 40 with progressive limitation of back motion and chest expansion
  - Diminished anterior flexion of lumbar spine, loss of lumbar lordosis, inflammation at tendon insertions
  - Peripheral arteritis and anterior uveitis in many
  - Aortic insufficiency with cardiac conduction defects in some
  - Cauda equina syndrome, apical pulmonary fibrosis are late complications
  - HLA-B27 histocompatibility antigen present in over 90% of patients; rheumatoid factor absent
  - Radiographic evidence of sacroiliac joint sclerosis; demineralization and squaring of the vertebral bodies with calcification of the anterior and lateral spinal ligaments (bamboo spine)

- ■ Differential Diagnosis
  - Rheumatoid arthritis
  - Osteoporosis
  - Reactive arthritis
  - Arthritis associated with inflammatory bowel disease
  - Psoriatic arthritis
  - Diffuse idiopathic skeletal hyperostosis (DISH)
  - Synovitis-acne-pustulosis-hyperostosis-osteitis (SAPHO) syndrome

- ■ Treatment
  - Physical therapy to maintain posture and mobility
  - NSAIDs (eg, indomethacin 50 mg three times daily) often marginally effective
  - Sulfasalazine reported effective in some patients
  - Intra-articular corticosteroids for synovitis; ophthalmic corticosteroids for uveitis
  - Surgery for severely affected joints; anti-TNF agents may be effective but are toxic

- ■ Pearl
  In a patient with burned-out ankylosing spondylitis and symptomatic "benign prostatic hyperplasia," test the cauda equina distribution neurologically before undertaking prostatectomy.

Reference

Koehler L et al: Managing seronegative spondarthritides. Rheumatology 2000; 39:360. [PMID: 10817767]

Psoriatic Arthritis

- **Essentials of Diagnosis**
  - Classically a destructive arthritis of distal interphalangeal joints; many patients also have peripheral arthritis involving shoulders, elbows, wrists, knees, and ankles, often asymmetrically
  - Sacroiliitis in B27-positive patients
  - Occurs in 15–20% of patients with psoriasis
  - Psoriatic arthritis associated with nail pitting, onycholysis, sausage digits, arthritis mutilans (severe deforming arthritis)
  - Rheumatoid factor negative; serum uric acid may be elevated
  - Radiographs may reveal irregular destruction of joint spaces and bone, pencil-in-cup deformity of the phalanges, sacroiliitis

- **Differential Diagnosis**
  - Rheumatoid arthritis
  - Ankylosing spondylitis
  - Arthritis associated with inflammatory bowel disease
  - Reactive arthritis
  - Juvenile spondyloarthropathy

- **Treatment**
  - NSAIDs (eg, ibuprofen, 800 mg three times daily) or COX-2 inhibitors
  - Intra-articular corticosteroid injection; sterilize skin carefully as psoriatic lesions are colonized with staphylococci and streptococci
  - Gold salts, methotrexate
  - Sulfasalazine reportedly effective in patients with symmetric poly-arthritis
  - Treatment of psoriasis helpful in many but not in sacroiliitis

- **Pearl**

In an arthritis of uncertain cause, examination of the intergluteal folds can give the diagnosis.

Reference

Gladman DD: Psoriatic arthritis. Rheum Dis Clin North Am 1998;24:829. [PMID: 9891713]

Reactive Arthritis

- ■ Essentials of Diagnosis
  - Predominantly found in young men
  - Triad of urethritis, conjunctivitis (or uveitis), and arthritis which may occur within a month of another sign or symptom; conjunctivitis may be subtle and evanescent
  - Follows dysenteric infection (with shigella, salmonella, yersinia, campylobacter) or sexually transmitted infection (with chlamydia)
  - Asymmetric, oligoarticular arthritis typically involving the knees and ankles
  - Associated with fever, mucocutaneous lesions, stomatitis, aortic regurgitation, optic neuritis, circinate balanitis, prostatitis, keratoderma blennorrhagicum, pericarditis
  - HLA-B27 histocompatibility antigen in most

- ■ Differential Diagnosis
  - Gonococcal arthritis
  - Rheumatoid arthritis
  - Ankylosing spondylitis
  - Psoriatic arthritis
  - Arthritis associated with inflammatory bowel disease
  - Juvenile spondyloarthropathy

- ■ Treatment
  - NSAIDs (eg, indomethacin, 50 mg three times daily); often ineffective
  - Tetracycline for associated *Chlamydia trachomatis* infection; obtain VDRL, consider HIV testing
  - Azathioprine, methotrexate in severe cases
  - Sulfasalazine may help in some patients
  - Intra-articular corticosteroids for arthritis, ophthalmic corticosteroids for uveitis

- ■ Pearl

Synovial fluid occasionally shows characteristic cells: large mononuclear cell with ingested polymorphonuclear leukocytes which may have inclusion bodies.

Reference

Barth WF et al: Reactive arthritis (Reiter's syndrome). Am Fam Physician 1999;60:499. [PMID: 10465225]

Arthritis Associated With Inflammatory Bowel Disease

- **Essentials of Diagnosis**

  - Peripheral arthritis: asymmetric oligoarthritis that typically involves the knees, ankles, and occasionally the upper extremities, usually parallels bowel disease in activity
  - Spondylitis: clinically identical to ankylosing spondylitis; HLA-B27 antigen present in most patients in a male:female ratio of 4:1
  - Articular features may precede intestinal symptoms, especially in Crohn's disease
  - Extra-articular manifestations may also occur in Crohn's disease (erythema nodosum) and in ulcerative colitis (pyoderma gangrenosum)

- **Differential Diagnosis**

  - Reactive arthritis
  - Ankylosing spondylitis
  - Psoriatic arthritis
  - Rheumatoid arthritis

- **Treatment**

  - Treat underlying intestinal inflammation
  - Aspirin, other NSAIDs (eg, indomethacin, 50 mg three times daily)
  - Physical therapy for spondylitis

- **Pearl**

The younger the patient, the less the gastrointestinal complaints; thus, arthritis in adolescence should prompt a search for inflammatory bowel disease despite absence of symptoms.

Reference

De Keyser F et al: Bowel inflammation and the spondyloarthropathies. Rheum Dis Clin North Am 1998;24:785. [PMID: 9891711]

Septic Arthritis (Nongonococcal Acute Bacterial Arthritis)

- **Essentials of Diagnosis**
  - Acute pain, swelling, erythema, warmth, and limited movement of joints
  - Typically monarticular; knee, hip, wrist, shoulder, or ankle most often involved
  - Infection usually occurs via hematogenous seeding of the synovium
  - Previous joint damage and intravenous drug abuse predispose
  - Most common organisms: *Staphylococcus aureus,* group A streptococci, *Escherichia coli,* and *Pseudomonas aeruginosa; Haemophilus influenzae* in children under 5; *Staphylococcus epidermidis* following arthroscopy or joint surgery
  - White cell count in synovial fluid > 100,000/μL; synovial fluid culture positive in 50–75%, blood culture in 50%

- **Differential Diagnosis**
  - Gonococcal arthritis
  - Microcrystalline synovitis
  - Rheumatoid arthritis
  - Still's disease
  - Infective endocarditis (may be associated)

- **Treatment**
  - Intravenous antibiotics should be administered empirically
  - Surgical evaluation for drainage and irrigation of the knee
  - Affected hip joint usually requires surgical drainage
  - Rest, immobilization, and elevation
  - Removal of prosthetic joint

- **Pearl**

Pneumococcal arthritis in the absence of pneumonia or endocarditis means multiple myeloma until proved otherwise.

Reference

Carreño Pérez L: Septic arthritis. Baillieres Best Pract Res Clin Rheumatol 1999;13:37. [PMID: 10052848]

Gonococcal Arthritis

■ **Essentials of Diagnosis**

- Most common in young women during menses or pregnancy
- Tenosynovitis in many joints followed by monarticular arthritis
- Characteristic purpuric skin lesions on the distal extremities
- White cell count in synovial fluid 50,000/µL; synovial fluid Gram stain and culture uncommonly positive; likewise blood cultures
- Urethral, cervical, throat, skin lesion and rectal cultures on chocolate or Thayer-Martin agar for *Neisseria gonorrhoeae* have higher yield, may be positive in the absence of symptoms
- Recurrent disseminated gonococcal infection seen with congenital complement component deficiencies

■ **Differential Diagnosis**

- Nongonococcal bacterial arthritis
- Reactive arthritis
- Lyme disease
- Sarcoidosis
- Infective endocarditis
- Meningococcemia with arthritis
- Seronegative spondyloarthropathy

■ **Treatment**

- Obtain VDRL, consider HIV testing
- Intravenous ceftriaxone or ceftizoxime for 7 days followed by oral cefixime or ciprofloxacin
- Daily reaspiration of the synovial fluid if it reaccumulates

■ **Pearl**

Surprisingly trivial destructive articular changes for a bacterial arthritis.

Reference

Cucurull E et al: Gonococcal arthritis. Rheum Dis Clin North Am 1998; 24:305. [PMID: 9606761]

Infectious Osteomyelitis

- ■ **Essentials of Diagnosis**
  - Infection usually occurs via hematogenous seeding of the bone; metaphyses of long bones and vertebrae most frequently involved
  - Subacute, vague pain and tenderness of affected bone or back with little or no fever in adults; more acute presentation in children
  - Organisms include *Staphylococcus aureus*, coagulase-negative staphylococci, group A streptococci, gram-negative rods, anaerobic and polymicrobial infections, tuberculosis, brucellosis, histoplasmosis, coccidioidomycosis, blastomycosis
  - Blood cultures may be positive; aspiration or biopsy of bone is diagnostic
  - Radiographs early in the course are often negative, but periarticular demineralization, erosion of bone, and periostitis may occur later
  - Radionuclide bone scan is 90% sensitive and may be positive within 2 days after onset of symptoms

- ■ **Differential Diagnosis**
  - Acute bacterial arthritis
  - Rheumatic fever
  - Cellulitis
  - Multiple myeloma
  - Ewing's sarcoma
  - Metastatic neoplasia

- ■ **Treatment**
  - Intravenous antibiotics after appropriate cultures have been obtained
  - Oral ciprofloxacin, 750 mg twice daily for 6–8 weeks, may be effective in limited osteomyelitis
  - In older patients, treat with broad-spectrum antibiotics as for a gram-negative bacteremia as a consequence of urinary, biliary, intestinal, and lower respiratory infections
  - Debridement if response to antibiotics is poor

- ■ **Pearl**

In re chronic osteomyelitis: once an osteo, always an osteo.

Reference

Lew DP et al: Osteomyelitis. N Engl J Med 1997;336:999. [PMID: 9077380]

Eosinophilic Fasciitis

- **Essentials of Diagnosis**
  - Occurs predominantly in men
  - Pain, swelling, stiffness, and tenderness of the hands, forearms, feet, or legs evolving to woody induration and retraction of subcutaneous tissue within days to weeks
  - Associated with peripheral eosinophilia, polyarthralgias, arthritis, carpal tunnel syndrome; no Raynaud's phenomenon
  - Biopsy of deep fascia is diagnostic
  - Association with aplastic anemia, thrombocytopenia

- **Differential Diagnosis**
  - Systemic sclerosis
  - Eosinophilia myalgia syndrome
  - Hypothyroidism
  - Trichinosis
  - Mixed connective tissue disease

- **Treatment**
  - NSAIDs
  - Short course of corticosteroids
  - Antimalarials

- **Pearl**

Perhaps the only systemic disease in medicine confined strictly to the fascia.

Reference

Varga J et al: Eosinophilia-myalgia syndrome, eosinophilic fasciitis, and related fibrosing disorders. Curr Opin Rheumatol 1997;9:562. [PMID: 9375286]

Fibrositis (Fibromyalgia)

- ### Essentials of Diagnosis
  - Most frequent in women ages 20–50
  - Chronic aching pain and stiffness of trunk and extremities, especially around the neck, shoulder, low back, and hips
  - Must have 11 of 18 bilateral tender points: occiput, low cervical, trapezius, supraspinatus, second rib at costochondral junction, lateral epicondyle, gluteal region, greater trochanter, and medial fat pad of the knee
  - Associated with fatigue, headaches, subjective numbness, sleep disorders, irritable bowel symptoms, and history of sexual or domestic abuse
  - Absence of objective signs of inflammation; normal laboratory studies, including erythrocyte sedimentation rate

- ### Differential Diagnosis
  - Chronic fatigue syndrome
  - Rheumatoid arthritis
  - SLE
  - Depression
  - Polymyalgia rheumatica
  - HIV disease

- ### Treatment
  - Patient education, supportive care, exercise programs
  - Aspirin, other NSAIDs
  - Tricyclics, cyclobenzaprine, chlorpromazine
  - Injection of trigger points with corticosteroids

- ### Pearl
A tender point is defined as pain elicited with application of 4 kg of pressure, the same amount required to cause a fingernail to blanch.

Reference

Leventhal LJ: Management of fibromyalgia. Ann Intern Med 1999;131:850. [PMID: 10610631]

Amyloidosis

■ **Essentials of Diagnosis**

- A group of disorders characterized by deposition in tissues of ordinarily soluble peptides
- Amyloid protein (with characteristic green birefringence under polarizing microscope after Congo red staining) may be found on biopsy of rectal mucosa, gingival mucosa, bone marrow, or aspiration of abdominal fat pad
- May be primary (idiopathic or myeloma-associated), familial, localized, or secondary to familial Mediterranean fever, chronic infectious or inflammatory disease, aging, hemodialysis; in each, a different protein is responsible
- Distribution depends on type of amyloid; most systemic, but localized amyloid found in Alzheimer's plaques, islet cells in diabetics, carpal ligaments in dialysis patients
- Associated variably and unpredictably with peripheral neuropathy, postural hypotension, nephrotic syndrome, cardiomyopathy, arrhythmias, esophageal hypomotility, hepatosplenomegaly, gastrointestinal malabsorption and obstruction, carpal tunnel syndrome, macroglossia, arthropathy, endocrine gland insufficiency, respiratory failure, cutaneous lesions, and ecchymoses
- M-spike in primary amyloidosis

■ **Differential Diagnosis**

- Hemochromatosis
- Sarcoidosis
- Waldenström's macroglobulinemia
- Metastatic neoplasm
- Other causes of nephrotic syndrome

■ **Treatment**

- Colchicine to prevent attacks of familial Mediterranean fever when present
- Melphalan, prednisone if myeloma-associated
- Treat underlying disease if present

■ **Pearl**

The combination of nephrotic syndrome and hepatosplenomegaly in a middle-aged patient is amyloidosis; only rarely can other single processes do it.

Reference

Gertz MA et al: Amyloidosis. Hematol Oncol Clin North Am 1999;13:1211. PMID: 10626146]

Reflex Sympathetic Dystrophy

- **Essentials of Diagnosis**
  - Usually follows direct trauma to the hand or foot, knee injury, stroke, peripheral nerve injury, or arthroscopic knee surgery
  - Severe pain and tenderness, most commonly of the hand or foot, associated with vasomotor instability, skin atrophy, and hyperhidrosis
  - Shoulder-hand variant with restricted ipsilateral shoulder movement common after neck or shoulder injuries or following myocardial infarction
  - Characteristic disparity between degree of injury (usually modest) and degree of pain (debilitating)
  - Triple phase bone scan reveals increased uptake in the early phases of the disease; radiographs show severe osteopenia (Sudeck's atrophy) late in the course

- **Differential Diagnosis**
  - Rheumatoid arthritis
  - Polymyositis
  - Scleroderma
  - Gout, pseudogout
  - Acromegaly
  - Multiple myeloma
  - Osteoporosis due to other causes

- **Treatment**
  - Supportive care
  - Physical therapy
  - Active and passive exercises combined with benzodiazepines
  - Stellate ganglion or lumbar sympathetic block
  - Short course of corticosteroids given early in course

- **Pearl**

A far more common disorder when prolonged bed rest was prescribed for myocardial infarction.

Reference

Lopez RF: Reflex sympathetic dystrophy. Timely diagnosis and treatment can prevent severe contractures. Postgrad Med 1997;101:185. [PMID: 9126211]

Carpal Tunnel Syndrome

- **Essentials of Diagnosis**
  - The most common entrapment neuropathy, caused by compression of median nerve (which innervates the flexor muscles of the wrist and fingers)
  - Middle aged women and those with a history of repetitive use of the hands commonly affected
  - Pain classically worse at night and exacerbated by hand movement
  - Initial symptoms of pain or paresthesias in thumb, index, middle, and lateral part of ring finger; progression to thenar eminence wasting
  - Pain radiation to forearm, shoulder, neck, chest, or other fingers of the hand not uncommon
  - Positive Tinel sign
  - Usually idiopathic; common secondary causes include rheumatoid arthritis, amyloidosis involving carpal ligament, sarcoidosis, hypothyroidism, diabetes, pregnancy, acromegaly, gout
  - Diagnosis is primarily clinical; electrodiagnostic testing (assessing nerve conduction velocity) helpful in some

- **Differential Diagnosis**
  - C6 or C7 cervical radiculopathy
  - Thoracic outlet syndrome leading to brachial plexus neuropathy
  - Mononeuritis multiplex
  - Syringomyelia
  - Multiple sclerosis
  - Angina pectoris, especially when left-sided

- **Treatment**
  - Conservative measures initially, including hand rest, splinting, anti-inflammatory medications
  - Steroid injection into the carpal tunnel occasionally
  - Surgical decompression in a few; best done prior to development of thenar atrophy

- **Pearl**

When obtaining a history of arm pain, remember that carpal tunnel syndrome affects the radial three and one-half fingers and myocardial ischemia the ulnar one and one-half—and hope it's the right arm.

Reference

Whitley JM et al: Carpal tunnel syndrome. A guide to prompt intervention. Postgrad Med 1995;97:89. [PMID: 7816719]

Endocrine Disorders

7

Panhypopituitarism

- **Essentials of Diagnosis**
  - Sexual dysfunction, weakness, easy fatigability; poor resistance to stress, cold, or fasting; axillary and pubic hair loss
  - Hypotension, often orthostatic; visual field defects if pituitary tumor present
  - Deficient cortisol response to ACTH; low serum T_4 with low or low-normal TSH; serum prolactin level may be elevated
  - Low serum testosterone in men; amenorrhea; FSH and LH are low or low-normal
  - MRI may reveal a pituitary or hypothalamic lesion

- **Differential Diagnosis**
  - Anorexia nervosa or severe malnutrition
  - Hypothyroidism
  - Addison's disease
  - Cachexia due to other causes (eg, carcinoma or tuberculosis)
  - Empty sella syndrome

- **Treatment**
  - Surgical removal of pituitary tumor if present; pituitary irradiation may be necessary for residual tumor but increases likelihood of permanent hypopituitarism
  - Lifelong endocrine replacement therapy with corticosteroids, thyroid hormone, sex hormones, and, if indicated, growth hormone

- **Pearl**

In a woman with panhypopituitarism, ask about a previous complicated pregnancy with postpartum bleeding; it could be Sheehan's syndrome.

Reference

Lissett CA et al: Management of pituitary tumours: strategy for investigation and follow-up. Horm Res 2000;53(Suppl 3):65. [PMID: 10971108]

Acromegaly & Gigantism

- **Essentials of Diagnosis**
  - Amenorrhea, headaches, excessive sweating
  - Excessive growth of hands (increased glove size), feet (increased shoe size), jaw (protrusion of lower jaw), face, and tongue; gigantism if prior to epiphysial closure; visual field loss, coarse facial features, deep voice
  - Hyperglycemia, hypogonadotropic hypogonadism
  - Elevated serum insulin-like growth factor-1 (IGF-1)
  - Elevated serum growth hormone with failure to suppress after an oral glucose load
  - Radiographic findings include enlarged sella, thickened skull, and terminal phalangeal tufting; MRI demonstrates pituitary tumor in 90%

- **Differential Diagnosis**
  - Physiologic growth spurt
  - Pseudoacromegaly
  - Familial coarse features
  - Myxedema

- **Treatment**
  - Transsphenoidal resection of adenoma is successful in many patients; medical therapy is necessary for those with residual disease
  - The majority of patients respond to treatment with somatostatin analogs (eg, octreotide)
  - Dopamine agonists (eg, bromocriptine, cabergoline) occasionally reduce growth hormone secretion
  - Pituitary irradiation may be necessary if patients are not cured by surgical and medical therapy
  - Residual panhypopituitarism may require hormonal replacement (burnout acromegaly)

- **Pearl**

Perfect application of the wallet biopsy: compare present appearance of the patient with photograph on the driver's license and you make the diagnosis.

Reference

Melmed S et al: Current treatment guidelines for acromegaly. J Clin Endocrinol Metab 1998;83:2646. [PMID: 9709926]

Hyperprolactinemia

- **Essentials of Diagnosis**
  - Women: menstrual disturbance (oligomenorrhea, amenorrhea), galactorrhea, infertility
  - Men: hypogonadism; decreased libido and erectile dysfunction; galactorrhea; infertility
  - Serum prolactin usually > 100 ng/mL
  - May be caused by primary hypothyroidism
  - Pituitary adenoma often demonstrated by MRI

- **Differential Diagnosis**
  - Primary hypothyroidism
  - Use of prolactin-stimulating drugs
  - Pregnancy or lactation
  - Hypothalamic disease
  - Cirrhosis; renal failure
  - Chronic nipple stimulation; chest wall injury

- **Treatment**
  - Dopamine agonists (eg, bromocriptine or cabergoline) usually shrink pituitary adenoma and restore fertility
  - Transsphenoidal resection for large tumors and for those causing visual compromise or refractory to dopamine agonists

- **Pearl**

Virtually every psychotropic drug causes hyperprolactinemia.

Reference

Kaye TB: Hyperprolactinemia. Causes, consequences, and treatment options. Postgrad Med 1996;99:265. [PMID: 8650091]

Diabetes Insipidus

- **Essentials of Diagnosis**
  - Polyuria with volumes of 2–20 L/d; polydipsia, intense thirst
  - Serum osmolality > urine osmolality
  - Urine specific gravity usually < 1.006 during ad libitum fluid intake
  - Inability to concentrate urine with fluid restriction, resulting in hypernatremia
  - Central diabetes insipidus (vasopressin-deficient) caused by hypothalamic or pituitary disease
  - Nephrogenic diabetes insipidus (vasopressin-resistant) may be familial or caused by lithium, chronic renal disease, hypokalemia, hypercalcemia, tetracycline
  - Vasopressin challenge establishes central cause

- **Differential Diagnosis**
  - Psychogenic polydipsia
  - Osmotic diuresis
  - Diabetes mellitus
  - Beer potomania

- **Treatment**
  - Ensure adequate free water intake
  - Intranasal desmopressin acetate for central diabetes insipidus
  - Hydrochlorothiazide or indomethacin for nephrogenic diabetes insipidus

- **Pearl**

Demeclocycline and other tetracyclines cause permanent if subtle nephrogenic diabetes insipidus; be cautious using them for acne during puberty.

Reference

Singer I et al: The management of diabetes insipidus in adults. Arch Intern Med 1997;157:1293. [PMID: 9201003]

Simple & Nodular Goiter

- **Essentials of Diagnosis**
  - Single or multiple thyroid nodules found on thyroid palpation
  - Large multinodular goiters may be associated with compressive symptoms (dysphagia, stridor)
  - Measurement of free thyroxine (FT_4) and TSH; radioiodine uptake scan helpful in selected cases for distinguishing cold from hot nodules

- **Differential Diagnosis**
  - Graves' disease (diffuse toxic goiter)
  - Autoimmune thyroiditis
  - Carcinoma of the thyroid

- **Treatment**
  - Fine-needle biopsy for single or dominant nodules; carcinomas or suspicious cold lesions require surgery
  - Levothyroxine treatment suppresses growth in benign nodules or multinodular goiter and may cause regression; contraindicated if TSH is low
  - Surgery for severe compressive symptoms

- **Pearl**

Pharmacologic iodine, as in contrast-enhanced radiographic studies, may result in hyperthyroidism via the jodbasedow phenomenon.

Reference

Hermus AR et al: Treatment of benign nodular thyroid disease. N Engl J Med 1998;338:1438. [PMID: 9589652]

Adult Hypothyroidism & Myxedema

- **Essentials of Diagnosis**
  - Cold intolerance, constipation, weight gain, hoarseness, altered mentation, depression, hypermenorrhea
  - Hypothermia, bradycardia, dry skin with yellow tone (carotenemia); nonpitting edema; macroglossia; delayed relaxation of deep tendon reflexes
  - Low serum FT_4; TSH elevated in primary hypothyroidism; macrocytic anemia
  - Myxedema coma may be associated with obtundation, profound hypothermia, hypoventilation, hypotension, striking bradycardia; pleural and pericardial effusions
  - Associated with other autoimmune endocrinopathies

- **Differential Diagnosis**
  - Chronic fatigue syndrome
  - Congestive heart failure
  - Primary amyloidosis
  - Depression
  - Exposure hypothermia
  - Parkinson's disease

- **Treatment**
  - Levothyroxine replacement starting with low doses and increasing gradually until euthyroid
  - Treat myxedema coma with intravenous levothyroxine; if adrenal insufficiency is suspected, add intravenous hydrocortisone

- **Pearl**

Treating myxedema may precipitate addisonian crisis because of subclinical concomitant adrenal insufficiency; add steroids to thyroid hormone until adrenocortical insufficiency has been ruled out.

Reference

Woeber, KA. Update on the management of hyperthyroidism and hypothyroidism. Arch Intern Med 2000;160:1067, [PMID: 10789598]

Hyperthyroidism

- **Essentials of Diagnosis**
  - Sweating, weight loss, heat intolerance, irritability, weakness, increased number of bowel movements, menstrual irregularity
  - Sinus tachycardia or atrial fibrillation, tremor, warm moist skin, eye findings (stare, lid lag); diffuse goiter, thyroid bruit and exophthalmos in Graves' disease
  - Serum FT_4 and T_3 increased; TSH low or undetectable
  - Radioiodine uptake scan will differentiate Graves' disease, toxic nodule, and thyroiditis; may also be useful in ectopic thyroid tissue (ovary)
  - Thyroid-stimulating immunoglobulin and thyroid autoantibodies are often positive in Graves' disease; common association with other endocrine gland autoantibodies

- **Differential Diagnosis**
  - Anxiety, neurosis, or mania
  - Pheochromocytoma
  - Exogenous thyroid administration
  - Catabolic illness
  - Chronic alcoholism

- **Treatment**
  - Supportive care for patients with thyroiditis
  - Propranolol for symptomatic relief of catecholamine-mediated symptoms
  - Antithyroid drugs (methimazole or propylthiouracil) for patients with mild Graves' disease or smaller goiters
  - Radioactive iodine ablation is indicated for more severe or refractory Graves' disease (contraindicated in pregnancy) and in patients with toxic nodular disease; in older patients or those with severe hyperthyroidism, treat first with antithyroid drugs
  - Subtotal thyroidectomy for failure of medical therapy if radioactive iodine is contraindicated (eg, pregnancy) or for very large nodular goiters; euthyroid state should be achieved medically before surgery

- **Pearl**

In patients over 60, when you think it's hyperthyroidism it's hypo- and when you think it's hypo- it's hyper-: the diseases become increasingly atypical with age.

Reference

Lazarus JH: Hyperthyroidism. Lancet 1997;349:339. [PMID: 9024389]

Thyroiditis

- **Essentials of Diagnosis**
  - Painful enlarged thyroid gland in acute and subacute forms; painless enlargement in chronic form
  - Generally classified as chronic lymphocytic (Hashimoto's) thyroiditis and subacute (granulomatous) thyroiditis; suppurative thyroiditis and Riedel's thyroiditis are uncommon
  - Thyroid function tests variable, with serum T_4 and T_3 levels often high in acute forms and low in chronic disease
  - Elevated erythrocyte sedimentation rate and reduced radioiodine uptake in subacute thyroiditis
  - Thyroid autoantibodies positive in Hashimoto's thyroiditis

- **Differential Diagnosis**
  - Endemic goiter
  - Graves' disease (diffuse toxic goiter)
  - Carcinoma of the thyroid
  - Pyogenic infections of the neck

- **Treatment**
  - Antibiotics for suppurative thyroiditis
  - Nonsteroid anti-inflammatory drugs for subacute thyroiditis; prednisone in severe cases; symptomatic treatment with propranolol
  - Levothyroxine replacement for Hashimoto's thyroiditis
  - Partial thyroidectomy for local severe pressure or adhesions in Riedel's thyroiditis

- **Pearl**

The patient can be hyper-, hypo-, or euthyroid depending on where the disease is when you test.

Reference

Slatosky J et al: Thyroiditis: differential diagnosis and management. Am Fam Physician 2000;61:1047. [PMID: 10706157]

Hypoparathyroidism

- **Essentials of Diagnosis**
  - Tetany, carpopedal spasms, tingling of lips and hands; altered mentation
  - Positive Chvostek sign (facial muscle contraction on tapping the facial nerve) and Trousseau phenomenon (carpal spasm after application of arm cuff); dry skin and brittle nails; cataracts
  - Serum calcium low; serum phosphate high; serum parathyroid hormone low to absent
  - Long ST segment resulting in long QT interval on ECG
  - History of previous thyroidectomy or neck surgery in patients with surgical hypoparathyroidism

- **Differential Diagnosis**
  - Pseudohypoparathyroidism
  - Vitamin D deficiency syndromes
  - Acute pancreatitis
  - Hypomagnesemia
  - Chronic renal failure
  - Hypoalbuminemia

- **Treatment**
  - For acute tetany, intravenous calcium gluconate, followed by oral calcium carbonate and vitamin D derivatives
  - Correct concurrent hypomagnesemia
  - Chronic therapy includes high-calcium diet in addition to calcium and vitamin D supplements
  - Avoid phenothiazines (prolonged QT) and furosemide (increases symptoms of hypocalcemia)

- **Pearl**

Radiotherapy causes hypothyroidism but never hypoparathyroidism—the parathyroids are among the most resistant tissues in the body to radiation.

Reference

Rude RK: Hypocalcemia and hypoparathyroidism. Curr Ther Endocrinol Metab 1997;6:546. [PMID: 9174804]

Primary Hyperparathyroidism

■ Essentials of Diagnosis

- Renal stones, bone pain, mental status changes, constipation ("stones, bones, moans, and abdominal groans"), polyuria; many patients are asymptomatic
- Serum and urine calcium elevated; low-normal to low serum phosphate; high-normal or elevated serum parathyroid hormone level; alkaline phosphatase often elevated
- Bone radiographs show cystic bone lesions (brown tumors) and subperiosteal resorption of cortical bone, especially the phalanges (osteitis fibrosa cystica); may have osteoporosis and pathologic fractures
- History of renal stones, nephrocalcinosis, recurrent peptic ulcer disease, or recurrent pancreatitis may be present

■ Differential Diagnosis

- Familial hypocalciuric hypercalcemia
- Hypercalcemia of malignancy
- Renal failure
- Vitamin D intoxication or milk-alkali syndrome
- Sarcoidosis, granulomatous disorders
- Hyperthyroidism
- Multiple myeloma

■ Treatment

- Parathyroidectomy for patients with symptomatic disease, markedly elevated calcium level, hypercalciuria, kidney stones, or bone disease
- Bisphosphonates (eg, pamidronate) for acute treatment of severe hypercalcemia while preparing for surgery
- For patients with mild asymptomatic disease: maintain adequate fluid intake and avoid immobilization, thiazide diuretics, and calcium-containing antacids; follow for disease progression
- Estrogen replacement for postmenopausal women

■ Pearl

The natural history of untreated hyperparathyroidism is benign; even superb centers have trouble obtaining follow-up of patients—because they do so well.

Reference

al Zahrani A et al: Primary hyperparathyroidism. Lancet 1997;349:1233. [PMID: 9130957]

Osteoporosis

- **Essentials of Diagnosis**
  - Asymptomatic or associated with back pain from vertebral fractures; loss of height; kyphosis
  - Demineralization of spine, hip, and pelvis by radiograph; vertebral compression fractures; spontaneous fractures often discovered incidentally
  - Bone mineral density more than 2.5 SD below the average value for a young adult

- **Differential Diagnosis**
  - Osteomalacia
  - Multiple myeloma
  - Metastatic carcinoma
  - Hypophosphatemic disorders
  - Osteogenesis imperfecta
  - Secondary osteoporosis due to steroids, hyperthyroidism, hypogonadism, alcoholism, or liver disease

- **Treatment**
  - Diet adequate in calcium and vitamin D with supplements to achieve 1000–1500 mg elemental calcium and 400 IU vitamin D daily
  - Regular exercise
  - Fall prevention strategies
  - Effective antiresorptive therapies include bisphosphonates (eg, alendronate, risedronate), estrogen replacement therapy, calcitonin, and selective estrogen receptor modulators (SERMS), eg, raloxifene
  - Men with hypogonadism are treated with testosterone

- **Pearl**

Easily the most debilitating nonmalignant disease of bone.

Reference

Lambing CL: Osteoporosis prevention, detection, and treatment. A mandate for primary care physicians. Postgrad Med 2000;107:37. [PMID: 10887444]

Paget's Disease (Osteitis Deformans)

- ### Essentials of Diagnosis
  - Often asymptomatic or associated with bone pain, fractures, and bone deformity (bowing, kyphosis)
  - Serum calcium and phosphate normal; alkaline phosphatase elevated; urinary hydroxyproline elevated
  - Dense, expanded bones on x-ray resulting from accelerated bone turnover and disruption of normal architecture; osteolytic lesions in the skull and extremities; vertebral fractures; fissure fractures in the long bones
  - May have neurologic sequelae due to nerve compression as pagetic bones enlarge (eg, deafness)

- ### Differential Diagnosis
  - Osteogenic sarcoma
  - Multiple myeloma
  - Fibrous dysplasia
  - Metastatic carcinoma
  - Osteitis fibrosa cystica (hyperparathyroidism)

- ### Treatment
  - No treatment for asymptomatic patients
  - Treat symptomatic disease with inhibitors of osteoclastic resorption (bisphosphonates or calcitonin)
  - The role of prophylactic treatment to prevent bone deformities or neurologic sequelae is not well established

- ### Pearl
  Was Paget's disease the cause of Beethoven's deafness? Only his pictures suggest it, as no alkaline phosphatase determinations were available between 1770 and 1828.

Reference

Delmas PD et al: The management of Paget's disease of bone. N Engl J Med 1997;336:558. [PMID: 9023094]

Primary Adrenal Insufficiency (Addison's Disease)

- **Essentials of Diagnosis**
  - Weakness, anorexia, weight loss, abdominal pain, nausea and vomiting; increased skin pigmentation
  - Hypotension, dehydration; postural symptoms
  - Hyponatremia, hyperkalemia, hypoglycemia, lymphocytosis, and eosinophilia; increased serum urea nitrogen and calcium may be present
  - Serum cortisol levels low to absent and ACTH elevated; cortisol level fails to rise after cosyntropin (ACTH) stimulation
  - Often associated with other autoimmune endocrinopathies; may also be due to trauma, infection (especially tuberculosis, histoplasmosis), adrenal hemorrhage, or adrenoleukodystrophy

- **Differential Diagnosis**
  - Secondary adrenal insufficiency
  - Anorexia nervosa
  - Malignancy
  - Infection
  - Salt-wasting nephropathy
  - Hemochromatosis

- **Treatment**
  - In acute adrenal crisis, treat immediately with intravenous hydrocortisone (100 mg intravenously every 8 hours) once the diagnosis is suspected; provide appropriate volume resuscitation and blood pressure support; consider empiric antibiotics
  - In chronic adrenal insufficiency, maintenance therapy includes glucocorticoids (hydrocortisone) and mineralocorticoids (fludrocortisone)
  - Increase glucocorticoid dose for trauma, surgery, infection, or stress

- **Pearl**

If the systolic blood pressure is over 100 mm Hg, consider other diseases.

Reference

Oelkers W: Adrenal insufficiency. N Engl J Med 1996;335:1206. [PMID: 8815944]

Hypercortisolism (Cushing's Syndrome)

- ### Essentials of Diagnosis
  - Weakness, muscle wasting, weight gain, central obesity, psychosis, hirsutism, acne, menstrual irregularity, hypogonadism
  - Hypertension, moon facies, buffalo hump, thin skin, easy bruisability, purple striae, poor wound healing, osteoporosis
  - Hyperglycemia, glycosuria, leukocytosis, lymphocytopenia; may have hypokalemia with ectopic ACTH secretion
  - Elevated plasma cortisol and urinary free cortisol; failure to suppress plasma cortisol with exogenous dexamethasone (overnight low-dose dexamethasone test)
  - A normal or high ACTH level indicates ACTH-dependent Cushing's disease (pituitary adenoma or ectopic ACTH syndrome); a low ACTH level indicates adrenal tumor
  - CT or MRI will reveal adrenal tumor if present

- ### Differential Diagnosis
  - Chronic alcoholism
  - Depression
  - Diabetes mellitus
  - Exogenous glucocorticoid administration
  - Severe obesity

- ### Treatment
  - Transsphenoidal resection of pituitary adenoma if present; radiation therapy for residual disease
  - Resection of adrenal tumor if present
  - Resection of ectopic ACTH-producing tumor if able to localize (eg, carcinoid, prostate small-cell)
  - Ketoconazole or metyrapone to suppress cortisol in unresectable cases
  - Bilateral adrenalectomy for adrenal hyperplasia in refractory cases of ACTH-dependent Cushing's syndrome

- ### Pearl

If you see the above picture in a man, the cortisol isn't from classic Cushing's syndrome; the incidence is 10:1 women to men.

Reference

Kirk LF Jr et al: Cushing's disease: clinical manifestations and diagnostic evaluation. Am Fam Physician 2000;62:1119. [PMID: 10997535]

Hirsutism & Virilizing Diseases of Women

- ■ Essentials of Diagnosis
  - • Menstrual disorders, hirsutism, acne
  - • Virilization may occur: increased muscularity, balding, deepening of the voice, enlargement of the clitoris
  - • Occasionally a pelvic mass is palpable
  - • Serum testosterone and androstenedione often elevated; serum DHEAS elevated in adrenal disorders
  - • May be due to polycystic ovary syndrome, congenital adrenal hyperplasia, ovarian or adrenal tumors, ACTH-dependent Cushing's syndrome

- ■ Differential Diagnosis
  - • Familial, idiopathic, or drug-related hirsutism
  - • Cushing's syndrome
  - • Exogenous androgen ingestion

- ■ Treatment
  - • Surgical removal of ovarian or adrenal tumor if present
  - • Oral contraceptives to suppress ovarian androgen excess and normalize menses
  - • Glucocorticoids for congenital adrenal hyperplasia
  - • Spironolactone and cyproterone acetate to ameliorate hirsutism; finasteride and flutamide may help in refractory cases
  - • Consider metformin for women with polycystic ovary syndrome

- ■ Pearl

Check the drug history in hirsutism—it's more likely than the above syndromes.

Reference

Rittmaster RS: Hirsutism. Lancet 1997;349:191. [PMID: 9111556]

Male Hypogonadism

- ■ Essentials of Diagnosis
    - Diminished libido and impotence
    - Sparse growth of male body hair
    - Testes may be small or normal in size; serum testosterone is usually decreased
    - Serum gonadotropins (LH and FSH) are decreased in hypogonadotropic hypogonadism; they are increased in primary testicular failure (hypergonadotropic hypogonadism)
    - Causes of hypogonadotropic hypogonadism include chronic illness, malnutrition, drugs, pituitary tumor, Cushing's syndrome, congenital syndromes, and Kallman's disease
    - Causes of hypergonadotropic hypogonadism include Klinefelter's syndrome, bilateral anorchia, testicular trauma, orchitis, and myotonic dystrophy

- ■ Differential Diagnosis
    - Cushing's syndrome
    - Hemochromatosis
    - Pituitary tumor
    - Androgen insensitivity

- ■ Treatment
    - Evaluate and treat underlying disorder
    - Testosterone replacement (intramuscular or transdermal)

- ■ Pearl

One of the reasons to check the first cranial nerve: anosmia is a feature of Kallman's syndrome.

Reference

Hayes FJ et al: Hypogonadotropic hypogonadism. Emerg Med Clin North Am 199827:739I. [PMID: 9922906]

Primary Hyperaldosteronism

- ### Essentials of Diagnosis
  - Hypertension (usually mild), polyuria, fatigue, and weakness
  - Hypokalemia, metabolic alkalosis
  - Elevated plasma and urine aldosterone levels with suppressed plasma renin level
  - May be associated with adrenocortical adenoma (75%) or bilateral adrenocortical hyperplasia (25%)
  - Rarely due to glucocorticoid-remediable aldosteronism
  - Adrenal mass often demonstrated by CT or MRI

- ### Differential Diagnosis
  - Essential hypertension
  - Periodic paralysis
  - Congenital adrenal hyperplasia
  - Pseudohyperaldosteronism; European licorice ingestion
  - Chronic diuretic use or laxative abuse
  - Unilateral renovascular disease
  - Cushing's syndrome

- ### Treatment
  - Surgical resection of unilateral adenoma secreting aldosterone (Conn's syndrome)
  - Spironolactone for bilateral adrenal hyperplasia; surgery does not cure hypertension in these cases and is not generally recommended
  - Dexamethasone for glucocorticoid-remediable aldosteronism
  - Antihypertensive therapy as necessary

- ### Pearl

If the sodium is less than 140 mg/dL and a spot urine potassium less than 40 mg/dL, consider something else.

Reference

Ganguly A: Primary aldosteronism. N Engl J Med 1998;339:1828. [PMID: 9854120]

Pheochromocytoma

- **Essentials of Diagnosis**
  - Paroxysmal or sustained hypertension; postural hypotension
  - Episodes of perspiration, palpitations, and headache; anxiety, nausea, chest or abdominal pain
  - Hypermetabolism with normal thyroid tests; hyperglycemia and glycosuria may be present
  - Elevated urinary catecholamines, metanephrines, and vanillyl-mandelic acid are diagnostic; serum epinephrine and norepinephrine elevated
  - CT or MRI can confirm and localize pheochromocytoma; ^{123}I-MIBG scan may help to localize tumors

- **Differential Diagnosis**
  - Essential hypertension
  - Thyrotoxicosis
  - Panic attacks
  - Preeclampsia-eclampsia
  - Acute intermittent porphyria

- **Treatment**
  - Surgical removal of tumor or tumors
  - Alpha blockade with phenoxybenzamine prior to surgery
  - Beta-adrenergic receptor blockade can be added after effective alpha blockade to help control tachycardia
  - Adequate volume replenishment mandatory prior to surgery
  - Oral phenoxybenzamine or metyrosine for symptomatic treatment in patients with inoperable tumors; metastatic pheochromocytoma may be treated with chemotherapy or ^{131}I-MIBG

- **Pearl**

Rule of tens: Approximately ten percent bilateral, ten percent malignant, ten percent extra-adrenal, ten percent familial, ten percent normotensive.

Reference

Werbel SS et al: Pheochromocytoma. Update on diagnosis, localization, and management. Med Clin North Am 1995;79:131. [PMID: 7808088]

Hypoglycemia in the Adult

- **Essentials of Diagnosis**
  - Blurred vision, diplopia, headache, slurred speech, weakness, sweating, palpitations, tremulousness, altered mentation; focal neurologic signs common
  - Plasma glucose < 40 mg/dL
  - Causes include alcoholism, postprandial hypoglycemia (eg, postgastrectomy), insulinoma, medications (insulin, sulfonylureas, pentamidine), adrenal insufficiency

- **Differential Diagnosis**
  - Central nervous system disease
  - Hypoxia
  - Psychoneurosis
  - Pheochromocytoma

- **Treatment**
  - Intravenous glucose (oral glucose for patients who are conscious and able to swallow)
  - Intramuscular glucagon if no intravenous access available
  - Treatment of underlying disease or removal of offending agent (eg, alcohol, pentamidine, sulfonylureas)
  - For patients with postprandial (reactive) hypoglycemia, eating small frequent meals with reduced proportion of carbohydrates may help

- **Pearl**

Remember neuroglycopenic hypoglycemia in hypothermia with altered mental status.

Reference

Service, FJ. Hypoglycemic disorders. N Engl J Med 1995;332:1144. [PMID: 7700289]

Type 1 Diabetes Mellitus

- **Essentials of Diagnosis**
  - Crisp onset, no family history
  - Polyuria, polydipsia, weight loss
  - Fasting plasma glucose > 126 mg/dL; random plasma glucose > 200 mg/dL with symptoms; glycosuria
  - Associated with ketosis in untreated state; may present as medical emergency (diabetic ketoacidosis)
  - Long-term risks include retinopathy, nephropathy, neuropathy, and cardiovascular disease

- **Differential Diagnosis**
  - Nondiabetic glycosuria (eg, Fanconi's syndrome)
  - Diabetes insipidus
  - Acromegaly
  - Cushing's disease or syndrome
  - Pheochromocytoma
  - Medications (eg, glucocorticoids, niacin)

- **Treatment**
  - Insulin treatment is required
  - Patient education is crucial, emphasizing dietary management, intensive insulin therapy, self-monitoring of blood glucose , hypoglycemia awareness, foot and eye care

- **Pearl**

The prognosis of diabetic ketoacidosis is better than that of a nonketotic hyperosmolar state (see page 196 for why).

Reference

Havas S: Educational guidelines for achieving tight control and minimizing complications of type 1 diabetes. Am Fam Physician 1999;60:1985. [PMID: 10569502]

Type 2 Diabetes Mellitus

- **Essentials of Diagnosis**
  - Most patients are older and tend to be obese
  - Gradual onset of polyuria, polydipsia; often asymptomatic
  - Candidal vaginitis in women, chronic skin infection, generalized pruritus, blurred vision
  - Fasting plasma glucose > 126 mg/dL; random plasma glucose > 200 mg/dL with symptoms; glycosuria; elevated glycosylated hemoglobin (A_{1c}); ketosis rare
  - Family history often present; frequently associated with hypertension, hyperlipidemia, and atherosclerosis
  - May present as medical emergency (especially in the elderly) as nonketotic hyperosmolar coma
  - Long-term risks include retinopathy, nephropathy, neuropathy, and cardiovascular disease

- **Differential Diagnosis**
  - Nondiabetic glycosuria (eg, Fanconi's syndrome)
  - Diabetes insipidus
  - Acromegaly
  - Cushing's disease or syndrome
  - Pheochromocytoma
  - Medications (eg, glucocorticoids, niacin)
  - Severe insulin resistance syndromes
  - Altered mental status due to other cause

- **Treatment**
  - Patient education is important, emphasizing dietary management, exercise, weight loss, self-monitoring of blood glucose, hypoglycemia awareness, foot and eye care
  - Mild cases may be controlled initially with diet, exercise, and weight loss
  - Oral hypoglycemic agents if diet is ineffective; insulin may be required if combination oral agents fail

- **Pearl**

  The cause of the most profound involuntary weight loss in medicine with a normal physical examination.

Reference

DeFronzo RA: Pharmacologic therapy for type 2 diabetes mellitus. Ann Intern Med 1999;131:281. [PMID: 10454950]

Diabetic Ketoacidosis

- **Essentials of Diagnosis**
  - Acute polyuria and polydipsia, marked fatigue, nausea and vomiting, coma
  - Fruity breath; dehydration, hypotension if severe volume depletion occurs; Kussmaul respirations
  - Hyperglycemia > 250 mg/dL, ketonemia, acidemia with blood pH < 7.3 and serum bicarbonate < 15 meq/L, elevated anion gap; glycosuria and ketonuria; total body potassium depleted despite elevation in serum potassium
  - Due to insulin deficiency or increased insulin requirements in a type 1 diabetic (eg, in association with myocardial ischemia, surgery, infection, gastroenteritis, intra-abdominal disease, or medical noncompliance)

- **Differential Diagnosis**
  - Alcoholic ketoacidosis
  - Uremia
  - Lactic acidosis
  - Sepsis

- **Treatment**
  - Aggressive volume resuscitation with saline; dextrose should be added to intravenous fluids once glucose reaches 250–300 mg/dL
  - Intravenous regular insulin replacement with frequent laboratory monitoring
  - Potassium, magnesium, and phosphate replacement
  - Identify and treat precipitating cause

- **Pearl**

Very low pH and severe hyperkalemia look bad and are bad, but osmolality determines the outcome.

Reference

Kitabchi AR et al: Management of diabetic ketoacidosis. Am Fam Physician 1999;60:455. [PMID: 10465221]

Hyperosmotic Nonketotic Diabetic Coma

- **Essentials of Diagnosis**
  - Gradual onset of polyuria, polydipsia, dehydration, and weakness; in severe cases, may progress to obtundation and coma
  - Occurs in patients with type 2 diabetes, typically in elderly patients with reduced fluid intake
  - Profound hyperglycemia (> 600 mg/dL), hyperosmolality (> 310 mosm/kg); pH > 7.3, serum bicarbonate > 15 meq/L; ketosis and acidosis are usually absent

- **Differential Diagnosis**
  - Cerebrovascular accident or head trauma
  - Diabetes insipidus
  - Hypoglycemia
  - Hyperglycemia

- **Treatment**
  - Aggressive volume resuscitation with normal saline until patient euvolemic, then with hypotonic saline
  - Regular insulin 15 units intravenously plus 15 units subcutaneously initially is usually effective, followed by subcutaneous insulin every 4 hours
  - Careful monitoring of serum sodium, osmolality, and glucose
  - Dextrose-containing fluids when glucose is 250–300 mg/dL
  - Potassium and phosphate replacement as needed

- **Pearl**

As for diabetic ketoacidosis, osmolality determines the outcome; it's the reason this condition's prognosis is worse than that of ketoacidosis, where osmolality is usually normal.

Reference

Lorber D: Nonketotic hypertonicity in diabetes mellitus. Med Clin North Am 1995;79:39. [PMID: 7808094]

Gynecomastia

- **Essentials of Diagnosis**
  - Glandular enlargement of the male breast
  - Often asymmetric or unilateral and may be tender
  - Nipple discharge may be present
  - Common in puberty and among elderly men
  - Multiple causes include obesity, androgen resistance, hyperprolactinemia, hyperthyroidism, hypogonadism, chronic liver disease, adrenal tumors, testicular tumors, bronchogenic carcinoma, and drugs (eg, alcohol, amiodarone, diazepam, digoxin, isoniazid, ketoconazole, marijuana, omeprazole, tricyclic antidepressants)

- **Differential Diagnosis**
  - Associations noted above
  - Benign or malignant tumors of the breast

- **Treatment**
  - Careful testicular examination; chest x-ray to rule out bronchogenic carcinoma; measurement of β-hCG, LH, testosterone, and estradiol may be indicated to rule out underlying disorder
  - Needle biopsy of suspicious areas of breast enlargement
  - Remove offending drug or treat underlying condition; reassurance if idiopathic
  - Consider surgical correction for severe cases

- **Pearl**

Remember that 1% of breast carcinoma occurs in men.

Reference

Neuman JF: Evaluation and treatment of gynecomastia. Am Fam Physician 1997;55:1835 [PMID: 9105209]

8

Infectious Diseases

VIRAL INFECTIONS

Herpes Simplex

- **Essentials of Diagnosis**
  - Recurrent grouped small vesicles on erythematous base, usually perioral or perigenital
  - Primary infection more severe and often associated with fever, regional lymphadenopathy, and aseptic meningitis
  - Recurrences precipitated by minor infections, trauma, stress, sun exposure
  - Oral and genital lesions highly infectious
  - Systemic infection may occur in immunosuppressed patients
  - Proctitis, esophagitis, and keratitis may complicate
  - Direct fluorescent antibody or culture of ulcer can be diagnostic

- **Differential Diagnosis**
  - Herpangina, hand-foot-and-mouth disease
  - Aphthous ulcers
  - Stevens-Johnson syndrome
  - Bacterial infection of the skin
  - Syphilis and other sexually transmitted diseases
  - Other causes of encephalitis, proctitis, or keratitis

- **Treatment**
  - Acyclovir, famciclovir, and valacyclovir may attenuate recurrent course of genital or oral lesions and are obligatory for systemic or central nervous system disease

- **Pearl**

In a smoker, a nonresolving "herpetic" ulcer on the lip suggests the diagnosis of squamous cell cancer.

Reference

Whitley RJ et al: Herpes simplex viruses. Clin Infect Dis 1998;26:541. [PMID: 9524821]

Measles (Rubeola)

- ■ **Essentials of Diagnosis**
  - • An acute systemic viral illness transmitted by inhalation of infective droplets
  - • Incubation period 10–14 days
  - • Prodrome of fever, coryza, cough, conjunctivitis, photophobia
  - • Progression of brick-red, irregular maculopapular rash 3 days after prodrome from face to trunk to extremities
  - • Koplik's spots (tiny "table salt crystals") on the buccal mucosa are pathognomonic but appear and disappear rapidly
  - • Leukopenia
  - • Encephalitis in 1–3%

- ■ **Differential Diagnosis**
  - • Other acute exanthems (eg, rubella, enterovirus, Epstein-Barr virus infection, varicella, roseola)
  - • Drug allergy
  - • Pneumonia or encephalitis due to other cause

- ■ **Treatment**
  - • Primary immunization preventive after age 15 months; revaccination of adults born after 1956 without documented immunity recommended
  - • Isolation for 1 week following onset of rash
  - • Specific treatment of secondary bacterial complications

- ■ **Pearl**

Of all the viral exanthems, systemic toxicity is most marked with measles.

Reference

Atkinson WL: Epidemiology and prevention of measles. Dermatol Clin 1995; 13:553. [PMID: 7554503]

Rubella

- **Essentials of Diagnosis**
  - A systemic illness transmitted by inhalation of infected droplets, with incubation period 14–21 days
  - No prodrome in children (mild in adults); fever, malaise, coryza coincide with eruption of fine maculopapular rash on face to trunk to extremities which rapidly fades
  - Arthralgias common, particularly in young women
  - Posterior cervical, suboccipital, and posterior auricular lymphadenopathy 5–10 days before rash
  - Leukopenia, thrombocytopenia
  - In one out of 6000 cases, postinfectious encephalopathy develops 1–6 days after the rash; mortality rate is 20%

- **Differential Diagnosis**
  - Other acute exanthems (eg, rubeola, enterovirus, Epstein-Barr virus infection, varicella)
  - Drug allergy

- **Treatment**
  - Active immunization after age 15 months; girls should be immunized before menarche though not during pregnancy
  - Symptomatic therapy only

- **Pearl**

Rubella-associated arthritis is more symptomatic after vaccination than with natural infection.

Reference

Rosa C: Rubella and rubeola. Semin Perinatol 1998;22:318. [PMID: 9738996]

Cytomegalovirus Disease

- **Essentials of Diagnosis**
  - Neonatal infection: hepatosplenomegaly, purpura, central nervous system abnormalities
  - Immunocompetent adults: mononucleosis-like illness characterized by fever, myalgias, hepatosplenomegaly, leukopenia with lymphocytic predominance, often following transfusion; no pharyngitis, however
  - Immunocompromised adults: retinitis (AIDS), pneumonia, meningoencephalitis, polyradiculopathy, chorioretinitis, chronic diarrhea
  - Fever may be prolonged in the latter group
  - In immunocompetent adults, IgM is diagnostic
  - In AIDS patients, funduscopic examination establishes the diagnosis; culture positivity does not establish the etiology of any symptom complex

- **Differential Diagnosis**
  - Infectious mononucleosis (Epstein-Barr virus)
  - Acute HIV infection
  - Other causes of prolonged fever (eg, lymphoma, endocarditis)
  - In immunocompromised patients: other causes of atypical pneumonia, meningoencephalitis, or chronic diarrhea
  - In infants: toxoplasmosis, rubella, herpes simplex, syphilis

- **Treatment**
  - Appropriate supportive care
  - Ganciclovir, foscarnet, or cidofovir intravenously in immunocompromised patients

- **Pearl**

Acute cytomegalovirus infection should always be considered in a patient with a mononucleosis-like illness and a negative heterophil agglutination test (Monospot), especially if pharyngitis is absent.

Reference

Nichols WG: Recent advances in the therapy and prevention of CMV infections. J Clin Virol 2000;16:25. [PMID: 10680738]

Varicella (Acute Chickenpox, Zoster [Shingles])

- ■ Essentials of Diagnosis
    - Acute varicella: fever, malaise with eruption of pruritic, centripetal, papular rash, vesicular and pustular before crusting; lesions in all stages at any given time; "drop on rose petal" is the first lesion
    - Incubation period 14–21 days
    - Bacterial infection, pneumonia, and encephalitis may complicate
    - Reactivation varicella (herpes zoster): dermatomal distribution, vesicular rash with pain often preceding eruption

- ■ Differential Diagnosis
    - Other viral infections
    - Drug allergy

- ■ Treatment
    - Supportive measures with topical lotions and antihistamines; antivirals (acyclovir, valacyclovir, famciclovir) for all adults with varicella
    - Immune globulin or antivirals for exposed susceptible immunosuppressed or pregnant patients
    - Acyclovir early for immunocompromised or pregnant patients, severe disease (eg, pneumonitis, encephalitis), or ophthalmic division of trigeminal nerve involvement with zoster
    - Corticosteroids combined with antiviral agent with rapid taper may diminish postherpetic neuralgia in older patients with zoster

- ■ Pearl

Epidemics are more frequent in winter and spring and in temperate climates.

Reference

Weller TH: Varicella: historical perspective and clinical overview. J Infect Dis 1996;174(Suppl 3):S306. [PMID: 8896536]

Mumps (Epidemic Parotitis)

- **Essentials of Diagnosis**
  - Painful, swollen salivary glands , usually parotid; may be unilateral
  - Incubation period 12–24 days
  - Orchitis or oophoritis, meningoencephalitis, or pancreatitis may occur
  - Cerebrospinal fluid shows lymphocytic pleocytosis in meningo-encephalitis with hypoglycorrhachia
  - Diagnosis confirmed by isolation of virus in saliva or appearance of antibodies after second week

- **Differential Diagnosis**
  - Parotitis or enlarged parotids due to other causes (eg, bacteria, sialolithiasis, cirrhosis, diabetes, starch ingestion, Sjögren's syndrome, sarcoidosis, tumor)
  - Aseptic meningitis, pancreatitis, or orchitis due to other causes

- **Treatment**
  - Immunization is preventive
  - Supportive care with surveillance for complications

- **Pearl**

Mumps is a treatable cause of sterility, associated with high blood FSH and low testosterone levels.

Reference

McQuone SJ: Acute viral and bacterial infections of the salivary glands. Otolaryngol Clin North Am 1999;32:793. [PMID: 10477787]

Viral Encephalitis

- **Essentials of Diagnosis**
  - Most common agents include enterovirus, Epstein-Barr virus, and viruses of herpes simplex, measles, rubella, rubeola, varicella, West Nile fever
  - Fever, malaise, stiff neck, nausea, altered mentation
  - Signs of upper motor neuron lesion: exaggerated deep tendon reflexes, absent superficial reflexes, spastic paralysis
  - Increased cerebrospinal fluid protein with lymphocytic pleocytosis, occasional hypoglycorrhachia
  - Isolation of virus from blood or cerebrospinal fluid; serology positive in paired specimens 3–4 weeks apart
  - Brain imaging shows temporal lobe abnormalities in herpetic encephalitis

- **Differential Diagnosis**
  - Other encephalitides (postvaccination, Reye's syndrome, toxins)
  - Lymphocytic choriomeningitis
  - Primary or secondary neoplasm
  - Bacterial meningitis or brain abscess

- **Treatment**
  - Vigorous supportive measures with attention to elevated central nervous system pressures
  - Mannitol in selected patients
  - Acyclovir for suspected herpes simplex encephalitis; other specific antiviral therapy is under study

- **Pearl**

In patients with suspected encephalitis, acyclovir is given until herpes is excluded.

Reference

Roos KL: Encephalitis. Neurol Clin 1999;17:813. [PMID: 10517930]

Poliomyelitis

- ■ **Essentials of Diagnosis**
  - Enterovirus acquired via fecal-oral route; vast majority of symptomatic cases are not neurologic
  - Muscle weakness, malaise, headache, fever, nausea, abdominal pain, sore throat
  - Signs of lower motor neuron lesions: asymmetric, flaccid paralysis with decreased deep tendon reflexes, muscle atrophy; may include cranial nerve abnormalities (bulbar form)
  - Cerebrospinal fluid lymphocytic pleocytosis with slight elevation of protein
  - Virus recovered from throat washings or stool

- ■ **Differential Diagnosis**
  - Other aseptic meningitides
  - Postinfectious polyneuropathy (Guillain-Barré syndrome)
  - Amyotrophic lateral sclerosis
  - Myopathy

- ■ **Treatment**
  - Vaccination is preventive and has eliminated the disease in the United States
  - Supportive care with particular attention to respiratory function, skin care, and bowel and bladder function

- ■ **Pearl**

Stiff neck after an enteric illness is a potential precursor of neurologic polio.

Reference

Melnick JL: Current status of poliovirus infections. Clin Microbiol Rev 1996;9:293. [PMID: 8809461]

Lymphocytic Choriomeningitis

- ■ Essentials of Diagnosis
  - • History of exposure to mice or hamsters
  - • "Influenza-like" prodrome with fever, chills, headache, malaise, and cough followed by headache, photophobia, or neck pain
  - • Kernig and Brudzinski signs positive
  - • Cerebrospinal fluid with lymphocytic pleocytosis and slight increase in protein
  - • Serology for arenavirus positive 2 weeks after onset of symptoms; virus recovered from blood and cerebrospinal fluid
  - • Illness usually lasts 1–2 weeks

- ■ Differential Diagnosis
  - • Other aseptic meningitides
  - • Bacterial or granulomatous meningitis

- ■ Treatment
  - • Supportive care

- ■ Pearl

One of the few causes of hypoglycorrhachia in a patient who appears to be well.

Reference

Barton LL et al: Lymphocytic choriomeningitis virus: reemerging central nervous system pathogen. Pediatrics 2000;105:E35. [PMID: 10699137]

Dengue (Breakbone Fever, Dandy Fever)

- **Essentials of Diagnosis**
    - A viral (togavirus, flavivirus) illness transmitted by the bite of the *Aedes* mosquito
    - Sudden onset of high fever, chills, severe myalgias, headache, sore throat
    - Biphasic fever curve with initial phase of 3–4 days, short remission, and second phase of 1–2 days
    - Rash is biphasic—first evanescent, followed by maculopapular, scarlatiniform, morbilliform, or petechial changes during remission or second phase of fever; first in the extremities and spreads to torso
    - Dengue hemorrhagic fever is a severe form in which gastrointestinal hemorrhage is prominent and patients often present with shock

- **Differential Diagnosis**
    - Malaria
    - Yellow fever
    - Influenza
    - Typhoid fever
    - Borreliosis
    - Other viral exanthems

- **Treatment**
    - Supportive care
    - Vaccine has been developed but not commercially available

- **Pearl**

Dengue should always be considered in the febrile returned traveler with presumed influenza.

Reference

Rigau-Pérez JG et al: Dengue and dengue haemorrhagic fever. Lancet 1998;352:971. [PMID: 9752834]

Colorado Tick Fever

- ■ Essentials of Diagnosis
  - A self-limited acute viral (coltivirus) infection transmitted by *Dermacentor andersoni* tick bites
  - Onset 3–6 days following bite
  - Abrupt onset of fever, chills, myalgia, headache, photophobia
  - Occasional faint rash
  - Second phase of fever after remission of 2–3 days common
  - Imbedded ticks, especially in children's scalps, may cause paresis

- ■ Differential Diagnosis
  - Borrelliosis
  - Influenza
  - Adult Still's disease
  - Other viral exanthems
  - Guillain-Barré syndrome (if paralysis present)

- ■ Treatment
  - Supportive for uncomplicated cases
  - With paresis, removal of tick results in prompt resolution of symptoms

- ■ Pearl

A tick-borne disease of the western mountains not associated with paralysis.

Reference

Attoui H: Serologic and molecular diagnosis of Colorado tick fever viral infections. Am J Trop Med Hyg 199859:763. [PMID: 9840594]

Rabies

- **Essentials of Diagnosis**
  - A rhabdovirus encephalitis transmitted by infected saliva
  - History of animal bite (bats, bears, skunks, foxes, raccoons; dogs and cats in developing countries)
  - Paresthesias, hydrophobia, rage alternating with calm
  - Convulsions, paralysis, thick tenacious saliva and muscle spasms

- **Differential Diagnosis**
  - Tetanus
  - Encephalitis due to other causes

- **Treatment**
  - Active immunization of household pets and persons at risk (eg, veterinarians)
  - Thorough, repeated washing of bite and scratch wounds
  - Postexposure immunization, both passive and active
  - Observation of healthy biting animals, examination of brains of sick or dead biting animals
  - Treatment is supportive only; disease is almost uniformly fatal

- **Pearl**

Bats are the most common vector for rabies in the United States, and even absent history of a bite, children exposed to bats indoors should be immunized.

Reference

Plotkin SA: Rabies. Clin Infect Dis 1998;59:763. [PMID: 10619725]

Influenza

- **Essentials of Diagnosis**
  - Caused by an orthomyxovirus transmitted via the respiratory route
  - Abrupt onset of fever, headache, chills, malaise, dry cough, coryza, and myalgias; constitutional signs out of proportion to catarrhal symptoms
  - Epidemic outbreaks in fall or winter, with short incubation period
  - Virus isolated from throat washings; serologic tests positive after second week of illness
  - Complications include bacterial sinusitis, otitis media, and pneumonia
  - Myalgias occur early in course, rhabdomyolysis late

- **Differential Diagnosis**
  - Other viral syndromes
  - Primary bacterial pneumonia
  - Meningitis
  - Dengue in returned travelers
  - Rhabdomyolysis of other cause

- **Treatment**
  - Yearly active immunization of persons at high risk (eg, chronic respiratory disease, pregnant women, cardiac disease, health care workers, immunosuppressed); also for all over 50
  - Chemoprophylaxis for epidemic influenza A effective with amantadine; zanamivir and oseltamivir effective against influenza A and B
  - Antivirals reduce duration of symptoms and infectivity if given within 48 hours
  - Avoid salicylates in children because of association with Reye's syndrome

- **Pearl**

Complicating staphylococcal pneumonia is the most common cause of death in epidemics.

Reference

Stamboulian D: Influenza. Infect Dis Clin North Am 2000;14:141. [PMID: 10738677]

Infectious Mononucleosis (Epstein-Barr Virus Infection)

- ## Essentials of Diagnosis
  - An acute viral illness due to EBV, usually occurring up to age 35 but any age possible
  - Transmitted by saliva; incubation period is 5–15 days or longer
  - Fever, severe sore throat, striking malaise, lymphadenopathy
  - Maculopapular rash, splenomegaly common
  - Leukocytosis and lymphocytosis with atypical large lymphocytes by smear; positive heterophil agglutination test (Monospot) by fourth week of illness; false-positive rapid plasma reagin test (RPR) in 10%
  - Clinical picture much less typical in older patients
  - Complications include splenic rupture, hepatitis, myocarditis, thrombocytopenia, and encephalitis

- ## Differential Diagnosis
  - Other causes of pharyngitis
  - Other causes of hepatitis
  - Toxoplasmosis
  - Rubella
  - Acute HIV, CMV, or rubella infections
  - Acute leukemia or lymphoma
  - Kawasaki syndrome
  - Hypersensitivity reaction due to carbamazepine

- ## Treatment
  - Supportive care only; fever usually disappears in 10 days, lymphadenopathy and splenomegaly in 4 weeks
  - Ampicillin apt to cause rash
  - Avoid vigorous abdominal activity or exercise

- ## Pearl

Mononucleosis is the most common cause of the otherwise rare anti-i hemolytic anemia.

Reference

Cohen JI: Epstein-Barr virus infection. N Engl J Med 2000;343:481. [PMID: 10944566]

RICKETTSIAL INFECTIONS

Rocky Mountain Spotted Fever *(Rickettsia rickettsii)*

- **Essentials of Diagnosis**
  - Exposure to tick bite in endemic area
  - Influenzal prodrome followed by chills, fever, severe headache, myalgias, occasionally delirium and coma
  - Red macular rash with onset between second and sixth days of fever; first on extremities, then centrally, may become petechial or purpuric
  - Leukocytosis, proteinuria, hematuria
  - Serologic tests positive by second week of illness, but diagnosis may be made earlier by skin biopsy with immunologic staining

- **Differential Diagnosis**
  - Meningococcemia
  - Endocarditis
  - Gonococcemia
  - Ehrlichiosis
  - Measles

- **Treatment**
  - Tetracyclines or chloramphenicol
  - Vaccine in development

- **Pearl**

Despite the name, Rocky Mountain spotted fever is far more common in the southeastern United States.

Reference

Thorner AR et al: Rocky Mountain spotted fever. Clin Infect Dis 1998;27:1353. [PMID: 9868640]

Q Fever *(Coxiella burnetii)*

- **Essentials of Diagnosis**
  - Infection following exposure to sheep, goats, cattle, or fowl
  - Acute or chronic febrile illness with severe headache, cough, and abdominal discomfort
  - Pulmonary infiltrates by chest x-ray; leukopenia
  - Serologic confirmation by third to fourth weeks of illness
  - Granulomatous hepatitis and culture-negative endocarditis in occasional cases

- **Differential Diagnosis**
  - Atypical pneumonia
  - Granulomatous hepatitis due to other cause
  - Brucellosis
  - Other causes of culture-negative endocarditis

- **Treatment**
  - Tetracyclines suppressive but not always curative, especially with endocarditis; surgery may be necessary
  - Vaccine being developed

- **Pearl**

Some recent outbreaks are laboratory-acquired where sheep are used in cardiovascular research.

Reference

Maurin M: Q fever. Clin Microbiol Rev 1999;12:518. [PMID: 10515901]

BACTERIAL INFECTIONS

Streptococcal Pharyngitis

- ■ Essentials of Diagnosis
  - • Abrupt onset of sore throat, fever, malaise, nausea, headache
  - • Pharynx erythematous and edematous with exudate; cervical adenopathy
  - • Strawberry tongue
  - • Throat culture or rapid antigen detection confirmatory
  - • If erythrotoxin (scarlet fever) is produced, scarlatiniform rash red and papular with petechiae and fine desquamation; prominent in axilla, groin, behind knees
  - • Glomerulonephritis, rheumatic fever may complicate

- ■ Differential Diagnosis
  - • Viral pharyngitis
  - • Mononucleosis
  - • Diphtheria
  - • With rash: meningococcemia, toxic shock syndrome, drug reaction, viral exanthem

- ■ Treatment
  - • For two or more clinical criteria (cervical adenopathy, fever, exudate, and absence of rhinorrhea): empiric penicillin
  - • If equivocal, await culture or antigen confirmation
  - • If history of rheumatic fever, continuous antibiotic prophylaxis for 5 years

- ■ Pearl

Despite the clinical severity of pharyngeal diphtheria, fever is higher in strep throat.

Reference

Bisno AL: Acute pharyngitis. N Engl J Med 2001;344:205. [PMID: 11172144]

Streptococcal Skin Infection

- **Essentials of Diagnosis**
  - Erysipelas: rapidly spreading cutaneous erythema and edema with sharp borders
  - Impetigo: rapidly spreading erythema with vesicular or denuded areas and salmon-colored crust
  - Culture of wound or blood grows group A beta hemolytic streptococci
  - Complication: glomerulonephritis

- **Differential Diagnosis**
  - Other causes of infectious cellulitis (eg, staphylococcal, *E coli*)
  - Toxic shock syndrome
  - Beriberi (in setting of thiamin deficiency)

- **Treatment**
  - Penicillin for culture-proved streptococcal infection
  - Staphylococcal coverage (dicloxacillin) for empiric therapy or uncertain diagnosis

- **Pearl**

Group A cutaneous infections can result in glomerulonephritis but not rheumatic fever.

Reference

Bisno AL et al: Streptococcal infections of skin and soft tissues. N Engl J Med 1996;334:240. [PMID: 8532002]

Pneumococcal Infections

- **Essentials of Diagnosis**
  - Pneumonia characterized by initial chill, severe pleuritis, fever without diurnal variation; signs of consolidation and lobar infiltrate on x-ray ensue rapidly
  - Leukocytosis, hyperbilirubinemia
  - Gram-positive diplococci on Gram-stained smear of sputum; lancet-shaped only on stained culture colonies
  - Meningitis: rapid onset of fever, altered mental status and headache; cerebrospinal fluid polymorphonuclear leukocytosis with elevated protein and decreased glucose; Gram-stained smear of fluid positive in 90% of cases
  - Endocarditis, empyema, pericarditis, and arthritis may also complicate, with empyema most common
  - Predisposition to bacteremia in children under 24 months of age or in asplenic or immunocompromised adults (eg, AIDS, elderly)

- **Differential Diagnosis**
  - Pneumonia, meningitis of other cause
  - Pulmonary embolism
  - Myocardial infarction
  - Acute exacerbation of chronic bronchitis
  - Acute bronchitis
  - Gram-negative septicemia

- **Treatment**
  - Blood culture prior to antibiotics
  - Third-generation cephalosporin for severe disease; add empiric vancomycin for meningitis pending culture results
  - Adults over 50 with any serious medical illness, patients with sickle cell disease, and asplenic patients should receive pneumococcal vaccine
  - Penicillin unreliable pending results of susceptibility testing

- **Pearl**

Rigors after the first day of infection in a patient with pneumonia suggest a different etiology or an extrapulmonary complication.

Reference

Harwell JI: The drug-resistant pneumococcus: clinical relevance, therapy, and prevention. Chest 2000;117:530. [PMID: 10669700]

Staphylococcal Soft Tissue or Skin Infections

- **Essentials of Diagnosis**
  - Painful, pruritic erythematous rash with golden crusts or discharge
  - Folliculitis, furunculosis, carbuncle, abscess, and cellulitis all seen
  - Culture of wound or abscess is diagnostic; Gram-stained smear positive for large gram-positive cocci *(Staphylococcus aureus)* in clusters

- **Differential Diagnosis**
  - Streptococcal skin infections

- **Treatment**
  - Penicillinase-resistant penicillin or cephalosporin; erythromycin may also be effective in some cases
  - Drainage of abscess
  - Persistence of blood culture positivity suggests endocarditis or osteomyelitis

- **Pearl**

Gram stain of material infected with staphylococci shows marked avidity of the organisms for the stain; they also thrive intracellularly—in contrast to pneumococci.

Reference

Thestrup-Pedersen K: Bacteria and the skin: clinical practice and therapy update. Br J Dermatol 1998;139(Suppl)53:1. [PMID: 9990405]

Staphylococcus aureus-Associated Toxic Shock Syndrome

- **Essentials of Diagnosis**
  - Abrupt onset of fever, vomiting, diarrhea, sore throat, headache, myalgia
  - Toxic appearance, with tachycardia and hypotension
  - Diffuse maculopapular erythematous rash with desquamation on the palms and soles; nonpurulent conjunctivitis
  - Association with tampon use; culture of nasopharynx, vagina, rectum, and wounds may yield staphylococci, but blood cultures usually negative
  - Usually caused by toxic shock syndrome toxin-1 (TSST-1)

- **Differential Diagnosis**
  - Streptococcal infection, particularly scarlet fever
  - Gram-negative sepsis
  - Rickettsial disease, especially Rocky Mountain spotted fever

- **Treatment**
  - Aggressive supportive care (eg, fluids, vasopressor medication, monitoring)
  - Antistaphylococcal antibiotics to eliminate source

- **Pearl**

Consider chronic staphylococcal osteomyelitis as a potential cause of toxic shock syndrome.

Reference

Bannan J et al: Structure and function of streptococcal and staphylococcal super-antigens in septic shock. Infect Dis Clinics North Am 1999;13:387. [PMID: 10340173]

Clostridial Myonecrosis (Gas Gangrene)

- **Essentials of Diagnosis**
  - Sudden onset of pain, swelling in an area of wound contamination
  - Severe systemic toxicity and rapid progression of involved tissue
  - Brown or blood-tinged watery exudate with surrounding skin discoloration
  - Gas in tissue by palpated or auscultated crepitus or x-ray
  - *Clostridium perfringens* in anaerobic culture or smear of exudate is the classic—but not the only—cause

- **Differential Diagnosis**
  - Other gas-forming infections (mixed aerobic and anaerobic enteric organisms)
  - Cellulitis due to staphylococcal or streptococcal infection

- **Treatment**
  - Immediate surgical debridement and exposure of infected areas
  - Hyperbaric oxygen of uncertain benefit
  - Intravenous penicillin with clindamycin
  - Tetanus prophylaxis

- **Pearl**

In a patient severely symptomatic and extremely toxic with the clinical picture noted, a relatively low-grade fever is virtually diagnostic of gas gangrene.

Reference

Chapnick EK: Necrotizing soft-tissue infections. Infect Dis Clinics North Am 1996;10:835.[PMID: 8958171])

Tetanus *(Clostridium tetani)*

- ■ Essentials of Diagnosis
  - History of nondebrided wound or contamination may or may not be obtained
  - Jaw stiffness followed by spasms (trismus)
  - Stiffness of neck or other muscles, dysphagia, irritability, hyper-reflexia; late, painful convulsions precipitated by minimal stimuli; fever is low-grade

- ■ Differential Diagnosis
  - Infectious meningitis
  - Rabies
  - Strychnine poisoning
  - Malignant neuroleptic syndrome
  - Hypocalcemia

- ■ Treatment
  - Active immunization preventive
  - Passive immunization with tetanus immune globulin and concurrent active immunization for all suspected cases
  - Chlorpromazine or diazepam for spasms or convulsions, with additional sedation by barbiturates as necessary
  - Vigorous supportive care with particular attention to airway and laryngospasm
  - Penicillin

- ■ Pearl
Tetanus should be high on the list in "skin-popping" illicit drug users with increased muscle tone.

Reference

Ernst ME et al: Tetanus: pathophysiology and management. Ann Pharmacother 1997;31:1507. [PMID: 9416389]

Botulism *(Clostridium botulinum)*

- **Essentials of Diagnosis**
  - Sudden onset of cranial nerve paralysis, diplopia, dry mouth, dysphagia, dysphonia, and progressive muscle weakness
  - Fixed and dilated pupils in 50%
  - In infants: irritability, weakness, and hypotonicity
  - History of recent ingestion of home-canned, smoked, or vacuum-packed foods
  - Demonstration of toxin in serum or food

- **Differential Diagnosis**
  - Bulbar poliomyelitis
  - Myasthenia gravis
  - Posterior cerebral circulation ischemia
  - Tick paralysis
  - Guillain-Barré syndrome or variant
  - Inorganic phosphorus poisoning

- **Treatment**
  - Removal of unabsorbed toxin from gut
  - Specific antitoxin (CDC Poison Control Hotline 800-292-6678)
  - Vigilant support, including attention to respiratory function
  - Penicillin

- **Pearl**

In intravenous drug users with cranial nerve findings, this picture is classic for wound botulism caused by black tar heroin.

Reference

Shapiro RL et al: Botulism in the United States: a clinical and epidemiologic review. Ann Intern Med 1998;129:221. [PMID: 9696731]

Anthrax *(Bacillus anthracis)*

- ### Essentials of Diagnosis
  - History of industrial or agricultural exposure (farmer, veterinarian, tannery or wool worker); a potential agent in biological warfare
  - Persistent necrotic ulcer on exposed surface
  - Regional adenopathy, fever, malaise, headache, nausea and vomiting
  - Inhalation of spores causes severe tracheobronchitis and pneumonia with dyspnea and cough
  - Hematologic spread with profound toxic and cardiovascular collapse may complicate either cutaneous or pulmonary form
  - Confirmation of diagnosis by culture or specific fluorescent antibody test, but clinical picture highly suggestive

- ### Differential Diagnosis
  - Skin lesions: staphylococcal or streptococcal infection
  - Pulmonary disease: tuberculosis, fungal infection, sarcoidosis, lymphoma with mediastinal adenopathy, plague

- ### Treatment
  - Therapy for post exposure prophylaxis is oral doxycyline or oral ciprofloxacin
  - Optimal therapy for confirmed disease due to a susceptible strain is oral amoxacillin or oral doxycyline for 60 days
  - Mortality rate is high despite proper therapy, especially in pulmonary disease

- ### Pearl
  A rare infectious disease in which the patient "dies sterile"—all organisms are eliminated, but the toxicity is lethal.

Reference

Swartz MN: Recognition and management of anthrax—an update. N Engl J Med 2001;345:1626. [PMID: 11757510]

Diphtheria *(Corynebacterium diphtheriae)*

- **Essentials of Diagnosis**
  - An acute infection spread by respiratory secretions
  - Sore throat, rhinorrhea, hoarseness, malaise, relatively unimpressive fever (usually < 37.8 °C)
  - Tenacious gray membrane at portal of entry
  - Toxin-induced myocarditis and neuropathy may complicate, due to an exotoxin
  - Smear and culture confirm diagnosis

- **Differential Diagnosis**
  - Other causes of pharyngitis (streptococcal, infectious mononucleosis, adenovirus)
  - Necrotizing gingivostomatitis
  - Candidiasis
  - Myocarditis from other causes
  - Myasthenia gravis
  - Botulism

- **Treatment**
  - Active immunization (usually as DTP) is preventive
  - Diphtheria antitoxin
  - Penicillin or erythromycin
  - Corticosteroids in selected patients with severe laryngeal involvement, myocarditis, or neuropathy
  - Exposures of susceptible individuals call for booster toxoid, active immunization, antibiotics, and daily throat inspections

- **Pearl**

Hypesthetic shallow skin ulcers in homeless patients suggest the diagnosis of cutaneous diphtheria.

Reference

Galazka A: The changing epidemiology of diphtheria in the vaccine era. J Infect Dis 2000;181(Suppl 1):S2. [PMID: 10657184]

Pertussis *(Bordetella pertussis)*

- **Essentials of Diagnosis**
    - An acute infection of the respiratory tract spread by respiratory droplets
    - History of declined DTP vaccination
    - Two-week prodromal catarrhal stage of malaise, cough, coryza, and anorexia; seen predominantly in infants under age 2
    - Paroxysmal cough ending in high-pitched inspiratory "whoop" (whooping cough)
    - Absolute lymphocytosis with extremely high white counts possible
    - Culture confirms diagnosis

- **Differential Diagnosis**
    - Viral pneumonia
    - Foreign body aspiration
    - Acute bronchitis
    - Acute leukemia (when leukocytosis marked)

- **Treatment**
    - Active immunization preventive (as part of DTP)
    - Erythromycin with immune globulin in selected patients
    - Treat secondary pneumonia and other complications

- **Pearl**

The cause of the highest benign white counts in clinical medicine.

Reference

Orenstein WA: Pertussis in adults: epidemiology, signs, symptoms, and implications for vaccination. Clin Infect Dis 1999;28(Suppl 2):S147. [PMID: 10447034]

Meningococcal Meningitis *(Neisseria meningitidis)*

- **Essentials of Diagnosis**
  - Fever, headache, vomiting, confusion, delirium, or seizures; typically epidemic in young adults; onset may be astonishingly abrupt
  - Petechial or ecchymotic rash of skin and mucous membranes
  - May have positive Kernig and Brudzinski signs
  - Purulent spinal fluid with gram-negative intracellular and extracellular cocci by Gram-stained smear
  - Culture of cerebrospinal fluid, blood, or petechial aspirate confirms diagnosis
  - Disseminated intravascular coagulation and shock may complicate

- **Differential Diagnosis**
  - Meningitis due to other causes
  - Petechial rash due to rickettsial, viral, or other bacterial infection
  - Idiopathic thrombocytopenic purpura

- **Treatment**
  - Active immunization available for selected susceptible groups (military recruits, college dormitory residents)
  - Penicillin, ceftriaxone, or chloramphenicol
  - Mannitol and corticosteroids for elevated intracranial pressure
  - Ciprofloxacin (single dose) or rifampin (2 days) therapy for intimate exposures

- **Pearl**

The most common bacterial meningitis in which organisms are not seen on cerebrospinal fluid Gram stain (50% of cases).

Reference

Salzman MB et al: Meningococcemia. Infect Dis Clin North Am 1996; 10:709. [PMID: 8958165]

Legionnaire's Disease

- **Essentials of Diagnosis**
  - Caused by *Legionella pneumophila* and a common cause of community-acquired pneumonia in some areas
  - Seen in patients who are immunocompromised or have chronic lung disease
  - Malaise, dry cough, fever, headache, pleuritic chest pain, toxic appearance, purulent sputum
  - Chest x-ray with patchy infiltrates often unimpressive early; subsequent development of effusion or multiple lobar involvement common
  - Purulent sputum without organisms seen by Gram stain; diagnosis confirmed by culture or special silver stains or direct fluorescent antibodies, urinary antigen

- **Differential Diagnosis**
  - Other infectious pneumonias
  - Pulmonary embolism
  - Pleurodynia
  - Myocardial infarction

- **Treatment**
  - Erythromycin with rifampin added in severe disease or immunocompromised patients
  - Newer macrolides and quinolones are also effective (but expensive) alternatives

- **Pearl**

The early assertion that hyponatremia and gastrointestinal symptoms are diagnostic is erroneous—many atypical pneumonias have the same problem.

Reference

Breiman RF et al: Legionnaires' disease: clinical, epidemiological, and public health perspectives. Semin Respir Infect 1998;13:84. [PMID: 9643385]

Enteric Fever (Typhoid Fever)

■ Essentials of Diagnosis

- Caused by several salmonella species; in "typhoid fever," serotype *Salmonella typhi* is causative and accompanied by bacteremia
- Transmitted by contaminated food or drink; incubation period is 5–14 days
- Gradual onset of malaise, headache, sore throat, cough, followed by diarrhea or, with *S typhi,* constipation; stepladder rise of fever to maximum of 40 °C over 7–10 days, then slow return to normal with little diurnal variation
- Rose spots, relative bradycardia, splenomegaly, abdominal distention and tenderness
- Leukopenia; blood, stool, and urine cultures positive for *S typhi* (group D) or other salmonellae

■ Differential Diagnosis

- Brucellosis
- Tuberculosis
- Infectious endocarditis
- Q fever and other rickettsial infections
- Yersiniosis
- Hepatitis
- Lymphoma
- Adult Still's disease

■ Treatment

- Active immunization helpful during epidemics for travelers to endemic areas or for household contacts of persons with the disease
- Ciprofloxacin or second-generation cephalosporin pending susceptibility results
- Cholecystectomy may be necessary for relapsed cases
- Complications in one-third of untreated patients include intestinal hemorrhage or perforation, cholecystitis, nephritis, and meningitis

■ Pearl

The development of tachycardia and leukocytosis in a patient with typhoid fever suggests ileal perforation until proved otherwise.

Reference

Magill AJ: Fever in the returned traveler. Infect Dis Clin North Am 1998;12:445. [PMID: 9658253]

Salmonella Gastroenteritis
(Various Salmonella Species)

- **Essentials of Diagnosis**
  - The most common form of salmonellosis
  - Nausea, headache, meningismus, fever, high-volume diarrhea, usually without blood, and abdominal pain 8–48 hours after ingestion of contaminated food or liquid
  - Positive fecal leukocytes
  - Culture of organism from stool; bacteremia less common

- **Differential Diagnosis**
  - Viral gastroenteritis, especially enterovirus
  - Dysenteric illness (shigella, campylobacter, amebic)
  - Enterotoxigenic *E coli* infection
  - Inflammatory bowel disease

- **Treatment**
  - Rehydration and potassium repletion
  - Antibiotics (ciprofloxacin or ceftriaxone) essential in those with sickle cell anemia or immunosuppression
  - In others, antimicrobials reduce symptoms by 1–2 days

- **Pearl**

All patients continuously bacteremic with salmonella should be suspected of having a mycotic aortic aneurysm.

Reference

Slutsker L et al: Foodborne diseases. Emerging pathogens and trends. Infect Dis Clin North Am 1998;12:199. [PMID: 9494839]

Bacillary Dysentery (Shigellosis)

- **Essentials of Diagnosis**
  - Fever, malaise, toxicity, diarrhea (typically bloody), cramping
  - Positive fecal leukocytes; organism isolated in stool; in immuno-suppressed patients, blood culture often positive—not so in others

- **Differential Diagnosis**
  - Campylobacter and salmonella infection
  - Amebiasis
  - Ulcerative colitis
  - Viral gastroenteritis
  - Food poisoning

- **Treatment**
  - Supportive care
  - Antibiotics determined based on sensitivies of local shigella species; trimethoprim-sulfamethoxazole and ciprofloxacin are the usual drugs of choice

- **Pearl**

The first organism associated with reactive arthritis.

Reference

Edwards BH: Salmonella and Shigella species. Clin Lab Med 1999;19:469. [PMID: 10549421]

Campylobacter Enteritis *(Campylobacter jejuni)*

- ■ Essentials of Diagnosis
  - Outbreaks associated with consumption of raw milk
  - Fever, vomiting, abdominal pain, bloody diarrhea
  - Fecal leukocytes present; presumptive diagnosis by darkfield or phase contrast microscopy of stool wet mount
  - Definitive diagnosis by stool culture

- ■ Differential Diagnosis
  - Shigellosis
  - Salmonellosis
  - Viral gastroenteritis
  - Amebic dysentery
  - Food poisoning
  - Ulcerative colitis

- ■ Treatment
  - Erythromycin or ciprofloxacin will shorten the duration of illness by approximately 1 day
  - Disease is self-limited but can be severe

- ■ Pearl

The most commonly isolated pathogen in dysentery.

Reference

Fields PI et al: *Campylobacter jejuni.* Clin Lab Med 1999;19:489. [PMID: 10549422]

Cholera *(Vibrio cholerae)*

- ■ Essentials of Diagnosis
    - • Acute diarrheal illness leading to profound hypovolemia and death if not addressed promptly
    - • Occurs in epidemics under conditions of crowding and famine; acquired via ingestion of contaminated food or water
    - • Sudden onset of frequent, high-volume diarrhea
    - • Liquid ("rice water") stool is gray, turbid
    - • Rapid development of hypotension, marked dehydration, acidosis, and hypokalemia
    - • History of travel to endemic area or contact with infected person
    - • Positive stool culture confirmatory; serologic testing useful in first to second weeks

- ■ Differential Diagnosis
    - • Other small intestinal diarrheal illness (eg, salmonellosis, enterotoxigenic *E coli*)
    - • Viral gastroenteritis
    - • VIP-producing pancreatic tumor (pancreatic cholera)

- ■ Treatment
    - • Vaccination preventive for travelers to endemic areas but is rarely indicated (www.cdc.gov/travel/)
    - • Rapid replacement of fluid and electrolytes, especially potassium
    - • Cola beverages inhibit cAMP, reduce diarrhea, in areas where standard volume repletion is unavailable
    - • Tetracycline and many other antibiotics may shorten duration of vibrio excretion

- ■ Pearl

In cholera, markedly elevated hematocrits from severe dehydration may lead to hyperviscosity of the circulation.

Reference

Kaper JB et al: Cholera. Clin Microbiol Rev 1995;8:48. [PMID: 7704895]

Brucellosis (Brucella Species)

- **Essentials of Diagnosis**
  - Invariable history of animal exposure (veterinarian, slaughterhouse) or ingestion of unpasteurized milk or cheese
  - Vectors are cattle, hogs, and goats
  - Insidious onset of fever, diaphoresis, anorexia, fatigue, headache, back pain
  - Cervical and axillary lymphadenopathy, hepatosplenomegaly
  - Lymphocytosis with normal total white cell count; positive blood, cerebrospinal fluid, or bone marrow culture after days to weeks; serologic tests positive in second week of illness
  - Osteomyelitis, epididymitis, meningitis, and endocarditis may complicate

- **Differential Diagnosis**
  - Lymphoma
  - Infective endocarditis
  - Tuberculosis
  - Q fever
  - Typhoid fever
  - Tularemia
  - Malaria
  - Other causes of osteomyelitis

- **Treatment**
  - Rifampin and doxycycline required for 21days

- **Pearl**

In clinically typical brucellosis, dilution of previously negative serum sample is ordered to exclude a prozone effect; drastically high titers are falsely negative unless diluted.

Reference

Corbel MJ: Brucellosis: an overview. Emerg Infect Dis 1997;3:213. [PMID: 9204307]

Tularemia *(Francisella tularensis)*

- ■ Essentials of Diagnosis
  - • History of contact with rabbits, other rodents, and biting arthropods (eg, ticks) in endemic areas; incubation period 2–10 days
  - • Fever, headache, nausea begin suddenly
  - • Papule progressing to ulcer at site of inoculation; the conjunctiva may be the site in occasional patients
  - • Prominent, tender regional lymphadenopathy, splenomegaly
  - • Diagnosis confirmed by culture of ulcerated lesion, lymph node aspirate, or blood; serologic confirmation positive after second week of illness
  - • Though primarily cutaneous, ocular, glandular, or typhoidal; only the very rare pneumonic form is transmissible between humans

- ■ Differential Diagnosis
  - • Cat-scratch disease
  - • Infectious mononucleosis
  - • Plague
  - • Typhoid fever
  - • Lymphoma
  - • Various rickettsial infections
  - • Meningococcemia

- ■ Treatment
  - • Combination antibiotics required; streptomycin and tetracycline are usually used

- ■ Pearl

Although named for the index case in Tulare County in California, the most prominent epidemic was on Martha's Vineyard in Massachusetts; it is rarely encountered in Tulare County.

Reference

Gill V et al: Tularemia pneumonia. Semin Respir Infect 1997;12:61. [PMID: 9097380]

Plague *(Yersinia pestis)*

- ■ Essentials of Diagnosis
  - History of exposure to rodents in endemic area of southwestern United States; by bites of fleas or contact with infected rodents; human-to-human transmission with pneumonic plague only
  - Sudden onset of high fever, severe malaise, myalgias; stunning systemic toxicity
  - Regional lymphangitis and lymphadenitis with suppuration of nodes
  - Bacteremia, pneumonitis, or meningitis complicate
  - Positive smear and culture from aspirate or blood; striking leukopenia with marked left shift

- ■ Differential Diagnosis
  - Tularemia
  - Lymphadenitis with bacterial disease of extremity
  - Lymphogranuloma venereum
  - Other bacterial pneumonia or meningitis
  - Typhoid fever
  - Various rickettsial diseases

- ■ Treatment
  - Combination antibiotics required (eg, streptomycin plus tetracycline)
  - Tetracycline prophylaxis for persons exposed to patients with pneumonic plague
  - Strict isolation of pneumonic disease patients

- ■ Pearl

Plague should be treated empirically in any case of meningitis encountered in the arid southwestern United States.

Reference

Titball RW et al: Plague. Br Med Bull 1998, 54:625. [PMID: 10326289] (UI: 99258139)

Gonorrhea *(Neisseria gonorrhoeae)*

- Essentials of Diagnosis
  - A common communicable venereal disease; incubation period is 2–8 days
  - Purulent profuse urethral discharge (men); vaginal discharge rare (women); may be asymptomatic in both sexes
  - Disseminated disease causes intermittent fever, skin lesions (few in number and peripherally located), tenosynovitis in numerous joints, and usually monarticular arthritis involving the knee, ankle, or wrist
  - Conjunctivitis, pharyngitis, proctitis, endocarditis, meningitis also occur
  - Gram-negative intracellular diplococci on urethral smear or culture from cervix, rectum, or pharynx; molecular testing of first 10 mL of urine superior to cervical or urethral cultures
  - Synovial fluid cultures seldom positive

- Differential Diagnosis
  - Cervicitis, vaginitis, or urethritis due to other causes
  - Other causes of pelvic inflammatory disease
  - Reactive arthritis
  - Meningococcemia

- Treatment
  - Rapid plasma reagin (RPR) obtained in all, HIV in selected cases
  - Ceftriaxone intramuscularly for suspected cases; treat all sexual partners
  - Oral antibiotics for concurrent chlamydial infection also recommended
  - Intravenous antibiotics required for salpingitis, prostatitis, arthritis, or endocarditis

- Pearl

Gonococcal endocarditis is one of medicine's few causes of a biquotidian fever spike.

Reference

Cohen MS et al: Human experimentation with *Neisseria gonorrhoeae:* progress and goals. J Infect Dis 1999;179(Suppl 2):S375. [PMID: 10081510]

Chancroid *(Haemophilus ducreyi)*

- **Essentials of Diagnosis**
  - A sexually transmitted disease with an incubation period of 3–5 days
  - Painful, tender genital ulcer
  - Inguinal adenitis with erythema or fluctuance and multiple genital ulcers often develop
  - Balanitis, phimosis frequent complications
  - Women have no external signs of infection

- **Differential Diagnosis**
  - Behçet's syndrome
  - Syphilis
  - Pyogenic infection of lower extremity with regional lymphadenitis
  - Genital ulcers of other cause

- **Treatment**
  - Appropriate antibiotic (azithromycin, ceftriaxone, erythromycin, or ciprofloxacin)
  - Rapid plasma reagin (RPR) for all, HIV when appropriate

- **Pearl**

Tender inguinal lymphadenopathy in overweight patients may not be nodes; an incarcerated femoral hernia may be the answer.

Reference

Eichmann A: Chancroid. Curr Probl Dermatol 1996;24:20. [PMID: 8743249]

Granuloma Inguinale
(Calymmatobacterium granulomatis)

- **Essentials of Diagnosis**
  - A chronic relapsing granulomatous anogenital infection; incubation period is 1–12 weeks
  - Ulcerative lesions on the skin or mucous membranes of the genitalia or perianal area
  - Donovan bodies revealed by Wright's or Giemsa's stain of ulcer scrapings

- **Differential Diagnosis**
  - Venereal ulcers of other cause
  - Syphilis
  - Herpes simplex
  - Reactive arthritis
  - Behçet's disease

- **Treatment**
  - Appropriate antibiotic (erythromycin or tetracycline) for at least 21 days
  - Surveillance and counseling for other STDs (eg, syphilis, gonorrhea, HIV)

- **Pearl**

The most indolent of the major venereal diseases.

Reference

Hart G: Donovanosis. Clin Infect Dis 1997;25:24. [PMID: 9243028]

Cat-Scratch Disease *(Bartonella henselae)*

- ■ Essentials of Diagnosis
  - History of cat scratch or contact with cats; may be forgotten by patient
  - Primary lesion (papule, pustule, conjunctivitis) at site of inoculation in one-third of cases
  - One to 3 weeks after scratch, fever, malaise, and headache accompanied by regional lymphadenopathy
  - Sterile pus from node aspirate
  - Biopsy consistent with cat-scratch disease with a necrotizing lymphadenitis; positive skin test; positive serology for bacteria
  - Bacillary angiomatosis and peliosis hepatis in immunosuppressed patients

- ■ Differential Diagnosis
  - Lymphadenitis due to other bacterial infections
  - Lymphoma
  - Tuberculosis
  - Toxoplasmosis
  - Kikuchi's disease

- ■ Treatment
  - Nonspecific; exclusion of similar diseases most important
  - Isoniazid, rifampin, or erythromycin in immunocompromised patients

- ■ Pearl

In a patient with isolated but bilateral axillary adenopathy and fever, go back and take a pet history: this is a rare distribution for lymphoma.

Reference

Spach DH et al: Bartonella-associated infections. Infect Dis Clin North Am 1998;12:137. [PMID: 9494835]

Actinomycosis

- **Essentials of Diagnosis**
  - Due to anaerobic gram-positive rod (actinomyces species) normally part of the mouth flora; becomes pathogenic when introduced into traumatized tissue
  - Chronic suppurative lesion of the skin (cervicofacial in 60%) with sinus tract formation; thoracic or abdominal abscesses seen; pelvic disease associated with intrauterine devices
  - Accelerated sedimentation rate; anemia, thrombocytosis
  - Isolation of actinomyces species or sulfur granule from pus by anaerobic culture
  - Sulfur granules show gram-positive hyphae on smear

- **Differential Diagnosis**
  - Lung cancer
  - Other causes of cervical adenitis
  - Scrofula
  - Nocardiosis
  - Crohn's disease
  - Pelvic inflammatory disease of other cause

- **Treatment**
  - Long-term penicillin
  - Surgical drainage necessary in selected cases

- **Pearl**

Poor dental hygiene in the face of the clinical scenario noted obligates consideration of actinomycosis.

Reference

Smego RA Jr et al: Actinomycosis. Clin Infect Dis 1998;26:1255. [PMID: 9686342]

Nocardiosis

- **Essentials of Diagnosis**
  - *Nocardia asteroides* and *Nocardia brasiliensis* are aerobic soil bacteria causing pulmonary and systemic disease
  - Malaise, weight loss, fever, night sweats, cough
  - Pulmonary consolidation or thin-walled abscess; invasion through chest wall possible
  - Lobar infiltrates, air-fluid level, effusion by chest x-ray
  - Delicate branching, gram-positive filaments by Gram stain, weakly positive acid-fast staining; culture identifies specifically
  - Disseminated form may occur with abscess in any organ; brain, subcutaneous nodules most frequent
  - Alveolar proteinosis, corticosteroid use, immunodeficiency predispose to infection
  - The above are all due to *N asteroides; N brasiliensis* causes lymphangitis after skin inoculation and is common among gardeners

- **Differential Diagnosis**
  - Actinomycosis
  - Tuberculosis or atypical mycobacterial infections
  - Other causes of pyogenic lung abscess
  - Lymphoma
  - Coccidioidomycosis
  - Histoplasmosis
  - Herpetic whitlow
  - Bacterial lymphangitis *(N brasiliensis)*

- **Treatment**
  - Parenteral and then oral trimethoprim-sulfamethoxazole for many months
  - Surgical drainage and resection may be needed

- **Pearl**

Lymphangitis unresponsive to beta-lactams, especially in a person with soil exposure, suggests N brasiliensis *infection—but also herpetic whitlow.*

Reference

Boiron P et al: Nocardia, nocardiosis and mycetoma. Med Mycol 1998,36(Suppl 1):26. [PMID: 9988489]

Tuberculous Meningitis *(Mycobacterium tuberculosis)*

- **Essentials of Diagnosis**
    - Insidious onset of listlessness, irritability, headaches
    - Meningeal signs, cranial nerve palsies
    - Tuberculous focus evident elsewhere in half
    - Cerebrospinal fluid with lymphocytic pleocytosis, low glucose, and high protein; culture positive for acid-fast bacilli in many but not all
    - Chest x-ray commonly reveals abnormalities compatible with pulmonary tuberculosis

- **Differential Diagnosis**
    - Chronic lymphocytic meningitis due to fungi, brucellosis, leptospirosis, HIV infection, neurocysticercosis
    - Carcinomatous meningitis
    - Unsuspected head trauma with subdural hematoma
    - Drug overdose
    - Psychiatric disorder
    - Sarcoidosis

- **Treatment**
    - Empiric antituberculous therapy essential in proper clinical setting
    - Concomitant corticosteroids reduce long-term complications

- **Pearl**

Striking hypoglycorrhachia in lymphocytic meningitis means tuberculous meningitis until disproved; acellular hypoglycorrhachia should be assumed to be hypoglycemia until proved otherwise by blood glucose.

Reference

Thwaites G et al: Tuberculous meningitis. J Neurol Neurosurg Psychiatry 2000;68:289. [PMID: 10675209]

Leprosy *(Mycobacterium leprae)*

- **Essentials of Diagnosis**
  - A chronic infection due to *M leprae*
  - Pale, anesthetic macular (tuberculoid) or infiltrative erythematous (lepromatous) skin lesions
  - Superficial nerve thickening with associated sensory changes; progression slow and symmetric (lepromatous) or sudden and asymmetric (tuberculoid)
  - Skin test negative (lepromatous) or positive (tuberculoid)
  - History of residence in endemic area during childhood; mode of transmission probably is respiratory
  - Acid-fast bacilli in skin lesions or nasal scrapings; characteristic histologic nerve biopsy
  - Lepromatous type occurs in patients with defective cellular immunity, organisms numerous in tissue specimens; bacilli sparse in tuberculoid disease

- **Differential Diagnosis**
  - Lupus erythematosus
  - Sarcoidosis
  - Syphilis
  - Erythema nodosum
  - Erythema multiforme
  - Vitiligo
  - Neuropathy due to other causes, particularly amyloidosis
  - Cutaneous tuberculosis
  - Scleroderma
  - Syringomyelia

- **Treatment**
  - Combination therapy for months or years, including dapsone, rifampin, and clofazimine

- **Pearl**

  M leprae *can be grown experimentally only in the armadillo foot pad.*

Reference

Haimanot RT et al: Leprosy. Curr Opin Neurol 2000;13:317. [PMID: 10871258]

9

Oncologic Diseases

Carcinoma of the Head and Neck

- **Essentials of Diagnosis**
  - Most common between ages 50 and 70; occurs in heavy smokers, with alcohol as an apparent cocarcinogen
  - Early hoarseness in true cord lesions; sore throat, otalgia fairly common; odynophagia, hemoptysis indicate more advanced disease
  - Comorbid lung cancer in some patients; may appear clinically up to several years later
  - Lesions found by physical examination or direct or indirect laryngoscopy; regional lymphadenopathy common at presentation

- **Differential Diagnosis**
  - Chronic laryngitis, including reflux laryngitis
  - Laryngeal tuberculosis
  - Myxedema
  - Vocal cord paralysis due to laryngeal nerve palsy caused by left hilar lesion
  - Serous otitis media
  - Herpes simplex

- **Treatment**
  - Treatment varies by stage and tumor location and may include surgery, radiation, radiosensitizing chemotherapy, or combinations of above
  - Chemotherapy may provide palliative benefit for metastatic or recurrent disease
  - Smoking cessation crucial for increasing treatment efficacy and preventing second malignancies

- **Pearl**

The typical head-neck squamous cancer remains undiagnosed for 9 months after patient or physician awareness of the first symptom or sign.

Reference

Correa AJ et al: Current options in management of head and neck cancer patients. Med Clin North Am 1999;83:235. [PMID: 9927972]

Colorectal Carcinoma

- **Essentials of Diagnosis**
  - Risk factors include colonic polyposis, Lynch syndrome (hereditary nonpolyposis colon cancer), and ulcerative colitis
  - Altered bowel habits, rectal bleeding from left-sided carcinoma; occult, blood in bowel movements; iron deficiency anemia in right-sided lesions
  - Palpable abdominal or rectal mass in minority
  - Characteristic barium enema or colonoscopic appearance; tissue biopsy is diagnostic
  - Elevated carcinoembryonic antigen (CEA) useful as marker of disease recurrence in patients with elevated CEA at diagnosis but is not useful as a diagnostic tool

- **Differential Diagnosis**
  - Hemorrhoids
  - Diverticular disease
  - Benign colonic polyps
  - Peptic ulcer disease
  - Ameboma
  - Functional bowel disease
  - Iron deficiency anemia due to other causes

- **Treatment**
  - Dukes staging predicts prognosis
  - Surgical resection for cure, also for palliation
  - Adjuvant chemotherapy recommended for those with significant risk of recurrence based on unfavorable Dukes stage after potentially curative surgery
  - Combination chemotherapy palliative for distant metastatic disease
  - Radiation with concurrent chemotherapy useful adjuvant to surgery for rectal cancer
  - Chemotherapy and radiotherapy curative in majority of localized anal cancers without need for surgery
  - Screening with colonoscopy will probably prove superior to flexible sigmoidoscopy

- **Pearl**

Patients with Streptococcus bovis *endocarditis have colonic neoplasia until proved otherwise.*

Reference

Rudy DR et al: Update on colorectal cancer. Am Fam Physician 2000;61:1759. [PMID: 10750881]

Hepatocellular Carcinoma

- **Essentials of Diagnosis**

  - Most common visceral malignancy worldwide; usually asymptomatic until disease advanced
  - Alcoholic cirrhosis, chronic hepatitis B or C, and hemochromatosis are risk factors
  - Abdominal enlargement, pain, jaundice, weight loss
  - Hepatomegaly, abdominal mass; rub or bruit heard over right upper quadrant in some
  - Anemia or erythrocytosis; liver function test abnormalities
  - Dramatic elevation in alpha-fetoprotein (AFP) helpful in diagnosis, though significant percentage have normal AFPs
  - Tendency to ascent hepatic vein and inferior vena cava
  - Angiography (though rarely performed) with characteristic abnormality; CT or MRI suggests diagnosis; tissue biopsy for confirmation

- **Differential Diagnosis**

  - Benign liver tumors: hemangioma, adenoma, focal nodular hyperplasia
  - Bacterial hepatic abscess
  - Amebic liver cyst
  - Metastatic tumor

- **Treatment**

  - Therapeutic options often limited by severe underlying liver disease; no surgical option if cirrhosis is present in remainder of liver
  - Surgical resection thought best curative option if lesions are resectable and patient is operative candidate
  - Liver transplant may be curative in small percentage of highly selected patients
  - Many intralesional therapies being developed for unresectable disease, though indications and timing of these interventions are not well established
  - Little benefit from chemotherapy in advanced disease

- **Pearl**

In a patient with known cirrhosis and a normal hematocrit, think hepatocellular carcinoma—it's the second most common tumor (after renal cell) to elaborate erythropoietin and pseudonormalizes the anemia typical of cirrhosis.

Reference

Ulmer SC: Hepatocellular carcinoma. A concise guide to its status and management. Postgrad Med 2000;107:117. [PMID: 10844947]

Malignant Tumors of the Bile Ducts

- **Essentials of Diagnosis**
  - Predisposing factors include choledochal cysts, primary sclerosing cholangitis, ulcerative colitis with sclerosing cholangitis, *Clonorchis sinensis* infection
  - Jaundice, pruritus, anorexia, right upper quadrant pain
  - Hepatomegaly, ascites, right upper quadrant tenderness
  - Dilated intrahepatic bile ducts by ultrasound or CT scan
  - Retrograde endoscopic cholangiogram characteristic; tissue biopsy is diagnostic
  - Hyperbilirubinemia (conjugated), markedly elevated alkaline phosphatase and cholesterol

- **Differential Diagnosis**
  - Choledocholithiasis
  - Drug-induced cholestasis
  - Cirrhosis
  - Chronic hepatitis
  - Metastatic hepatic malignancy
  - Pancreatic or ampullary carcinoma
  - Biliary stricture

- **Treatment**
  - Palliative surgical bypass of biliary flow
  - Stent bypass of biliary flow in selected patients
  - Pancreaticoduodenectomy for resectable distal duct tumors curative in minority

- **Pearl**

Half of cholangiocarcinoma patients have had ulcerative colitis, though colectomy doesn't reduce the risk; a far smaller number of patients with ulcerative colitis have bile duct tumors.

Reference

Molmenti EP et al: Hepatobiliary malignancies. Primary hepatic malignant neoplasms. Surg Clin North Am 1999;79:43. [PMID: 10073181]

Carcinoma of the Pancreas

- **Essentials of Diagnosis**
  - Peak incidence in seventh decade; more common in blacks, patients with chronic pancreatitis, and, debatably, diabetes mellitus
  - Upper abdominal pain with radiation to back, weight loss, diarrhea, pruritus, thrombophlebitis; painless jaundice, with symptoms depending on where tumor is located, most being in the head of the pancreas
  - Palpable gallbladder or abdominal mass in some
  - Elevated amylase with liver function abnormalities; anemia, hyperglycemia, or frank diabetes in minority
  - Dilated common hepatic ducts by ultrasound or endoscopic retrograde cholangiogram
  - CT, MRI, and endoscopic ultrasound may delineate extent of disease and guide biopsy
  - Often, true extent of disease not appreciated before exploratory laparotomy

- **Differential Diagnosis**
  - Choledocholithiasis
  - Drug-induced cholestasis
  - Hepatitis
  - Cirrhosis
  - Carcinoma of ampulla of Vater

- **Treatment**
  - Surgical diversion for palliation in most cases
  - Radical pancreaticoduodenal resection for disease limited to head of pancreas or periampullary zone (Whipple procedure) curative in rare cases, but more so in ampullary tumors
  - Chemotherapy, radiation, or combination in patients with advanced local disease may improve outcomes
  - Chemotherapy for metastatic disease may improve quality of life

- **Pearl**

A palpable periumbilical node—Sister Mary Joseph's node—was described by a scrub nurse at the Mayo Clinic, who noticed it while preoperatively sterilizing the abdominal walls of afflicted patients.

Reference

Lillemoe KD et al: Pancreatic cancer: state-of-the-art care. CA Cancer J Clin 2000;50:241. [PMID: 10986966]

Carcinoma of the Female Breast

- ■ Essentials of Diagnosis
    - Increased incidence in those with a family history of breast cancer and in nulliparous or late-childbearing women
    - Painless lump, often found by the patient; nipple or skin changes over breast (peau d'orange, redness, ulceration) later findings; axillary mass, malaise, or weight loss even later findings
    - Minority found by mammography
    - Metastatic disease to lung, bone, or central nervous system may dominate clinical picture
    - Staging based on size of tumor, involvement of lymph nodes, and presence of metastases

- ■ Differential Diagnosis
    - Mammary dysplasia (fibrocystic disease)
    - Benign tumor (fibroadenoma, ductal papilloma)
    - Fat necrosis
    - Mastitis
    - Thrombophlebitis (Mondor's disease)

- ■ Treatment
    - Treatment decisions require careful consideration of stage and other prognostic factors
    - Resection (lumpectomy plus radiation therapy versus modified radical mastectomy) in early-stage disease
    - Adjuvant chemotherapy or hormonal therapy recommended for many with completely resected disease except those at very low risk for recurrence
    - Menopausal and tumor hormone receptor status dictate best adjuvant therapy
    - Metastatic disease is incurable, but treatment with hormonal manipulation, chemotherapy, radiation, and monoclonal antibody therapy; may provide long-term remission or disease stabilization

- ■ Pearl

This is the most feared disease among American women; emotional support is as crucial as therapeutic care.

Reference

Sainsbury JR et al: ABC of breast diseases: breast cancer. BMJ 2000;321:745. [PMID: 10999911]

Carcinoma of the Male Breast

- ■ Essentials of Diagnosis
  - Painless lump or skin changes of breast
  - Nipple discharge, retraction or ulceration, palpable mass, gynecomastia
  - Staging as in women

- ■ Differential Diagnosis
  - Gynecomastia due to other causes
  - Benign tumor

- ■ Treatment
  - Modified radical mastectomy with staging as in women
  - For metastatic disease, endocrine manipulation (physical or chemical castration) with tamoxifen or related compounds, aminoglutethimide, or corticosteroids often quite effective

- ■ Pearl

This constitutes 1% of all breast cancer, but it is invariably diagnosed later in its course because men are neither suspected nor screened.

Reference

Donegan WL et al: Breast cancer in men. Surg Clin North Am 1996;76:343. [PMID: 8610268]

Cervical Intraepithelial Neoplasia (Dysplasia or Carcinoma in Situ of the Cervix)

- **Essentials of Diagnosis**
  - Associated in some with human papillomavirus infection, excessive sexual activity
  - Asymptomatic in many
  - Cervix appears grossly normal with dysplastic or carcinoma in situ cells by cytologic smear preparation
  - Culdoscopic examination with coarse punctate or mosaic pattern of surface capillaries, atypical transformation zone, and thickened white epithelium
  - Iodine-nonstaining (Schiller-positive) squamous epithelium is typical

- **Differential Diagnosis**
  - Cervicitis

- **Treatment**
  - Varies depending upon degree and extent of cervical or intraepithelial neoplasia; thus, staging crucial
  - Observation for mild dysplasia
  - Cryosurgery or CO_2 laser vaporization for moderate dysplasia
  - Cone biopsy or hysterectomy for severe dysplasia or carcinoma in situ
  - Repeat examinations to detect recurrence

- **Pearl**

One of the few disorders for which screening with Pap smear has made an important difference.

Reference

Cox JT: Management of cervical intraepithelial neoplasia. Lancet 1999;353:857. [PMID: 10093973]

Cancer of the Cervix

- ■ Essentials of Diagnosis
  - Abnormal uterine bleeding, vaginal discharge, pelvic or abdominal pain
  - Cervical lesion may be visible on inspection as tumor or ulceration
  - Vaginal cytology is usually positive; must be confirmed by biopsy
  - CT or MRI of abdomen and pelvis, examination under anesthesia useful for staging disease

- ■ Differential Diagnosis
  - Cervicitis
  - Chronic vaginitis or infection (tuberculosis, actinomycosis)
  - Sexually transmitted diseases (syphilis, lymphogranuloma venereum, chancroid, granuloma inguinale)
  - Aborted cervical pregnancy

- ■ Treatment
  - Stage-dependent and requires input of surgeons, medical oncologists, and radiation oncologists
  - Radical or extended hysterectomy curative in patients with early-stage disease
  - Combination of radiation therapy and radiosensitizing chemotherapy curative in majority of patients with localized disease not amenable to primary resection
  - Role of surgery following chemotherapy and radiotherapy still being defined
  - Combination chemotherapy for metastatic disease has significant response rate, but unclear magnitude of benefit on survival

- ■ Pearl

Adherence to screening guidelines can prevent the invasive stage of this disease.

Reference

Canavan TP et al: Cervical cancer. Am Fam Physician 2000;61:1369. [PMID: 10735343]

Endometrial Carcinoma

- **Essentials of Diagnosis**
  - Higher incidence in obesity, diabetes, nulliparity, polycystic ovaries, and women receiving tamoxifen as adjuvant therapy for breast cancer
  - Abnormal uterine bleeding, pelvic or abdominal pain
  - Uterus frequently not enlarged on palpation
  - Endometrial biopsy or curettage is required to confirm diagnosis after negative pregnancy test; vaginal cytologic examination is negative in high percentage of cases
  - Examination under anesthesia, chest x-ray, CT, or MRI required in staging

- **Differential Diagnosis**
  - Pregnancy, especially ectopic
  - Atrophic vaginitis
  - Exogenous estrogens
  - Endometrial hyperplasia or polyps
  - Other pelvic or abdominal neoplasms

- **Treatment**
  - Hysterectomy and salpingo-oophorectomy for well-differentiated or localized tumors
  - Combined surgery and radiation for poorly differentiated tumors, cervical extension, deep myometrial penetration, and regional lymph node involvement
  - Radiotherapy for unresectable localized malignancies
  - Palliative chemotherapy may benefit those with metastatic disease, though role and optimal regimen still being defined
  - Progestational agents may help some women with metastatic disease

- **Pearl**

Unlike cervical cancers, screening is less helpful than having a high index of suspicion in at-risk patients.

Reference

Canavan TP et al: Endometrial cancer. Am Fam Physician 1999;59:3069. [PMID: 10392590]

Carcinoma of the Vulva

- **Essentials of Diagnosis**
  - Prolonged vulvar irritation, pruritus, local discomfort, slight bloody discharge
  - History of genital warts common; association with human papillomavirus established
  - Early lesions may suggest chronic vulvitis
  - Late lesions may present as a mass, exophytic growth, or firm ulcerated area in vulva
  - Biopsy makes diagnosis

- **Differential Diagnosis**
  - Sexually transmitted diseases (syphilis, lymphogranuloma venereum, chancroid, granuloma inguinale)
  - Crohn's disease
  - Benign tumors (granular cell myoblastoma)
  - Reactive or eczematoid dermatitis
  - Vulvar dystrophy

- **Treatment**
  - Local resection for cases of in situ squamous cell carcinoma
  - Wide surgical excision with lymph node dissection for invasive carcinoma

- **Pearl**

This disorder may be diagnosed late because of its similarity to sexually transmitted diseases.

Reference

Homesley HD: Management of vulvar cancer. Cancer 1995;76(10 Suppl):2159. [PMID: 8635016]

Ovarian Tumors

- **Essentials of Diagnosis**
  - Abdominal distention, pelvic pain, vaginal bleeding
  - Ascites, abdominal mass or pelvic pain
  - Ultrasonography or CT scan of the abdomen or pelvis delineates extent of disease
  - Laparoscopy or laparotomy to obtain tissue from mass or ascites for cytologic examination
  - CA 125 (a tumor marker) useful to monitor for recurrence, less valuable for screening

- **Differential Diagnosis**
  - Uterine leiomyoma
  - Endometriosis
  - Tubal pregnancy
  - Pelvic kidney
  - Retroperitoneal tumor or fibrosis
  - Colorectal carcinoma
  - Chronic pelvic inflammatory disease (especially tuberculosis)
  - Benign ovarian masses

- **Treatment**
  - Premenopausal women with small ovarian masses can be observed with a trial of ovulation suppression for two cycles followed by repeat examination
  - Simple excision with ovarian preservation for many benign cell types
  - Unilateral salpingo-oophorectomy for certain cell types in younger women
  - Hysterectomy with bilateral salpingo-oophorectomy in postmenopausal women, or premenopausal women with resectable disease not candidates for more conservative surgery
  - Adjuvant chemotherapy for most patients with resected disease
  - Cytoreductive surgery followed by combination chemotherapy for women with advanced disease without distant metastases
  - Combination chemotherapy has high response rate and may provide durable remissions in women with metastatic disease

- **Pearl**

Be aware of this illness in overweight women—ascites may be difficult to detect on examination.

Reference

Nahhas WA: Ovarian cancer. Current outlook on this deadly disease. Postgrad Med 1997;102:112. [PMID: 9300021]

Gestational Trophoblastic Neoplasia (Hydatidiform Mole & Choriocarcinoma)

- ■ **Essentials of Diagnosis**
  - Uterine bleeding in first trimester
  - Uterus larger than expected for duration of pregnancy
  - No fetus demonstrated by ultrasound with sometimes characteristic findings of mole; excessively elevated levels of serum β-hCG for gestational duration of pregnancy
  - Vesicles may be passed from vagina
  - Preeclampsia seen in first trimester

- ■ **Differential Diagnosis**
  - Multiple pregnancy
  - Threatened abortion
  - Ectopic pregnancy

- ■ **Treatment**
  - Suction curettage for hydatidiform mole
  - For nonmetastatic malignant disease, single-agent chemotherapy (eg, methotrexate or dactinomycin) very effective, but the role of hysterectomy is uncertain
  - For metastatic disease, single-agent or combination chemotherapy depending upon clinical setting
  - Follow quantitative β-hCG until negative and then frequently for surveillance of tumor recurrence

- ■ **Pearl**

Remember an ectopic mole source in a young woman who has hyperthyroidism without a palpable thyroid gland.

Reference

Berkowitz RS et al: Gestational trophoblastic disease. Cancer 1995;76(10 Suppl):2079. [PMID: 8635004]

Thyroid Cancer

- **Essentials of Diagnosis**
  - History of irradiation to neck in some patients
  - Often hard, painless nodule; dysphagia or hoarseness occasionally
  - Cervical lymphadenopathy when local metastases present
  - Thyroid function tests normal; nodule is characteristically stippled with calcium on x-ray, cold by radioiodine scan, and solid by ultrasound; does not regress with thyroid hormone administration

- **Differential Diagnosis**
  - Thyroiditis
  - Other neck masses and other causes of lymphadenopathy
  - Thyroglossal duct cyst
  - Benign thyroid nodules

- **Treatment**
  - Fine-needle aspiration biopsy best differentiates benign from malignant nodules
  - Total thyroidectomy for carcinoma; radioactive iodine postoperatively for selected patients with iodine-avid metastases; combination chemotherapy in anaplastic tumors
  - Prognosis related to cell type and histology; papillary carcinoma offers excellent outlook, anaplastic the worst
  - Medullary thyroid cancer is typically refractory to chemotherapy and radiation; diagnosable by calcitonin elevation in MEN syndromes

- **Pearl**

In patients who had thymus radiation during childhood—a common practice in past years—a thyroid nodule is malignant until proved otherwise.

Reference

Rossi RL et al: Thyroid cancer. Surg Clin North Am 2000;80:571. [PMID: 10836007]

Carcinoma of the Prostate

- **Essentials of Diagnosis**
  - More common and seemingly more aggressive in blacks
  - Exact role of screening uncertain; may prove to be more useful in middle-aged men, especially blacks
  - Symptoms of prostatism more often absent than present; bone pain (especially back) if metastases present; asymptomatic in many, however
  - Stony, hard, irregular prostate palpable, usually lateral part of gland
  - Osteoblastic osseous metastases visible by plain radiograph
  - Prostate-specific antigen (PSA) is age-dependent and is elevated in older patients with benign prostatic hyperplasia and also acute prostatitis; reliably predicts extent of neoplastic disease and recurrence after prostatectomy

- **Differential Diagnosis**
  - Benign prostatic hyperplasia (may be associated)
  - Scarring secondary due to tuberculosis or calculi
  - Urethral stricture
  - Neurogenic bladder

- **Treatment**
  - Providers must apprise patients of the probability of post-therapeutic erectile dysfunction, urinary incontinence
  - Radiation therapy (external beam, brachytherapy, or combination) or radical prostatectomy, ideally nerve-sparing for localized disease
  - Radiation or surgical therapy for local nodal metastases in selected patients after prostatectomy
  - Androgen ablation (chemical or surgical) for metastatic disease, though exact timing of initiation of therapy (at diagnosis or at onset of symptoms) is unclear
  - Combination chemotherapy may benefit selected patients with hormone-refractory metastatic disease

- **Pearl**

About 1% of prostate tumors—most of these are small-cell carcinomas—are not adenocarcinoma and thus do not express PSA.

Reference

Klotz L: Hormone therapy for patients with prostate carcinoma. Cancer 2000;88(12 Suppl):3009. [PMID: 10898345]

Tumors of the Testis

- ■ Essentials of Diagnosis
  - Painless testicular nodule; peak incidence at age 20–35
  - Testis does not transilluminate
  - Gynecomastia, premature virilization in occasional patients
  - Tumor markers (AFP, LDH, hCG) useful in diagnosis, monitoring response to therapy, and surveillance for relapse
  - Pure seminoma produces hCG only, while nonseminomatous germ cell tumors may produce hCG and AFP

- ■ Differential Diagnosis
  - Genitourinary tuberculosis
  - Syphilitic orchitis
  - Hydrocele
  - Spermatocele
  - Epididymitis

- ■ Treatment
  - Orchiectomy, with lumbar and inguinal lymph nodes examined for staging
  - Additional radical resection of iliolumbar nodes indicated unless tumor is a seminoma for which radiation therapy is treatment of choice following surgery
  - Postsurgical radiation therapy also useful for other malignant cell types
  - Platinum-based chemotherapy curative in appreciable majority of patients with advanced or metastatic disease

- ■ Pearl

One of the great stories in oncology, with remarkable therapies resulting in many years of life saved.

Reference

Kinkade S: Testicular cancer. Am Fam Physician 1999;59:2539. [PMID: 10323360]

Carcinoma of the Bladder
(Transitional Cell Carcinoma)

- **Essentials of Diagnosis**
  - More common in men over 40 years of age; predisposing factors include smoking and alcohol as well as chronic *Schistosoma haematobium* infection, exposure to certain industrial toxins, or previous cyclophosphamide therapy
  - Microscopic or gross hematuria with no other symptoms is the most common presentation
  - Suprapubic pain, urgency, and frequency when concurrent infection present
  - Occasional uremia if both ureterovesical orifices obstructed
  - Tumor visible by cystoscopy

- **Differential Diagnosis**
  - Other urinary tract tumor
  - Acute cystitis
  - Renal tuberculosis
  - Urinary calculi
  - Glomerulonephritis or interstitial nephritis

- **Treatment**
  - Endoscopic transurethral resection for superficial or submucosal tumors; intravesical chemotherapy reduces the likelihood of recurrence
  - Radical cystectomy standard with muscle-invasive tumors, though less morbid procedures with intensive follow-up may provide similar outcomes
  - Role of adjuvant chemotherapy or radiation for completely resected patients unclear, but generally offered to those at high risk of recurrence
  - Combination chemotherapy for metastatic disease has a high response rate and may be curative in a small percentage of patients

- **Pearl**

Remember Kaposi's sarcoma of the bladder in an AIDS patient with a urinary catheter and gross hematuria; it usually (not always) presents in association with cutaneous disease.

Reference

van der Meijden AP: Bladder cancer. BMJ 1998;317:1366. [PMID: 99030215]

Adenocarcinoma of the Kidney
(Renal Cell Carcinoma; Hypernephroma)

- **Essentials of Diagnosis**
  - Dubbed the internist's tumor because of its pleomorphic clinical manifestations
  - Gross or microscopic hematuria, back pain, fever, weight loss, night sweats
  - Flank or abdominal mass may be palpable
  - When flank pain, hematuria, and palpable mass—the "too-late triad"—are present, only 15% are curable
  - Anemia in 30%, erythrocytosis in 3%; hypercalcemia, hypoglycemia sometimes seen
  - Frequent tumor or tumor thrombus invasion of renal vein and ascending inferior vena cava, on occasion causing superior vena cava syndrome
  - Renal ultrasound, CT, or MRI reveals characteristic lesion

- **Differential Diagnosis**
  - Simple cyst
  - Polycystic kidney disease
  - Single complex renal cyst; but 70% of these are malignant
  - Renal tuberculosis
  - Renal calculi
  - Renal infarction
  - Endocarditis

- **Treatment**
  - Nephrectomy curative for patients with early stage lesions
  - Poor response to chemotherapy or radiation in metastatic disease
  - Small response rate to combination bio-chemotherapy (interleukin 2 plus cytotoxic agents), though very toxic
  - Resection of primary lesion has been documented to result in regression of metastases on rare occasions
  - Nonmyeloablating allogeneic bone marrow transplantation has significant response rate in highly selected patients

- **Pearl**

A small proportion of patients have a nonmetastatic hepatopathy, with elevation of alkaline phosphatase; this abnormality does not imply inoperability and disappears with resection of the tumor.

Reference

Motzer RJ et al: Renal-cell carcinoma. N Engl J Med 1996;335:865. [PMID: 8778606]

Malignant Tumors of the Esophagus

■ Essentials of Diagnosis

- Progressive dysphagia—initially during ingestion of solid foods, later with liquids; progressive weight loss and inanition ominous
- Smoking, alcoholism, chronic esophageal reflux with Barrett's esophagus, achalasia, caustic injury, and asbestos are risk factors
- Noninvasive imaging (barium swallow, CT scan) suggestive, diagnosis confirmed by endoscopy and biopsy
- Staging of disease aided by endoscopic ultrasound
- Squamous histology more common, though incidence of adenocarcinoma increasing rapidly in Western countries for unclear reasons

■ Differential Diagnosis

- Benign tumors of the esophagus
- Benign esophageal stricture or achalasia
- Esophageal diverticulum
- Esophageal webs
- Achalasia (may be associated)
- Globus hystericus

■ Treatment

- Combination chemotherapy and radiotherapy or surgery for localized disease, though long-term remission or cure is achieved in only 10–15%
- Dilation or esophageal stenting may palliate advanced disease; little role for chemotherapy or radiation in advanced or metastatic disease

■ Pearl

Dysphagia is one of the few symptoms in medicine for which anatomic correlation always exists—too often it represents carcinoma.

Reference

Lerut T et al: Treatment of esophageal carcinoma. Chest 1999;116(6 Suppl):463S. [PMID: 10619509]

Carcinoma of the Stomach

- **Essentials of Diagnosis**
  - Few early symptoms, but abdominal pain not unusual; late complaints include dyspepsia, anorexia, nausea, early satiety, weight loss
  - Palpable abdominal mass (late)
  - Iron deficiency anemia, fecal occult blood positive; achlorhydria present in minority of patients
  - Mass or ulcer visualized radiographically; endoscopic biopsy and cytologic examination diagnostic
  - Associated with atrophic gastritis, *Helicobacter pylori;* role of diet, previous partial gastrectomy controversial

- **Differential Diagnosis**
  - Benign gastric ulcer
  - Gastritis
  - Functional or irritable bowel syndrome
  - Other gastric tumors, eg, leiomyosarcoma, lymphoma

- **Treatment**
  - Resection for cure; palliative resection with gastroenterostomy in selected cases
  - Adjuvant chemotherapy may improve long-term survival in high-risk patients post surgery and may achieve remission in a minority of patients with metastatic disease

- **Pearl**

A gastric ulcer with histamine-fast achlorhydria is adenocarcinoma in 100% of cases.

Reference

Scheiman JM et al: *Helicobacter pylori* and gastric cancer. Am J Med 1999;106:222. [PMID: 10230753]

Bronchogenic Carcinoma

- ■ Essentials of Diagnosis
  - Smoking most important cause, concomitant asbestos exposure synergistic; also associated with second-hand smoke
  - Chronic cough, dyspnea; chest pain, hoarseness, hemoptysis, weight loss; may be asymptomatic, however
  - Examination depends on disease stage; localized wheezing, clubbing, superior vena cava syndrome in some
  - Enlarging mass, infiltrate, atelectasis, pleural effusion, or cavitation by chest x-ray; peripheral coin lesions in a minority
  - Diagnostic: presence of malignant cells by sputum or pleural fluid cytology or on histologic examination of tissue biopsy
  - Metastases to other organs or paraneoplastic effects may produce the initial symptoms
  - Central nervous system metastases at time of diagnosis common with small cell histology

- ■ Differential Diagnosis
  - Tuberculosis
  - Pulmonary mycoses
  - Pyogenic lung abscess
  - Metastasis from extrapulmonary primary tumor
  - Benign lung tumor, eg, hamartoma
  - Noninfectious granulomatous disease

- ■ Treatment
  - Resection for appropriate non-small-cell carcinomas and all coin lesions, assuming no evidence of spread or other primary
  - Combination chemotherapy and radiation for limited-stage small-cell carcinoma; may be curative
  - Prophylactic cranial radiation probably beneficial for those achieving complete remission or excellent response with initial therapy
  - Palliative chemotherapy and radiation for metastatic non-small-cell carcinoma

- ■ Pearl

Of nonsmokers who develop this disorder, middle-aged women with non-small cell cancer are the most common; take pulmonary symptoms very seriously in this group.

Reference

Hoffman PC et al: Lung cancer. Lancet 2000;355:479. [PMID: 10841143]

Pleural Mesothelioma

- **Essentials of Diagnosis**
  - Insidious dyspnea, nonpleuritic chest pain, weight loss
  - Dullness to percussion, diminished breath sounds, pleural friction rub, clubbing
  - Nodular or irregular unilateral pleural thickening, often with effusion by chest radiograph; CT scan often helpful
  - Pleural biopsy usually necessary for diagnosis, though malignant nature of tumor only confirmed by natural history; pleural fluid exudative and usually hemorrhagic
  - Strong association with asbestos exposure, with usual latency from time of exposure 20 years or more

- **Differential Diagnosis**
  - Primary pulmonary parenchymal malignancy
  - Empyema
  - Benign pleural inflammatory conditions (posttraumatic, asbestosis)

- **Treatment**
  - No consistently effective therapy currently available, though investigations with combination surgery, radiotherapy, and chemotherapy are under way
  - One-year mortality rate > 75%

- **Pearl**

Consider this when empyema develops in patients irradiated for malignancy years earlier—it's a rare complication.

Reference

Sterman DH et al: Advances in the treatment of malignant pleural mesothelioma. Chest 1999;116:504. [PMID: 10453882]

Primary Intracranial Tumors

- **Essentials of Diagnosis**
  - Many different cell types; prognosis upon which one; half are gliomas
  - Most present with generalized or focal disturbances of cerebral function: generalized symptoms include nocturnal headache, seizures, and projectile vomiting; focal deficits relate to location of the tumor
  - CT or MRI with gadolinium enhancement defines the lesion; posterior fossa tumors are better visualized by MRI
  - Biopsy is the definitive diagnostic procedure, distinguishes primary brain tumors from brain abscess and other intracranial space-occupying lesions such as metastases

  Specific types:
  - Glioblastoma multiforme: in strictest sense an astrocytoma, but rapidly progressive with a poor prognosis
  - Astrocytoma: More chronic course than glioblastoma, with a variable prognosis
  - Medulloblastoma: seen primarily in children and arises from roof of fourth ventricle
  - Cerebellar hemangioblastoma: patients usually present with disequilibrium and ataxia, and occasional erythrocytosis
  - Meningioma: compresses rather than invades adjacent neural structures; usually benign
  - Primary cerebral lymphoma: usually in AIDS and other immunodeficient states, though may occur rarely in immunocompetent individuals

- **Treatment**
  - Treatment depends upon the type and site of the tumor and the condition of the patient
  - Resection to maximal extent possible is important predictor of outcome in most central nervous system malignancies
  - Radiation post surgery is mainstay of therapy
  - Herniation treated with intravenous corticosteroids, mannitol, and surgical decompression if possible
  - Prophylactic anticonvulsants are also commonly given

- **Pearl**

  A headache that awakens a patient from sleep should put this diagnosis at the top of the list.

Reference

DeAngelis LM: Brain tumors. N Engl J Med 2001;344:114. [PMID: 11150363]

10

Fluid, Acid-Base, & Electrolyte Disorders

Dehydration (Simple & Uncomplicated)

- ■ Essentials of Diagnosis
    - • Thirst, oliguria
    - • Decreased skin turgor, especially on anterior thigh; dry mucous membrane, postural hypotension, tachycardia
    - • Impaired renal function (BUN to creatinine ratio > 20), elevated urinary osmolality and specific gravity, decreased urinary sodium (fractional excretion of sodium is usually < 1%)

- ■ Differential Diagnosis
    - • Hemorrhage
    - • Sepsis
    - • Gastrointestinal fluid losses
    - • Skin sodium losses associated with burns or sweating
    - • Renal sodium loss
    - • Adrenal insufficiency
    - • Nonketotic hyperosmolar state in type 2 diabetics

- ■ Treatment
    - • Identify source of volume loss if present
    - • Replete with normal saline, blood, or colloid as indicated
    - • Half-normal saline may be substituted when blood pressure normalizes

- ■ Pearl

Dry mucous membranes are more indicative of mouth breathing than of dehydration.

Reference

Kleiner SM: Water: an essential but overlooked nutrient. J Am Diet Assoc 1999;99:200. [PMID: 9972188]

Shock

- ■ **Essentials of Diagnosis**
  - • History of hemorrhage, myocardial infarction, sepsis, trauma, or anaphylaxis
  - • Tachycardia, hypotension, hypothermia, tachypnea
  - • Cool, sweaty skin with pallor; may be warm or flushed, however, with early sepsis; clouded sensorium, altered level of consciousness, seizures
  - • Oliguria, increased urinary osmolality and specific gravity, anemia, disseminated intravascular coagulation, metabolic acidosis may complicate
  - • Hemodynamic measurements depend upon underlying cause

- ■ **Differential Diagnosis**
  - • Numerous causes of the syndrome, as noted above
  - • Adrenal insufficiency

- ■ **Treatment**
  - • Correct cause of shock (ie, control hemorrhage, treat infection, correct metabolic disease)
  - • Empiric broad-spectrum antibiotics often necessary
  - • Restore hemodynamics with fluids; vasopressor medications may be required
  - • Maintain urine output
  - • Treat contributing disease (eg, diabetes mellitus)

- ■ **Pearl**

The patient appearing to be in shock but who is hypertensive may have aortic dissection.

Reference

Dabrowski GP et al: A critical assessment of endpoints of shock resuscitation. Surg Clin North Am 2000;80:825. [PMID: 10897263]

Hypernatremia

- **Essentials of Diagnosis**
  - Usually severe thirst unless mentation altered; oliguria
  - If hypovolemic, loose skin with poor turgor, tachycardia, hypotension
  - Serum sodium > 145 meq/L, serum osmolality > 300 meq/L caused by free water loss
  - Affected patients usually include the very old, very young, critically ill, or neurologically impaired

- **Differential Diagnosis**
  - Diabetes insipidus, either idiopathic or drug-induced (eg, by lithium)
  - Loss of hypotonic fluid (insensible, diuretics, vomiting, diarrhea, nasogastric suctioning)
  - Salt intoxication
  - Volume resuscitation and continuation of normal saline (155 meq/L) after euvolemia achieved

- **Treatment**
  - Relatively rapid volume replacement followed by free water replacement over 48–72 hours (beware of cerebral edema)
  - Desmopressin acetate for central diabetes insipidus

- **Pearl**

In-patient mortality for a sodium > 150 mg/dL is approximately 50%.

Reference

Adrogue HJ et al: Hypernatremia. N Engl J Med 2000;342:1493. [PMID: 10816188]

Hyponatremia

- **Essentials of Diagnosis**
  - Nausea, headache, weakness, irritability, mental confusion (especially with serum sodium < 120 meq/L)
  - Generalized seizures, lethargy, coma, respiratory arrest and death may result
  - Serum sodium < 130 meq/L; osmolality < 270 meq/L (hypotonic hyponatremia); hypouricemia if SIADH or primary polydipsia is the cause

- **Differential Diagnosis**
  - Hypovolemic causes (thiazide diuretics, osmotic diuresis, adrenal insufficiency, vomiting, diarrhea, fluid sequestration or third-spacing)
  - Hypervolemic causes (congestive heart failure, cirrhosis, nephrotic syndrome, renal failure, pregnancy)
  - Euvolemic causes (hypothyroidism, SIADH, adrenocortical insufficiency, reset osmostat, primary polydipsia)
  - Hypertonic or isotonic hyponatremia (hyperglycemia, intravenous mannitol)
  - Pseudohyponatremia (hypertriglyceridemia, paraproteinemia): laboratory artifact

- **Treatment**
  - Treat underlying disorder
  - Corticosteroids empirically if adrenal insufficiency suspected
  - Gradual correction (24–48 hours) of sodium unless severe central nervous system signs present (beware of central pontine myelinolysis)
  - If hypovolemic, use saline
  - If hypervolemic, use water restriction, diuretics, and normal saline volume replacement of urine output
  - Demeclocycline in selected patients with SIADH

- **Pearl**

A sodium less than 130 mg/dL, BUN less than 10 mg/dL, and hypouricemia in a patient without liver, heart, or kidney disease is virtually diagnostic of SIADH.

Reference

Adrogue HJ et al: Hyponatremia. N Engl J Med 2000;342:1581. [PMID: 10824078]

Hyperkalemia

- **Essentials of Diagnosis**
  - Weakness or flaccid paralysis, abdominal distention, diarrhea
  - Serum potassium > 5 meq/L
  - Electrocardiographic changes: peaked T waves, loss of P wave with sinoventricular rhythm, QRS widening, ventricular asystole, cardiac arrest

- **Differential Diagnosis**
  - Renal failure with oliguria
  - Hypoaldosteronism (hyporeninism, potassium-sparing diuretics, ACE inhibitors, adrenal disease, interstitial renal disease)
  - Acidemia
  - Burns, hemolysis
  - Digitalis overdose
  - Spurious from thrombocytosis, leukocytosis

- **Treatment**
  - Emergency (cardiac toxicity, paralysis): intravenous bicarbonate, calcium gluconate, glucose, and insulin
  - Dietary potassium restriction and sodium polystyrene sulfonate or diuretic to lower body potassium subacutely
  - Dialysis if oliguric renal failure or severe acidosis complicates

- **Pearl**

A "junctional" rhythm in a patient with marked renal insufficiency is in all likelihood sinus rhythm with failure of atrial depolarization.

Reference

Halperin ML et al: Potassium. Lancet 1998;352:135. [PMID: 98336038]

Hypokalemia

- **Essentials of Diagnosis**
  - Usually asymptomatic
  - Muscle weakness, lethargy, paresthesias, polyuria, anorexia, constipation
  - May progress to weakness, muscle necrosis, ascending flaccid paralysis, ileus
  - Electrocardiographic changes: T wave flattening and ST depression → development of prominent u waves → AV block → cardiac arrest
  - Serum potassium < 3.5 meq/L; metabolic alkalosis sometimes concurrent

- **Differential Diagnosis/Causes**
  - Diuretic use
  - Alkalemia
  - Hyperaldosteronism (adrenal adenoma, primary hyperreninism, mineralocorticoid use, and European licorice ingestion)
  - Magnesium depletion
  - Hyperthyroidism
  - Diarrhea
  - Renal tubular acidosis (types I, II)
  - Bartter's, Gitelman's, and Liddle's syndromes
  - Familial hypokalemic periodic paralysis
  - Severe dietary potassium restriction

- **Treatment**
  - Identify and treat underlying cause
  - Oral or intravenous potassium supplementation

- **Pearl**

Think of hypokalemia in unexplained orthostatic hypotension.

Reference

Cohn JN et al: New guidelines for potassium replacement in clinical practice: a contemporary review by the National Council on Potassium in Clinical Practice. Arch Intern Med 2000;160:2429. [PMID: 10979053]

Hypercalcemia

- ■ Essentials of Diagnosis
  - Polyuria and constipation; abdominal pain in some
  - Thirst and dehydration
  - Mild hypertension
  - Altered mentation, hyporeflexia, stupor, coma
  - Serum calcium > 10.2 mg/dL (corrected with concurrent serum albumin)
  - Renal insufficiency or azotemia, isosthenuria
  - Shortened QT interval due to short ST segment, ventricular extrasystoles

- ■ Differential Diagnosis
  - Primary hyperparathyroidism
  - Adrenal insufficiency
  - Malignancy (multiple myeloma with osteoclast-activating factor; other primary tumor or metastasis releasing parathyroid hormone-related peptide)
  - Vitamin D intoxication
  - Milk-alkali syndrome
  - Sarcoidosis
  - Tuberculosis
  - Paget's disease of bone, especially with immobilization
  - Familial hypocalciuric hypercalcemia

- ■ Treatment
  - Identify and treat underlying disorder
  - Volume expansion, loop diuretics (once euvolemic)
  - Glucocorticoids, calcitonin, bisphosphonates, and dialysis all useful in certain instances
  - Resection of parathyroid adenoma, if present

- ■ Pearl

All hypercalcemia of malignancy is humoral in origin; bone metastases not elaborating such humoral factors do not elevate calcium.

Reference

Body JJ: Current and future directions in medical therapy: hypercalcemia. Cancer, 2000;88(12 Suppl):3054. [PMID: 10898351]

Hypocalcemia

- ■ Essentials of Diagnosis
  - • Abdominal and muscle cramps, stridor; tetany and seizures
  - • Diplopia, facial paresthesias
  - • Positive Chvostek and Trousseau signs
  - • Cataracts if chronic, likewise basal ganglion calcifications
  - • Serum calcium < 8.5 mg/dL (corrected with concurrent serum albumin); phosphate usually elevated; hypomagnesemia may cause or complicate
  - • Electrocardiographic changes: prolonged QT interval; ventricular arrhythmias, including ventricular tachycardia

- ■ Differential Diagnosis
  - • Vitamin D deficiency and osteomalacia
  - • Malabsorption
  - • Hypoparathyroidism
  - • Hyperphosphatemia
  - • Hypomagnesemia
  - • Chronic renal failure
  - • Alcoholism
  - • Drugs (loop diuretics, aminoglycosides, foscarnet)

- ■ Treatment
  - • Identify and treat underlying disorder
  - • For tetany, seizures, or arrhythmias, give calcium gluconate intravenously
  - • Magnesium replacement if indicated
  - • Oral calcium and vitamin D supplements
  - • Phosphate-binding antacids if phosphate elevated

- ■ Pearl

The prolonged QT of hypocalcemia results from a lengthened ST segment; T waves are normal.

Reference

Reber PM et al: Hypocalcemic emergencies. Med Clin North Am 1995;79: 93. [PMID: 7808098]

Hyperphosphatemia

- **Essentials of Diagnosis**
  - Few distinct symptoms
  - Cataracts, basal ganglion calcifications in hypoparathyroidism
  - Serum phosphate > 5 mg/dL; renal failure, hypocalcemia occasionally seen

- **Differential Diagnosis**
  - Renal failure
  - Hypoparathyroidism
  - Excess phosphate intake, vitamin D toxicity
  - Phosphate-containing laxative use
  - Cell destruction, rhabdomyolysis, respiratory or metabolic acidosis
  - Multiple myeloma

- **Treatment**
  - Treat underlying disease when possible
  - Oral calcium carbonate to reduce phosphate absorption
  - Hemodialysis if refractory

- **Pearl**

Overshoot hyperphosphatemia from therapy of hypophosphatemia may precipitate the acute onset of tetany.

Reference

Weisinger JR et al: Magnesium and phosphorus. Lancet, 1998;352:391. [PMID: 9717944]

Hypophosphatemia

- **Essentials of Diagnosis**
  - Seldom an isolated abnormality
  - Anorexia, myopathy, arthralgias
  - Irritability, confusion, seizures, coma
  - Rhabdomyolysis if severe
  - Serum phosphate < 2.5 mg/dL, severe < 1 mg/dL; elevated creatine kinase if rhabdomyolysis
  - Hemolysis in severe cases

- **Differential Diagnosis**
  - Hyperparathyroidism, hyperthyroidism
  - Alcoholism
  - Vitamin D-resistant osteomalacia
  - Malabsorption, starvation
  - Hypercalcemia, hypomagnesemia
  - Correction of hyperglycemia
  - Recovery from catabolic state

- **Treatment**
  - Intravenous phosphate replacement when severe
  - Oral phosphate supplements (unless hypercalcemic); be cautious about overshooting
  - Correct magnesium deficit, if present

- **Pearl**

  Phosphate levels even as low as 0–0.1 mg/dL are possible without clinical manifestations.

Reference

Subramanian R et al: Severe hypophosphatemia. Pathophysiologic implications, clinical presentations, and treatment. Medicine 2000;79:1. [PMID: 10670405]

Hypermagnesemia

- **Essentials of Diagnosis**
  - Weakness, hyporeflexia, respiratory muscle paralysis
  - Confusion, altered mentation
  - Serum magnesium > 3 mg/dL; renal insufficiency common; increased uric acid, phosphate, potassium, and decreased calcium may be seen
  - Increased PR interval → heart block → cardiac arrest

- **Differential Diagnosis**
  - Renal insufficiency
  - Excessive magnesium intake (food, antacids, laxatives, intravenous administration)

- **Treatment**
  - Correct renal insufficiency, if possible (volume expansion)
  - Intravenous calcium chloride for severe manifestations (eg, electrocardiographic changes, respiratory arrest)
  - Dialysis

- **Pearl**

Be cautious about magnesium-containing antacids—available OTC— in patients with renal insufficiency.

Reference

Weisinger JR et al: Magnesium and phosphorus. Lancet 1998;352:391. [PMID: 9717944]

Hypomagnesemia

- **Essentials of Diagnosis**

  - Muscle restlessness or cramps, athetoid movements, twitching or tremor, convulsions or delirium
  - Muscle wasting, hyperreflexia, positive Babinski sign, nystagmus, hypertension
  - Serum magnesium < 1.5 meq/L; decreased calcium, potassium often seen
  - Electrocardiographic changes: tachycardia, premature atrial or ventricular beats, increased QT interval, ventricular tachycardia or fibrillation

- **Differential Diagnosis**

  - Inadequate dietary intake (ie, malnutrition)
  - Hypervolemia
  - Diuretics, cisplatin, aminoglycosides, amphotericin B
  - Malabsorption or diarrhea
  - Alcoholism
  - Hyperaldosteronism, hyperthyroidism, hyperparathyroidism
  - Respiratory alkalosis

- **Treatment**

  - Identify and treat underlying cause
  - Intravenous magnesium replacement followed by oral maintenance
  - Calcium and potassium supplements if needed

- **Pearl**

Many manifestations of hypomagnesemia relate to the hypocalcemia induced by resistance to parathyroid hormone.

Reference

Agus ZS: Hypomagnesemia. J Am Soc Nephrol 1999;10:1616. [PMID: 10405219]

Respiratory Acidosis

- **Essentials of Diagnosis**
  - Central to all is alveolar hypoventilation
  - Confusion, altered mentation, somnolence
  - Dyspnea, respiratory distress, pulmonary abnormalities with or without cyanosis and asterixis
  - Arterial P_{CO_2} increased; arterial pH decreased
  - Lung disease may be acute (pneumonia, asthma) or chronic (COPD)
  - May occur in the absence of lung disease

- **Differential Diagnosis**
  - Chronic obstructive lung disease or airway obstruction
  - Central nervous system depressants
  - Structural disorders of the thorax
  - Myxedema
  - Neurologic disorders, eg, Guillain-Barré syndrome

- **Treatment**
  - Address underlying cause
  - Artificial ventilation if necessary to oxygenate, invasive or non-invasive

- **Pearl**

Hypoxemia must be corrected before ascribing mental status changes to an elevated P_{CO_2}; it's the case in most hypercapnic patients.

Reference

Adrogue HJ et al: Management of life-threatening acid-base disorders. First of two parts. N Engl J Med 1998;338:26. [PMID: 9414329]

Respiratory Alkalosis

- ■ Essentials of Diagnosis
  - Lightheadedness, numbness or tingling of extremities, circumoral paresthesias
  - Tachypnea; positive Chvostek and Trousseau signs in acute hyperventilation; carpopedal spasm and tetany
  - Arterial pH > 7.45, P_{CO_2} < 30 mm Hg

- ■ Differential Diagnosis
  - Restrictive lung disease or hypoxia
  - Central nervous system lesion
  - Pulmonary embolism
  - Salicylate toxicity
  - Anxiety
  - End-stage cirrhosis
  - Sepsis
  - Pregnancy
  - High-altitude residence

- ■ Treatment
  - Correct hypoxia or underlying ventilatory stimulant
  - Increase ventilatory dead space (eg, breathe into paper bag, but only in anxiety-induced hyperventilation)

- ■ Pearl

A lowered P_{CO_2} is a dependable early sign of bacteremia and sepsis syndrome.

Reference

Adrogue HJ et al: Management of life-threatening acid-base disorders. Second of two parts. N Engl J Med 1998;338:107. [PMID: 9420343]

Metabolic Acidosis

- **Essentials of Diagnosis**
  - Dyspnea, hyperventilation, respiratory fatigue
  - Tachycardia, hypotension, shock (depending on cause)
  - Acetone breath (in ketoacidosis)
  - Arterial pH < 7.35, serum bicarbonate decreased; anion gap may be normal or high; ketonuria

- **Differential Diagnosis**
  - Ketoacidosis (diabetic, alcoholic, starvation)
  - Lactic acidosis
  - Poisons (methyl alcohol, ethylene glycol, salicylates, isopropyl alcohol)
  - Uremia
  - Normal anion gap causes (diarrhea, renal tubular acidosis)

- **Treatment**
  - Identify and treat underlying cause
  - Correct volume, electrolyte status
  - Bicarbonate therapy indicated in ethylene glycol or methanol toxicity, renal tubular acidosis, debated for other causes
  - Hemodialysis, mechanical ventilation if necessary

- **Pearl**

A low pH in diabetic ketoacidosis is not the cause of an altered mental status—hyperosmolality is.

Reference

Forsythe SM et al: Sodium bicarbonate for the treatment of lactic acidosis. Chest 2000;117:260. [PMID: 10631227]

Metabolic Alkalosis

- ■ Essentials of Diagnosis

  - Weakness, malaise, lethargy; other symptoms depend on cause
  - Hyporeflexia, tetany, ileus, muscle weakness
  - Arterial pH > 7.45, P_{CO_2} up to 45 mm Hg, and serum bicarbonate > 30 meq/L; serum potassium and chloride usually low; hypo-ventilation is seldom prominent irrespective of pH

- ■ Differential Diagnosis

  - Loss of acid (vomiting or nasogastric aspiration)
  - Diuretic overuse or any volume contraction
  - Exogenous bicarbonate or base load
  - Primary hyperaldosteronism states (hyperreninemia, ingestion of some types of licorice, adrenal tumor or hyperplasia, Bartter's or Gitelman's syndrome)

- ■ Treatment

  - Identify and correct underlying cause
  - Replenish volume and electrolytes (use 0.9% sodium chloride)
  - Hydrochloric acid rarely if ever needed
  - Supplemental KCl in most

- ■ Pearl

Vomiting causes mild metabolic alkalosis—only if associated with gastric outlet obstruction are abnormalities marked.

Reference

Galla JH: Metabolic alkalosis. J Am Soc Nephrol 2000;11:369. [PMID: 10665945]

11

Genitourinary & Renal Disorders

GENITOURINARY DISORDERS

Tuberculosis of the Genitourinary Tract

- ■ Essentials of Diagnosis
  - Fever, malaise, night sweats, weight loss; evidence of pulmonary tuberculosis in 50%
  - Symptoms or signs of urinary tract infection may be present
  - Nodular, indurated epididymis, testes, or prostate
  - Sterile pyuria or hematuria without bacteriuria; white blood cell casts can be seen with renal parenchymal involvement
  - Positive culture of morning urine on one of three consecutive samples
  - Plain radiographs may show renal and lower tract calcifications
  - Excretory urogram reveals "moth-eaten" calices, papillary necrosis, and beading of ureters
  - Occasionally, ulcers or granulomas of bladder wall at cystoscopy

- ■ Differential Diagnosis
  - Other causes of chronic urinary tract infections
  - Interstitial nephritis, especially drug-induced
  - Nonspecific urethritis
  - Urinary calculi
  - Epididymitis
  - Bladder cancer

- ■ Treatment
  - Standard combination antituberculosis therapy
  - Surgical procedures for obstruction and severe hemorrhage
  - Nephrectomy for extensive destruction of the kidney

- ■ Pearl

Tuberculosis of the genitourinary tract is the only descending urinary tract infection; all others ascend.

Reference

Weiss SG 2nd et al: Genitourinary tuberculosis. Urology 1998;51:1033. [PMID: 9609647]

Bacterial Prostatitis

- **Essentials of Diagnosis**
  - Acute bacterial prostatitis: fever, dysuria, urinary urgency and frequency, perineal or suprapubic pain; very tender prostate; leukocytosis, pyuria, bacteriuria, and hematuria
  - Caused by *Escherichia coli* most commonly, also by *Neisseria gonorrhoeae, Chlamydia trachomatis,* other gram-negative rods (eg, proteus, pseudomonas) or gram-positive organisms (eg, enterococcus)
  - Prostatic massage may produce septicemia
  - Chronic prostatitis: usually in older men, may be asymptomatic; in some, urgency and frequency, dysuria, perineal or suprapubic pain; prostate boggy, not tender; pathogenic organisms can persist despite treatment
  - Expressed prostatic secretions demonstrate increased numbers of leukocytes; culture often sterile

- **Differential Diagnosis**
  - Urethritis
  - Cystitis
  - Epididymitis
  - Prostatodynia
  - Nonbacterial prostatitis
  - Perirectal abscess

- **Treatment**
  - Symptomatic treatment with hot sitz baths, NSAIDs, and stool softeners
  - For acute bacterial prostatitis in men under 35 years of age, treat for *N gonorrhoeae* and *C trachomatis* infection
  - For acute bacterial prostatitis in men over age 35 years or homosexual men, treat for Enterobacteriaceae with oral or intravenous antibiotics (eg, trimethoprim-sulfamethoxazole or ciprofloxacin) for 21 days
  - For chronic bacterial prostatitis, treat for Enterobacteriaceae with oral antibiotics (eg, trimethoprim-sulfamethoxazole or ciprofloxacin) for 6–12 weeks; cure rate is often less than 50%

- **Pearl**

Trimethoprim-sulfamethoxazole achieves one of the highest intraprostatic levels of all antibiotics; an ideal drug for this process.

Reference

Nickel JC: Prostatitis: evolving management strategies. Urol Clin North Am 1999;26:737. [PMID: 10584615]

Urinary Calculi

- **Essentials of Diagnosis**
  - Most common in the stone belt, extending from central Ohio through mid Florida
  - Sudden, severe colicky pain localized to the flank, commonly associated with nausea, vomiting, and fever; marked urinary urgency and frequency if stone lodged at ureterovesical junction
  - Occasionally asymptomatic
  - Hematuria in 90%, pyuria with concurrent infection; presence of crystals in urine may be diagnostically helpful
  - Plain films of the abdomen (stone seen in 90%), spiral computerized tomography, or sonography may be used to visualize location of stone
  - Depending on the metabolic abnormality, stones can be composed of calcium oxalate or phosphate, struvite, uric acid, or cystine; over 50% of patients develop recurrent stones

- **Differential Diagnosis**
  - Acute pyelonephritis
  - Chronic prostatism
  - Tumor of genitourinary system
  - Renal tuberculosis
  - Renal infarction

- **Treatment**
  - Stones usually pass spontaneously with analgesia and hydration
  - Antibiotics if concurrent infection present
  - Patient should filter urine and save stone for analysis
  - Hydration is mainstay to prevent recurrence; also dietary change, thiazides, allopurinol, citrate, or a combination of these may be used to prevent recurrence, depending on composition of the stone
  - Refer to specialist for recurrent stones
  - Lithotripsy or surgical lithotomy may be necessary in refractory cases

- **Pearl**

Analyze all stones: it is a rare noninvasive way to understand fully the pathophysiology of a disease process.

Reference

Saklayen MG: Medical management of nephrolithiasis. Med Clin North Am 1997;81:785. [PMID: 9167658]

Acute Epididymitis

- **Essentials of Diagnosis**
  - Sudden pain and swelling of epididymis, with fever, dysuria, urinary urgency, and frequency of less than 6 weeks duration
  - Marked epididymal, testicular, or spermatic cord tenderness with symptomatic relief upon elevation of scrotum (Prehn's sign)
  - Leukocytosis, pyuria, bacteriuria
  - Usually caused by *Neisseria gonorrhoeae* or *Chlamydia trachomatis* in heterosexual men under age 40 and by Enterobacteriaceae in homosexual men of all ages and heterosexual men over age 40
  - Doppler ultrasonography differentiates from testicular torsion

- **Differential Diagnosis**
  - Testicular torsion
  - Testicular tumor
  - Orchitis
  - Prostatitis
  - Testicular trauma

- **Treatment**
  - Empiric antibiotics after culture of urine obtained
  - In men under age 40, treat for *N gonorrhoeae* and *C trachomatis* infection for 10–21 days
  - Consider examination and treatment of sexual partners
  - In men over age 40, treat for Enterobacteriaceae for 21–28 days
  - Analgesics and bed rest with elevation and support of scrotum

11

- **Pearl**

  Have a low threshold for ordering a VDRL and testing for HIV.

Reference

National guideline for the management of epididymo-orchitis. Clinical Effectiveness Group (Association of Genitourinary Medicine and the Medical Society for the Study of Venereal Diseases). Sex Transm Infect 1999; 75(Suppl 1):S51. [PMID: 10616385]

Testicular Torsion

- ■ **Essentials of Diagnosis**
  - Usually occurs in males under 25 years of age; may present as an acute abdomen
  - Sudden onset of severe, unilateral scrotal or inguinal pain
  - Exquisitely tender and swollen testicle and spermatic cord; pain worsened with elevation
  - Leukocytosis and pyuria
  - Technetium Tc 99m sodium pertechnetate scan shows decreased uptake on the affected side (versus increased uptake with epididymitis)
  - Doppler ultrasonography confirms diagnosis

- ■ **Differential Diagnosis**
  - Epididymitis
  - Orchitis
  - Testicular trauma
  - Testicular tumor

- ■ **Treatment**
  - Inability to rule out testicular torsion requires surgical consult
  - Diagnostic confirmation requires immediate surgery

- ■ **Pearl**

Probably the diagnosis least easily forgotten by the affected patient in all of medicine.

Reference

Galejs LE: Diagnosis and treatment of the acute scrotum. Am Fam Physician 1999;59:817. [PMID: 10068706]

Benign Prostatic Hyperplasia

- **Essentials of Diagnosis**
  - Urinary hesitancy, intermittent stream, straining to initiate micturition, reduced force and caliber of the urinary stream, nocturia, frequency, urgency
  - Palpably enlarged prostate
  - Hematuria, pyuria when infection complicates
  - High postvoid residual volume as determined by ultrasonography or excretory urography; not always prognostic of outcome
  - May be complicated by acute urinary retention or azotemia following prolonged obstruction

- **Differential Diagnosis**
  - Urethral stricture
  - Vesicular stone
  - Neurogenic bladder
  - Prostate cancer
  - Bladder tumor

- **Treatment**
  - Treat associated infection if present; trimethoprim-sulfamethoxazole is usually best
  - Minimize evening fluid intake
  - Alpha$_1$-blockers for symptom relief; androgen suppression (finasteride) in certain populations
  - Utilization of symptom scoring instruments to follow success of treatment
  - Transurethral resection for intolerable symptoms, refractory urinary retention, recurrent gross hematuria, and progressive renal insufficiency with demonstrated obstruction

- **Pearl**

In acute urinary retention in older men, ask about recent upper respiratory infections; anticholinergic medications in over-the-counter remedies may be the answer.

Reference

Ramsey EW: Office treatment of benign prostatic hyperplasia. Urol Clin North Am 1998;25:571. [PMID: 10026766]

RENAL DISORDERS

Acute Renal Failure

- ■ Essentials of Diagnosis
  - When not otherwise qualified, usually synonymous with acute tubular necrosis
  - Anorexia with nausea, lethargy, headache, confusion
  - History can include exposure to nephrotoxic agents, sepsis, trauma, surgery, shock, or hemorrhage
  - Oliguria in many patients
  - Pericardial friction rub, asterixis may be present
  - Azotemia with increased potassium and phosphate, decreased serum bicarbonate
  - Inability to retain sodium
  - Kidneys of normal size or enlarged on imaging studies; renal osteodystrophy absent
  - Hematuria, proteinuria, and isosthenuria with renal tubular casts

- ■ Differential Diagnosis
  - Prerenal azotemia (eg, cirrhosis, nephrosis, heart failure, hypovolemia)
  - Postrenal azotemia (eg, obstructive uropathy)

- ■ Treatment
  - Volume resuscitation with isotonic fluid for hypovolemia
  - Ultrasonography to rule out obstructive process
  - Possible renal biopsy (eg, if cause unknown or glomerulonephritis suspected)
  - Supportive care for uncomplicated cases: minimize fluid intake, follow potassium and bicarbonate levels
  - Oliguric renal failure with worse prognosis than a nonoliguric process; role of diuretics to convert to latter process recommended but unproved
  - Dialysis for fluid overload, hyperkalemia, pericarditis, symptoms of uremia
  - Adjust dosage of medications for reduced glomerular filtration rate

- ■ Pearl

If a contrast study is performed in acute renal failure (however inappropriately), capture the first specimen thereafter—it has the highest yield for casts, which are diagnostic.

Reference

Agrawal M et al: Acute renal failure. Am Fam Physician 2000;61:2077. [PMID: 10779250]

11

Chronic Renal Insufficiency

■ Essentials of Diagnosis
- End stage of many glomerular or interstitial diseases
- Malaise, headaches, anorexia, nausea, hiccups, pruritus, occasional polyuria and nocturia
- Hypertension, hyperpnea, pallor; signs of congestive heart failure common
- Progressive azotemia over weeks to years
- Anemia, azotemia, and metabolic acidosis; hyperkalemia in oliguric patients, hyperphosphatemia, hypocalcemia, isosthenuria; benign urinary sediment with possible broad waxy casts
- Bilateral shrunken kidneys on imaging studies; exceptions include polycystic kidney disease, diabetic nephropathy, myeloma kidney, HIV-associated nephropathy
- Renal osteodystrophy

■ Differential Diagnosis
- Obstructive uropathy
- Acute renal failure
- Prerenal azotemia
- Drug toxicity

■ Treatment
- Attention to comorbid factors, especially hypertension
- Low-protein diet, salt and water restriction for patients with hypertension and edema, multivitamin and folic acid supplements
- Potassium, phosphorus, and magnesium restriction once GFR is below approximately mL/min
- Phosphorus binders for associated hyperphosphatemia with avoidance of chronic aluminum hydroxide if possible; calcium and vitamin D supplements if needed to prevent osteodystrophy; aim for intact parathyroid hormone of two to three times normal values
- Dialysis (peritoneal or hemodialysis) for end-stage renal disease
- Renal transplantation for all eligible patients

■ Pearl

Untreated chronic renal insufficiency is the cause of the highest PTH levels in clinical medicine.

Reference

McCarthy JT: A practical approach to the management of patients with chronic renal failure. Mayo Clin Proc 1999;74:269. [PMID: 10089997]

Acute Glomerulonephritis

- **Essentials of Diagnosis**
  - History of preceding streptococcal or other infection, evidence of systemic vasculitis may be present
  - Malaise, headache, fever, dark urine
  - Hypertension, edema, and retinal hemorrhages typical
  - Azotemia in all save mesangial nephropathy; moderate proteinuria, low fractional excretion of sodium, and hematuria with or without dysmorphic red cells and red cell casts
  - Depending on the history, further tests may include complement levels (CH50, C3, C4), antistreptolysin O (ASO) titer, antideoxyribonuclease B (anti-DNA B) titer, antinuclear antibody (ANA) titers, anti-GBM antibody levels, anti-neutrophil cytoplasmic antibodies, hepatitis B and C antibodies, cryoglobulins, and renal biopsy to establish cause

- **Differential Diagnosis**
  - IgA nephropathy
  - Goodpasture's syndrome (anti-GBM antibody syndrome)
  - Other vasculitides (eg, polyarteritis nodosa, SLE)
  - Membranoproliferative glomerulonephritis
  - Hepatitis B- or C-associated glomerulonephritis, other post-infectious glomerulonephritides
  - Infective endocarditis
  - Wegener's granulomatosis
  - Henoch-Schönlein purpura

- **Treatment**
  - Steroids and cytotoxic agents are used for rapidly progressive glomerulonephritis, more effective at higher GFRs
  - Plasmapheresis occasionally of value in anti-GBM disease
  - Lower blood pressure slowly to prevent sudden decreases in renal perfusion
  - Supportive therapy with fluid and sodium restriction
  - Monitor for malignant hypertension, congestive heart failure

- **Pearl**

A red cell cast indicates glomerulonephritis; a urine specimen after 1000 mL of water and an hour of lordosis increases the yield.

Reference

Couser WG: Glomerulonephritis. Lancet 1999;353:1509. (PMID: 99247293)

Nephrotic Syndrome

- **Essentials of Diagnosis**
  - May be primary or secondary: systemic infections (such as secondary syphilis, malaria, endocarditis), diabetes, multiple myeloma with or without amyloidosis, heavy metals, and autoimmune diseases
  - Anorexia, dyspnea, anasarca, foamy urine
  - Proteinuria (> 3.5 g/24h), hypoalbuminemia (< 3 g/dL), edema, hyperlipidemia in < 50% upon presentation
  - Hypoalbuminemia may cause ascites, hydrothorax, anasarca, and pulmonary edema, particularly when serum albumin < 2 g/dL
  - Hypercoagulability with peripheral renal vein thrombosis
  - Lipiduria with oval fat bodies, Maltese crosses, and fatty and waxy casts in urinary sediment
  - Depending on the history, further tests may include complement levels (CH50, C3, C4), serum and urine electrophoresis, antinuclear antibody (ANA), renal ultrasound, and renal biopsy if treatment implications present

- **Differential Diagnosis**
  - Congestive heart failure
  - Cirrhosis
  - Constrictive pericarditis
  - Hypothyroidism

- **Treatment**
  - Supportive therapy with fluid and sodium restriction, lipid-lowering agents
  - Low-protein diet (unless urinary protein loss exceeds 10 g/24 h; then, additional dietary protein to match losses)
  - When diabetes is present, consider ACE inhibitor even if renal function is decreased
  - Corticosteroids for minimal change disease (lipoid nephrosis); in focal and segmental glomerular sclerosis, longer courses of steroid therapy are beneficial; membranous nephropathy is best treated with corticosteroids and cytotoxic agents; in membranoproliferative glomerulonephropathy, steroid use is less well established

- **Pearl**

Unexplained membranous glomerulonephritis in patients over 50 suggests a paraneoplastic response to a visceral malignancy.

Reference

Orth SR et al: The nephrotic syndrome. N Engl J Med 1998;338:1202. [PMID: 9554862]

IgA Nephropathy (Berger's Disease)

■ Essentials of Diagnosis

- Most common form of acute and chronic glomerulonephritis in the USA and Asian countries
- Focal proliferative glomerulonephritis of unknown cause
- First episode: macroscopic hematuria, often associated with a viral infection, with or without upper respiratory and gastrointestinal symptoms
- Recurrent hematuria and mild proteinuria over decades, with same precipitants
- Serum IgA increased in 30–50%; renal biopsy reveals inflammation and deposition of IgA with or without C3 and IgM in the mesangium of all glomeruli
- Usually indolent; 20–30% of patients progress to end-stage renal disease over 2–3 decades

■ Differential Diagnosis

- Poststreptococcal acute glomerulonephritis
- Infective endocarditis
- Goodpasture's syndrome
- Other vasculitides (eg, polyarteritis nodosa, SLE)
- Wegener's granulomatosis
- Henoch-Schönlein purpura

■ Treatment

- Supportive therapy for patients with < 1 g/d of proteinuria with yearly monitoring of renal function
- In patients with proteinuria > 1g/d, decrease with ACE inhibitors
- Fish oil of questionable benefit but not harmful
- Steroids in selected causes

■ Pearl

Berger's disease is not Buerger's disease—the latter is thromboangiitis obliterans.

Reference

Julian BA: Treatment of IgA nephropathy. Semin Nephrol 2000;20:277. [PMID: 10855937]

Anti-Glomerular Basement Membrane Nephritis (Goodpasture's Syndrome)

- **Essentials of Diagnosis**
  - Triad of pulmonary hemorrhage with hemoptysis, circulating anti-GBM antibody, and glomerulonephritis due to anti-GBM
  - Most common in young (18–30) and middle-aged (50–60s) white men; smokers also have a predilection
  - Extrarenal manifestations may be absent
  - On immunofluorescence, renal biopsy reveals linear deposition of IgG with or without C3 deposition along the glomerular basement membrane
  - Serum anti-GBM antibody is pathognomonic

- **Differential Diagnosis**
  - Wegener's granulomatosis
  - Other vasculitides (eg, polyarteritis nodosa, SLE)
  - Endocarditis
  - Postinfectious glomerulonephritis
  - Primary pulmonary hemorrhage

- **Treatment**
  - Plasmapheresis to remove circulating anti-GBM antibody
  - Prednisone and cyclophosphamide for at least 3 months
  - Recovery of renal function more likely if treatment is begun prior to a serum creatinine of 6–7 mg/dL; hemodialysis as necessary
  - Renal transplant delayed for 3–6 months after disappearance of antibody from the serum

- **Pearl**

One of the few causes in medicine of a dramatically elevated D_{LCO}.

Reference

Kalluri R: Goodpasture syndrome. Kidney Int 1999;55:1120. [PMID: 10027952]

Acute & Chronic Tubulointerstitial Nephritis

- **Essentials of Diagnosis**
  - Responsible for 10–15% of cases of acute renal failure
  - Most drug-related (beta-lactam antibiotics or NSAIDs), but may be idiopathic or, rarely, associated with infections such as legionellosis and leptospirosis
  - Sudden decrease in renal function, associated with fever, maculopapular rash, and eosinophilia; flank pain may be present
  - Hematuria, pyuria, proteinuria, white blood cell casts, and occasionally eosinophils in urine (Wright's stain necessary)
  - Chronic tubulointerstitial nephritis characterized by polyuria and nocturia, salt wasting, mild proteinuria, small kidneys, isosthenuria, hyperchloremic metabolic acidosis
  - Chronic form may result from prolonged obstruction, analgesic abuse, sickle cell trait, chronic hypercalcemia, uric acid nephropathy, or exposure to heavy metals

- **Differential Diagnosis**
  - Acute or chronic glomerulonephritis
  - Prerenal azotemia
  - Primary obstructive uropathy

- **Treatment**
  - Discontinue all possible offending drugs or treat associated infection in patients with acute tubulointerstitial nephritis
  - Corticosteroids of debatable benefit but often used if renal function does not improve shortly after discontinuation of drug
  - Temporary dialysis may be necessary in up to one-third of patients with drug-induced acute interstitial nephritis

- **Pearl**

In ill-defined pain syndromes (headache, low back pain) with moderate renal insufficiency, over-the-counter analgesics used to great excess by the patient may be the culprit.

Reference

Rastegar A et al: The clinical spectrum of tubulointerstitial nephritis. Kidney Int 1998;54:313. [PMID: 9690108]

Uric Acid Nephropathy

- **Essentials of Diagnosis**
  - Three distinct syndromes; terminology confusing
  - Uric acid nephrolithiasis: Radiolucent urate stones in 3% of patients with gout
  - Gouty kidney: interstitial sodium urate crystals of uncertain significance in patients with gout and interstitial nephropathy; no correlation with degree of elevation of serum uric acid
  - Uric acid nephropathy: uric acid sludge within nephron due to cellular necrosis, typically after chemotherapy, in patients without previous gout

- **Differential Diagnosis**
  - Renal failure due to other cause
  - Hypertensive nephrosclerosis
  - Nephrolithiasis due to other cause
  - Myeloma kidney

- **Treatment**
  - Depends upon syndrome
  - Intravenous hydration and alkalinization of urine for uric acid stones
  - Pretreatment with allopurinol and intravenous hydration for selected patients receiving chemotherapy; maintain urine pH > 6.5 and urine output > 2 L/d
  - In patients with gout, allopurinol and colchicine adjusted for renal function; NSAID use minimized in patients with renal dysfunction

- **Pearl**

Remember aspirin and uric acid; at low dose (< 3 g/d), aspirin causes hyperuricemia because of blockage of secretion; at higher doses, all transport is impaired and extreme hypouricemia ensues.

Reference

Reiter L et al: Familial hyperuricemic nephropathy. Am J Kidney Dis 1995; 25:235. [PMID: 7847350]

Obstructive Nephropathy

- **Essentials of Diagnosis**
  - Most cases are postvesical and usually of prostatic origin
  - A few cases result from bilateral ureteral obstruction, usually from stones
  - Postvesical obstruction presents with nocturia, incontinence, malaise, nausea, with normal 24-hour urine output but in swings
  - Renal ultrasound localizes site of obstruction with proximal tract dilation and hydronephrosis
  - Spectrum of causes includes anatomic abnormalities, stricture, tumor, prostatic hypertrophy, bilateral renal stones, drug effect (methysergide), and neuromuscular disorders

- **Differential Diagnosis**
  - Prerenal azotemia
  - Interstitial nephritis
  - Acute or chronic renal failure due to any cause

- **Treatment**
  - Urinary catheter or ultrasonography to rule out obstruction secondary to enlarged prostate
  - Nephrostomy tubes if significant bilateral hydronephrosis present with bilateral ureteral obstruction
  - Treatment of concurrent infection if present
  - Observe for postobstructive diuresis; can be brisk

- **Pearl**

One stone can cause obstructive nephropathy—in the one in 500 patients born with a single kidney.

Reference

Klahr S: Obstructive nephropathy. Intern Med 2000;39:355. [PMID: 10830173]

Myeloma Kidney

- ■ Essentials of Diagnosis
  - • May be initial presentation of multiple myeloma
  - • The systemic disease with easily the most renal and metabolic complications
  - • Classic definition: Light chain of immunoglobulins (Bence Jones proteins) directly toxic to tubules, or causing tubular obstruction by precipitation
  - • Myeloma may also be associated with glomerular amyloidosis, hypercalcemia, nephrocalcinosis, nephrolithiasis, plasma cell infiltration of the renal parenchyma, hyperviscosity syndrome compromising renal blood flow, proximal (Fanconi-like syndrome) or distal renal tubular acidosis, type IV renal tubular acidosis, and progressive renal insufficiency
  - • Serum anion gap is low in the majority due to positively charged paraprotein
  - • Serum and urinary electrophoresis reveals monoclonal spike in over 90% of patients; some cases are nonsecretory and are very aggressive clinically

- ■ Differential Diagnosis
  - • Interstitial nephritis
  - • Prerenal azotemia
  - • Obstructive nephropathy
  - • Nephrotic syndrome of other cause
  - • Drug-induced nephropathy

- ■ Treatment
  - • Therapy for myeloma; prognosis for renal survival is better if serum creatinine is < 2 mg/dL prior to treatment
  - • Treat hypertension and hypercalcemia if present
  - • Avoid contrast agents and other nephrotoxins
  - • Avoid dehydration and maintain adequate intravascular volume; remember that hypercalcemia causes nephrogenic diabetes insipidus, and this worsens dehydration

- ■ Pearl

The urine dipstick detects only albumin and intact globulin; light chains are missed even when present in large amounts.

Reference

Goldschmidt H et al: Multiple myeloma and renal failure. Nephrol Dial Transplant 2000;15:301. [PMID: 10652511]

11

Polycystic Kidney Disease

- **Essentials of Diagnosis**
  - Autosomal dominant inheritance and nearly complete penetrance, thus strikingly positive family history
  - Abdominal or flank pain associated with hematuria, frequent urinary tract infections, and positive family history
  - Hypertension, large palpable kidneys, positive family history
  - Renal insufficiency in 50% of patients by age 70; unlikely to develop renal disease if no cystic renal lesions by age 30
  - Normal hematocrits common: the cysts may elaborate erythropoietin
  - Diagnosis confirmed by ultrasonography or CT scan
  - Increased incidence of cerebral aneurysms (10% of affected patients), aortic aneurysms, and abnormalities of the mitral valve; 40–50% have concomitant hepatic cysts

- **Differential Diagnosis**
  - Renal cell carcinoma
  - Simple renal cysts
  - Other causes of chronic renal failure

11

- **Treatment**
  - Treat hypertension and nephrolithiasis
  - Observe for urinary tract infection
  - Low-protein diet
  - High fluid intake
  - Patients with family history of cerebral aneurysm should have screening abdominal CT
  - Occasional nephrectomy required for repeated episodes of pain and infection
  - Excellent outcome with transplant

- **Pearl**

Hypertension, an abdominal mass, and azotemia is polycystic disease until proved otherwise.

Reference

Torres VE: New insights into polycystic kidney disease and its treatment. Curr Opin Nephrol Hypertens 1998;7:159. [PMID: 9529618]

Renal Tubular Acidosis

- **Essentials of Diagnosis**
  - Unexplained metabolic acidosis with a normal anion gap
  - Type I (distal): inability to acidify urine, hypokalemia, abnormal (positive) urinary anion gap; may be familial (autosomal dominant) or secondary to autoimmune disease, obstructive uropathy, drugs (eg, amphotericin B), hyperglobulinemia, hypercalciuria, or sickle cell anemia
  - Type II (proximal): bicarbonaturia, glycosuria, hypokalemia, aminoaciduria, phosphaturia, and uricosuria due to impaired absorption; may be secondary to myeloma, drugs, or renal transplant
  - Type IV: low renin and aldosterone; hyperkalemia, abnormal (positive) urinary anion gap; typical of renal insufficiency; others due to diabetes mellitus, drugs (eg, ACE inhibitors, NSAIDs, cyclosporine), chronic interstitial nephritis, or nephrosclerosis

- **Differential Diagnosis**
  - Fanconi's syndrome
  - Diarrhea
  - Ileal loop constriction after surgery for bladder cancer
  - Hypokalemia or hyperkalemia from other causes

- **Treatment**
  - Discontinue offending drug or treat underlying disease if present
  - Bicarbonate or citrate and potassium replacement for types I and II
  - Vitamin D analogs for type I to prevent osteomalacia, not type II because of possible hypercalcemia and further damage to the distal tubule
  - Thiazides may increase bicarbonate reabsorption for type II
  - Fludrocortisone for type IV only if volume repletion is difficult

- **Pearl**

Along with SIADH, type II renal tubular acidosis is one of the few causes of hypouricemia in all of medicine.

Reference

Smulders YM et al: Renal tubular acidosis. Pathophysiology and diagnosis. Arch Intern Med 1996;156:1629. [PMID: 8694660]

Acute Cystitis & Pyelonephritis

- **Essentials of Diagnosis**
  - Dysuria with urinary frequency and urgency, abdominal or flank pain
  - Fever, flank or suprapubic tenderness, and vomiting with pyelonephritis
  - Pyuria, bacteriuria, hematuria, positive urine culture, white cell casts on urinalysis (latter in pyelonephritis)
  - Usually caused by gram-negative bacteria (eg, *E coli*, proteus, klebsiella, Enterobacteriaceae) but may be due to gram-positive organisms (eg, *Enterococcus faecalis, Staphylococcus saprophyticus*)

- **Differential Diagnosis**
  - Urethritis
  - Nephrolithiasis
  - Prostatitis
  - Pelvic inflammatory disease or vaginosis
  - Lower lobe pneumonia
  - Surgical abdomen due to any cause, eg, appendicitis

- **Treatment**
  - Empiric oral antibiotics (eg, trimethoprim-sulfamethoxazole, cephalexin, or ciprofloxacin) for 3 days for uncomplicated cystitis
  - Oral or intravenous antibiotics (eg, fluoroquinolone or cephalosporin) for 7–14 days for pyelonephritis
  - Intravenous antibiotics and fluids if dehydration or vomiting present
  - Pyridium for early symptomatic relief
  - Consider hospitalization for patients with single kidney or immunosuppression
  - Pursue evaluation for anatomic abnormalities in men who develop cystitis or pyelonephritis
  - Recurrent episodes of cystitis (more than two per year) often treated with low-dose prophylactic antibiotics

- **Pearl**

Pyelonephritis is one of the reasons no one should have an exploratory laparotomy without a urinalysis.

Reference

Roberts JA: Management of pyelonephritis and upper urinary tract infections. Urol Clin North Am 1999;26:753. [PMID: 10584616]

Asymptomatic Bacteriuria

- **Essentials of Diagnosis**
  - History of recurring urinary tract infections may be present
  - Bacteriuria with absence of symptoms or signs referable to the urinary tract
  - May be associated with obstruction, anatomic or neurologic abnormalities, pregnancy, indwelling catheter, urologic procedures, diverted urinary stream (eg, ileal loop conduit), diabetes, or old age
  - Usually caused by Enterobacteriaceae, pseudomonas, or enterococci

- **Differential Diagnosis**
  - Drug-induced nephropathy, especially analgesics
  - Contaminated urine specimen

- **Treatment**
  - Indications for treatment include pregnancy, persistent bacteriuria in certain patients and prior to urologic procedures
  - Urine culture to guide antimicrobial therapy
  - Surgical relief of obstruction if present
  - In selected cases, chronic antibiotic suppression

- **Pearl**

Most patients with asymptomatic bacteriuria should not *be given antibiotics.*

Reference

Nicolle LE: Asymptomatic bacteriuria in the elderly. Infect Dis Clin North Am 1997;11:647. [PMID: 9378928]

Lupus Nephritis

- **Essentials of Diagnosis**
  - Can be the initial presentation of systemic lupus erythematosus
  - WHO classification of renal biopsy: normal renal biopsy (class I); mesangial proliferation (class II); focal proliferation (class III); diffuse proliferation (class IV); membranous (class V)
  - Proteinuria or hematuria of glomerular origin; hypocomplementemic common
  - Glomerular filtration rate need not be depressed
  - Chronic changes on biopsy portend a worse prognosis

- **Differential Diagnosis**
  - Glomerulonephritis due to other diseases, including anti-GBM disease, microscopic polyarteritis, Wegener's membranous nephropathy, IgA nephropathy
  - Nephrotic syndrome due to other causes

- **Treatment**
  - Follow serial measures of renal function and urinalysis
  - Strict control of hypertension
  - ACE inhibitor to reduce proteinuria
  - Steroids and cytotoxic agents for severe class III or any class IV
  - Repeat biopsy for flare of renal disease
  - Upon reaching end-stage renal disease, renal transplantation is an excellent alternative to dialysis

- **Pearl**

The kidney is not involved when SLE is drug-induced.

Reference

Mojcik CF et al: End-stage renal disease and systemic lupus erythematosus. Am J Med 1996;101:100. [PMID: 8686702]

Hypertensive Nephrosclerosis

- ■ Essentials of Diagnosis
  - Poorly controlled hypertension for over 15 years; alternatively, severe, aggressive hypertension, especially in young blacks
  - With extreme blood pressure elevation, papilledema and encephalopathy may occur
  - Ultrasound reveals bilateral small, echogenic kidneys
  - Proteinuria is usual
  - Biopsy can show thickened vessels and sclerotic glomeruli; malignant nephrosclerosis reveals characteristic onion-skinning

- ■ Differential Diagnosis
  - Atheroembolic or atherosclerotic renal disease
  - Renal artery stenosis, especially bilateral
  - End-stage renal disease due to any other cause

- ■ Treatment
  - Strict sodium restriction
  - Aggressive control of hypertension, including ACE inhibitor if possible
  - If patient presents with hypertensive urgency or emergency, decrease blood pressure slowly over several days to prevent decreased renal perfusion
  - May take up to 6 months of adequate blood pressure control to achieve improved baseline of renal function

- ■ Pearl

In benign nephrosclerosis, the rule is for serum creatinine to rise after beginning therapy. Stay the course with blood pressure control and improved renal function will follow.

Reference

Luke RG: Hypertensive nephrosclerosis: pathogenesis and prevalence. Essential hypertension is an important cause of end-stage renal disease. Nephrol Dial Transplant 199914:2271. [PMID: 10568241]

Diabetic Nephropathy

- **Essentials of Diagnosis**
  - Seen in diabetes mellitus of 15–20 years' duration
  - Diabetic retinopathy almost always present
  - GFR increases initially, returns to normal as further renal damage occurs, then continues to fall
  - Proteinuria > 1 g/d, often nephrotic range
  - Normal to enlarged kidneys on ultrasound
  - Biopsy can show mesangial matrix expansion, diffuse glomerulosclerosis and nodular intercapillary glomerulosclerosis, the latter pathognomonic

- **Differential Diagnosis**
  - Nephrotic syndrome due to other cause, especially amyloidosis
  - Glomerulonephritis with nephrotic features such as that seen in systemic lupus erythematosus, membranous glomerulonephritis, or IgA nephropathy

- **Treatment**
  - ACE inhibition or, probably, angiotensin II receptor blockade early may reduce hyperfiltration
  - Strict glycemic and blood pressure control
  - Supportive care for progression of chronic renal insufficiency—includes treatment of anemia, avoidance of renal osteodystrophy
  - Protein restriction has been advocated but not proved in clinical trials
  - Transplantation an alternative to dialysis at end stage, but comorbid vasculopathy can be daunting

- **Pearl**

One of medicine's few causes of massive albuminuria sustained in the end stages of renal function.

Reference

Ritz E et al: Nephropathy in patients with type 2 diabetes mellitus. N Engl J Med 1999;341:1127. [PMID:10511612]

12

Neurologic Diseases

Migraine Headache

- **Essentials of Diagnosis**
  - Onset in adolescence or early adulthood
  - Classic pattern: lateralized, unilateral throbbing pain, with prodrome including nausea, photophobia, scotomas
  - May be triggered by stress, foods (chocolate, red wine), birth control pills
  - Basilar artery variant: profound visual disturbances, dysequilibrium, followed by occipital headache
  - Ophthalmic variant: painless loss of vision, scotomas, usually unilateral

- **Differential Diagnosis**
  - Tension headache
  - Cluster headache
  - Giant cell arteritis
  - Subarachnoid hemorrhage
  - Mass lesion, eg, tumor or abscess

- **Treatment**
  - Avoidance of precipitating factors
  - Acute treatment: triptans, ergotamine with caffeine; analgesics (preferably at onset of prodrome)
  - Maintenance therapy includes NSAIDs, propranolol, amitriptyline, ergotamine, valproic acid

- **Pearl**

Interesting etymology: hemi *(mi)* cranium *(graine), a linguistic corruption here indicating the unilaterality of the process.*

Reference

Ferrari MD: Migraine. Lancet 1998;351:1043. [PMID: 9546526]

Idiopathic Epilepsy

- **Essentials of Diagnosis**
  - Abrupt onset of paroxysmal, transitory, recurrent alterations of central nervous system function, often accompanied by alteration in consciousness
  - Family history may be present
  - Generalized tonic-clonic (grand mal): loss of consciousness, generalized motor convulsions; altered mentation or focal abnormalities may persist for up to 48 hours postictally
  - Partial seizures: focal motor convulsions or altered consciousness (complex); may become generalized
  - Absence seizures may be manifested only as episodic inattention, usually in children
  - Characteristic EEG during seizures; often abnormal during interictal periods

- **Differential Diagnosis**
  - Seizures due to metabolic disorders (electrolyte disturbance), toxins (alcohol, cocaine), or vascular, infectious, neoplastic, or immunologic disease
  - Syncope
  - Narcolepsy
  - Psychiatric abnormalities (hysteria, panic attack)
  - Stroke (when patient first seen postictally)
  - Hypoglycemia

- **Treatment**
  - Phenytoin, carbamazepine, and valproic acid for most types of epilepsy
  - Newer generation anticonvulsants and phenobarbital may be helpful in patients unresponsive to other medications
  - For absence seizures, ethosuximide, valproic acid, and clonazepam are useful
  - Status epilepticus is treated as a medical emergency with intravenous diazepam or lorazepam and phenytoin; general anesthesia with barbiturates or halothane may be necessary in refractory cases

- **Pearl**

Remember subclinical epilepsy in critically ill and unconscious patients. EEG may reveal status epilepticus.

Reference

Feely M: Fortnightly review: drug treatment of epilepsy. BMJ 1999; 318:106. [PMID: 9880286]

Ischemic & Hemorrhagic Stroke

- **■ Essentials of Diagnosis**
  - May have history of atherosclerotic heart disease, hypertension, diabetes, valvular heart disease, or atrial fibrillation
  - Sudden onset of neurologic complaint, variably including focal weakness, sensory abnormalities, visual change, language defect, or altered mentation
  - Neurologic signs dependent on vessels involved: hemiplegia, hemianopia, and aphasia in anterior circulatory involvement; cranial nerve abnormalities, quadriplegia, cerebellar findings in posterior circulatory disease; hyperreflexia in both, but may be delayed
  - Deficits persist > 24 hours; if resolution in < 24 hours, transient ischemic attack or other process is present
  - CT of the head may be normal in the first 24 hours, depending on cause; hemorrhage visible immediately; MRI a superior imaging modality in posterior fossa

- **■ Differential Diagnosis**
  - Primary or metastatic brain tumor
  - Subdural or epidural hematoma
  - Brain abscess
  - Multiple sclerosis
  - Any metabolic abnormality, especially hypoglycemia
  - Neurosyphilis
  - Seizure (and postictal state)
  - Migraine

- **■ Treatment**
  - Control of contributing factors, especially hypertension and hypercholesterolemia
  - Tissue plasminogen activator (t-PA) for selected patients with ischemic stroke who can be treated within 3 hours after onset
  - Anticoagulation for stroke due to cardiac emboli
  - Aspirin, clopidogrel, or the combination dipyridamole and aspirin for thrombotic stroke
  - Carotid endarterectomy may be considered later in selected patients

- **■ Pearl**

A stroke is never a stroke unless it's had 50 of D50.

Reference

Brott T et al: Treatment of acute ischemic stroke. N Engl J Med 2000;343:710. [PMID: 10974136]

Intracranial Aneurysms & Subarachnoid Hemorrhage

- **Essentials of Diagnosis**
  - Asymptomatic until expansion or rupture; sometimes preceded by abrupt onset of headaches that resolve (sentinel leaks)
  - Rupture characterized by sudden, severe headache, altered mental status, photophobia, nuchal rigidity, and vomiting
  - Focal neurologic signs unusual except for third nerve palsy with posterior communicating artery aneurysm
  - Multiple in 20% of cases; associated with polycystic renal disease, coarctation of aorta, fibromuscular dysplasia
  - CT scan or bloody cerebrospinal fluid confirmatory; MRI or MRA may reveal aneurysm; cerebral angiography indicates size, location, and number

- **Differential Diagnosis**
  - Primary or metastatic intracranial tumor
  - Hypertensive intraparenchymal hemorrhage
  - Ruptured arteriovenous malformation
  - Tension headache
  - Migraine headache
  - Meningitis

- **Treatment**
  - Nimodipine (calcium channel blocker) may reduce neurologic deficits
  - Induced hypertension and intracranial angioplasty may be useful for treating vasospasm, which often accompanies subarachnoid hemorrhage
  - Definitive therapy with surgical clipping or endovascular coil embolization of aneurysm if anatomy suitable and if patient's functional status is otherwise acceptable
  - Small unruptured aneurysms may not require treatment

- **Pearl**

When a patient complains of "the worst headache I ever had in my life," it's a ruptured berry aneurysm.

Reference

Edlow JA et al: Avoiding pitfalls in the diagnosis of subarachnoid hemorrhage. N Engl J Med 2000;342:29. [PMID: 10620647]

Arteriovenous Malformations

- **Essentials of Diagnosis**
  - Congenital vascular malformations that consist of arteriovenous communications without intervening capillaries
  - Patients typically under age 30 and normotensive
  - Initial symptoms include acute headache, seizures, abrupt onset of coma—the latter with rupture
  - May also present as transverse myelitis (spinal cord arteriovenous malformation)
  - Up to 70% of arteriovenous malformations bleed during their natural history, most commonly before age 40
  - CT of the brain suggests diagnosis; angiography characteristically diagnostic, but some types (eg, cavernous malformations) may not be visualized; MRI often helpful

- **Differential Diagnosis**
  - Dural arteriovenous fistulas
  - Seizures due to other causes
  - Hypertensive intracerebral hemorrhage
  - Ruptured intracranial aneurysm
  - Intracranial tumor
  - Meningitis or brain abscess
  - Transverse myelopathy due to other causes

- **Treatment**
  - Excision if malformation accessible and neurologic risk not great
  - Endovascular embolization in selected malformations
  - Radiosurgery for small malformations

- **Pearl**

The most common cause of intracranial hemorrhage between ages 15 and 30.

Reference

Arteriovenous malformations of the brain in adults. N Engl J Med 1999; 340:1812. [PMID: 10362826]

Brain Abscess

- **Essentials of Diagnosis**
  - History of sinusitis, otitis, endocarditis, chronic pulmonary infection, or congenital heart defect common
  - Headache, focal neurologic symptoms, seizures may occur
  - Examination may confirm focal findings
  - The most common organisms are streptococci, staphylococci, and anaerobes; toxoplasma in AIDS patients; commonly polymicrobial
  - Ring-enhancing lesion on CT scan or MRI; lumbar puncture potentially dangerous because of mass effect

- **Differential Diagnosis**
  - Primary or metastatic tumor
  - Cerebral infarction
  - Encephalitis
  - Subdural empyema
  - Neurosyphilis

- **Treatment**
  - Intravenous broad-spectrum antibiotics (with coverage to include anaerobic organisms) may be curative if abscess smaller than 2 cm in diameter
  - Surgical aspiration through burr hole if no response to antibiotic drugs, either clinically or by CT scan

- **Pearl**

Frank brain abscess is the least common neurologic manifestation of endocarditis.

Reference

Treatment of brain abscess. Lancet 1988;1:219. [PMID: 2893043]

Pseudotumor Cerebri
(Benign Intracranial Hypertension)

- ■ Essentials of Diagnosis
  - Headache, diplopia, nausea
  - Papilledema, sixth nerve palsy
  - CT scan shows normal or small ventricular system
  - Lumbar puncture with elevated pressure but normal cerebrospinal fluid
  - Associations include sinus thrombosis (transverse or sagittal), endocrinopathy (hypoparathyroidism, Addison's disease), hypervitaminosis A, drugs (tetracyclines, oral contraceptives), chronic pulmonary disease, obesity; often idiopathic
  - Untreated pseudotumor cerebri may lead to secondary optic atrophy and permanent visual loss

- ■ Differential Diagnosis
  - Primary or metastatic tumor
  - Optic neuritis
  - Neurosyphilis
  - Brain abscess or basilar meningitis
  - Chronic meningitis (eg, coccidioidomycosis or cryptococcosis)
  - Vascular headache, migraine headache

- ■ Treatment
  - Treat underlying cause if present
  - Acetazolamide or furosemide to reduce cerebrospinal fluid formation
  - Repeat lumbar puncture with removal of cerebrospinal fluid
  - Oral corticosteroids may be helpful; weight loss in obese patients
  - Surgical therapy with placement of ventriculoperitoneal shunt or optic nerve sheath fenestration in refractory cases

- ■ Pearl

Pseudotumor may not be "pseudo" in women—mammography may indicate a primary breast cancer.

Reference

Radhakrishnan K et al: Idiopathic intracranial hypertension. Mayo Clinic Proc 1994;69:169. [PMID: 8309269]

Parkinson's Disease

- **Essentials of Diagnosis**
  - Insidious onset in older patient of pill-rolling tremor (3–5/s), rigidity, bradykinesia, and progressive postural instability; tremor is the least disabling feature
  - Mask-like facies, cogwheeling of extremities on passive motion; cutaneous seborrhea characteristic
  - Absence of tremor—not uncommon—may delay diagnosis
  - Reflexes normal
  - Mild intellectual deterioration often noted, but concurrent Alzheimer's disease may account for this in many

- **Differential Diagnosis**
  - Essential tremor
  - Phenothiazine, metoclopramide toxicity; also carbon monoxide, manganese poisoning
  - Hypothyroidism
  - Wilson's disease
  - Multiple system atrophy, progressive supranuclear palsy
  - Diffuse Lewy body disease
  - Depression
  - Normal pressure hydrocephalus

- **Treatment**
  - Carbidopa-levodopa is most effective medical regimen in patients with definite disability; dose should be reduced if dystonias occur
  - Dopamine agonists and bromocriptine may be of value as first-line therapy or in permitting reduction of carbidopa-levodopa dose
  - Anticholinergic drugs and amantadine are useful adjuncts
  - Inhibition of monoamine oxidase B with selegiline (L-deprenyl) offers theoretical advantage of preventing progression but not yet established for this indication
  - Surgical options remain highly controversial

- **Pearl**

Autonomic abnormalities early in the course of a parkinsonian syndrome mean the diagnosis is not *Parkinson's disease.*

Reference

Young R: Update on Parkinson's disease. Am Fam Physician 1999;59:2155. [PMID: 10221302]

Huntington's Disease

- **Essentials of Diagnosis**
  - Family history usually present (autosomal dominant)
  - Onset at age 30–50, with gradual progressive chorea and dementia; death usually occurs within 20 years after onset
  - Caused by a trinucleotide-repeat expansion in a gene located on the short arm of chromosome 4
  - The earliest mental changes are often behavioral, including hypersexuality
  - CT scan shows cerebral atrophy, particularly in the caudate

- **Differential Diagnosis**
  - Sydenham's chorea
  - Tardive dyskinesia
  - Lacunar infarcts of subthalamic nuclei
  - Other causes of dementia

- **Treatment**
  - Principally supportive
  - Antidopaminergic agents (eg, haloperidol) or reserpine may reduce severity of movement abnormality
  - Genetic counseling for offspring

- **Pearl**

All movement abnormalities in Huntington's disease disappear when the patient is asleep.

Reference

Ross CA et al: Huntington disease and the related disorder, dentatorubral-pallidoluysian atrophy (DRPLA). Medicine 1997;76:305. [PMID: 9352736]

Tourette's Syndrome

- **Essentials of Diagnosis**
  - Motor and phonic tics; onset in childhood or adolescence
  - Compulsive utterances, often of obscenities, are typical
  - Hyperactivity, nonspecific electroencephalographic abnormalities in 50%
  - Obsessive-compulsive disorder common

- **Differential Diagnosis**
  - Simple tic disorder
  - Wilson's disease
  - Focal seizures

- **Treatment**
  - Haloperidol is the drug of choice
  - Clonazepam, clonidine, phenothiazine, pimozide if intolerant of or resistant to haloperidol
  - Serotonin-specific reuptake inhibitors for obsessive-compulsive symptoms

- **Pearl**

When a child has no neurologic signs other than tics and Wilson's disease has been excluded, think Tourette's syndrome.

Reference

Bagheri MM et al: Recognition and management of Tourette's syndrome and tic disorders. Am Fam Physician 1999;59:2263. [PMID: 10221310]

12

Multiple Sclerosis

- **Essentials of Diagnosis**

  - Patient usually under 50 years of age at onset
  - Episodic symptoms that may include sensory abnormalities, blurred vision due to optic neuritis, sphincter disturbances, and weakness with or without spasticity
  - Neurologic progression to fixed abnormalities occurs variably
  - Single pathologic lesion cannot explain clinical findings
  - Multiple foci in white matter best demonstrated radiographically by MRI
  - Finding of oligoclonal bands or elevated Ig index on lumbar puncture is nonspecific

- **Differential Diagnosis**

  - Vasculitis or systemic lupus erythematosus
  - Small-vessel infarctions
  - Neurosyphilis
  - Optic neuritis due to other causes
  - Primary or metastatic central nervous system neoplasm
  - Cerebellar ataxia due to other causes
  - Pernicious anemia
  - Spinal cord compression or radiculopathy due to mechanical compression
  - Syringomyelia

- **Treatment**

  - Beta-interferon reduces exacerbation rate; copolymer 1 (a random polymer-simulating myelin basic protein) may also be beneficial
  - Steroids may hasten recovery from relapse
  - Treatment with other immunosuppressants may be effective, but role is controversial
  - Symptomatic treatment of spasticity and bladder dysfunction

- **Pearl**

If you diagnose multiple sclerosis in a patient over age 50, diagnose something else.

Reference

Noseworthy JH et al: Multiple sclerosis. N Engl J Medicine 2000;343: 938. [PMID: 11006371]

Syringomyelia

- **Essentials of Diagnosis**
  - Characterized by destruction or degeneration of the gray and white matter adjacent to the central canal of the cervical spinal cord
  - Initial loss of pain and temperature sense with preservation of other sensory function; unrecognized burning or injury of hands a characteristic presentation
  - Weakness, hyporeflexia or areflexia, atrophy of muscles at level of spinal cord involvement (usually upper limbs and hands); hyperreflexia and spasticity at lower levels
  - Thoracic kyphoscoliosis common; associated with Arnold-Chiari malformation
  - Secondary to trauma in some cases
  - MRI confirms diagnosis

- **Differential Diagnosis**
  - Spinal cord tumor or arteriovenous malformation
  - Transverse myelitis
  - Multiple sclerosis
  - Neurosyphilis
  - Degenerative arthritis of the cervical spine

- **Treatment**
  - Surgical decompression of the foramen magnum
  - Syringostomy in selected cases

- **Pearl**

One of the few causes of disassociation of pain and temperature on neurologic examination.

Reference

Schwartz ED et al: Posttraumatic syringomyelia: pathogenesis, imaging, and treatment. AJR Am J Roentgenol 1999;173:487. [PMID: 10430159]

Guillain-Barré Syndrome (Acute Inflammatory Polyneuropathy)

- **Essentials of Diagnosis**
  - Associated with viral infections, stress, and preceding *Campylobacter jejuni* enteritis, but most cases do not have any definite link to pathogens
  - Progressive, usually ascending, symmetric weakness with variable paresthesia or dysesthesia; autonomic involvement (eg, cardiac irregularities, hypertension, or hypotension) may be prominent
  - Electromyography consistent with demyelinating injury; also a less common axonal form
  - Lumbar puncture, normal in early or mild disease, shows high protein, normal cell count later in course

- **Differential Diagnosis**
  - Diphtheria, poliomyelitis (where endemic)
  - Porphyria
  - Heavy metal poisoning
  - Botulism
  - Transverse myelitis of any origin
  - Familial periodic paralysis

- **Treatment**
  - Plasmapheresis or intravenous immunoglobulin
  - Pulmonary functions closely monitored, with intubation of forced vital capacity < 15 mL/kg
  - Respiratory toilet with physical therapy
  - Up to 20% of patients are left with persisting disability

- **Pearl**

The occasional Guillain-Barré may start in the stem and descend—the C. Miller Fischer variant.

Reference

Hahn AF: Guillain-Barré syndrome. Lancet 1998;352:635. [PMID: 9746040]

Bell's Palsy (Idiopathic Facial Paresis)

- **Essentials of Diagnosis**
  - An idiopathic facial paresis
  - Abrupt onset of hemifacial (including the forehead) weakness, difficulty closing eye; ipsilateral ear pain may precede or accompany weakness
  - Unilateral peripheral seventh nerve palsy on examination; taste lost on the anterior two-thirds of the tongue, and hyperacusis may occur

- **Differential Diagnosis**
  - Carotid distribution stroke
  - Intracranial mass lesion
  - Basilar meningitis, especially that associated with sarcoidosis

- **Treatment**
  - Treatment with corticosteroids and acyclovir when it can be initiated early
  - Supportive measures with frequent eye lubrication and nocturnal eye patching
  - Only 10% of patients are dissatisfied with the final outcome of their disability or disfigurement

- **Pearl**

The Bell phenomenon: the eye on the affected side moves superiorly and laterally when the patient closes his eyes.

Reference

Jackson CG et al: The facial nerve. Current trends in diagnosis, treatment, and rehabilitation. Med Clin North Am 1999;83:179. [PMID: 9927969]

Combined System Disease
(Posterolateral Sclerosis)

- ■ Essentials of Diagnosis
  - Numbness (pins and needles), tenderness, weakness; feeling of heaviness in toes, feet, fingers, and hands
  - Stocking and glove distribution of sensory loss in some patients
  - Extensor plantar response and hyperreflexia typical, as is loss of position and vibratory senses
  - Serum vitamin B_{12} level low
  - Megaloblastic anemia may be present but does not parallel neurologic dysfunction

- ■ Differential Diagnosis
  - Tabes dorsalis
  - Multiple sclerosis
  - Transverse myelitis of viral or other origin
  - Epidural tumor or abscess
  - Cervical spondylosis
  - Polyneuropathy due to toxin or metabolic abnormality

- ■ Treatment
  - Vitamin B_{12}

- ■ Pearl

When B_{12} deficiency is the cause, pharmacologic amounts of folic acid may worsen the neurologic picture.

Reference

Clementz GL et al: The spectrum of vitamin B_{12} deficiency. Am Fam Physician 1990;41:150. [PMID: 2278553]

Myasthenia Gravis

- **Essentials of Diagnosis**
  - Symptoms due to a variable degree of block of neuromuscular transmission
  - Fluctuating weakness of most-commonly used muscles; diplopia, dysphagia, ptosis, facial weakness with chewing and speaking
  - Short-acting anticholinesterases transiently increase strength
  - Electromyography and nerve conduction studies demonstrate decremental muscle response to repeated stimuli
  - Associations include thymic tumors, thyrotoxicosis, rheumatoid arthritis, and SLE
  - Elevated acetylcholine receptor antibody assay confirmatory but not completely sensitive

- **Differential Diagnosis**
  - Botulism
  - Lambert-Eaton syndrome
  - Polyneuropathy due to other causes
  - Amyotrophic lateral sclerosis
  - Bulbar poliomyelitis
  - Neuromuscular blocking drug toxicity (aminoglycosides)
  - Primary myopathy, eg, polymyositis

- **Treatment**
  - Anticholinesterase drugs—particularly pyridostigmine—may be effective
  - Thymectomy in an otherwise healthy patient under age 60 if weakness not restricted to extraocular muscles
  - Corticosteroids and immunosuppressants if response to above measures not ideal
  - Plasmapheresis or intravenous immunoglobulin therapy provides short-term benefit in selected patients
  - Avoid aminoglycosides
  - Many other medications may lead to exacerbations

- **Pearl**

Given the day-to-day variability of symptoms, many patients are labeled with a psychiatric diagnosis before myasthenia gravis is considered, let alone diagnosed.

Reference

Keesey J: Myasthenia gravis. Arch Neurol 1998;55:745. [PMID: 9605737]

Periodic Paralysis Syndromes

- **Essentials of Diagnosis**
  - Episodes of flaccid weakness or paralysis with strength normal between attacks
  - Hypokalemic variety: attacks may be prolonged upon awakening, after exercise or after carbohydrate meals; hyperthyroidism commonly associated in Asian men
  - Hyperkalemic variety or normokalemic variety: brief attacks after exercise

- **Differential Diagnosis**
  - Myasthenia gravis
  - Polyneuropathies due to other causes, especially Guillain-Barré syndrome

- **Treatment**
  - Hypokalemic variant: potassium replacement for acute episode; low-carbohydrate, low-salt diet chronically, perhaps acetazolamide prophylactically; treatment of hyperthyroidism, when associated, reduces attacks, as does therapy with beta-blockers
  - Hyperkalemic-normokalemic variant: intravenous calcium, intravenous diuretics useful for acute therapy; prophylactic acetazolamide or thiazides also beneficial

- **Pearl**

Potassium levels as low as can be observed in medicine, yet commonly rise spontaneously before treatment is given.

Reference

Griggs RC et al: Mutations of sodium channels in periodic paralysis: can they explain the disease and predict treatment? Neurology 1999;52:1309. [PMID: 10227611]

Trigeminal Neuralgia (Tic Douloureux)

- **Essentials of Diagnosis**
  - Characterized by momentary episodes of lancinating facial pain that arises from one side of the mouth and shoots toward the ipsilateral eye, ear, or nostril
  - Commonly affects women more than men in mid and later life
  - Triggered by touch, movement, and eating
  - Symptoms are confined to the distribution of the ipsilateral trigeminal nerve (usually the second or third division)
  - Occasionally caused by multiple sclerosis or a brain stem tumor

- **Differential Diagnosis**
  - Atypical facial pain syndrome
  - Glossopharyngeal neuralgia
  - Postherpetic neuralgia
  - Temporomandibular joint dysfunction
  - Angina pectoris
  - Giant cell arteritis
  - Brain stem gliosis

- **Treatment**
  - Either carbamazepine or gabapentin is the drug of choice; if this is ineffective or poorly tolerated, phenytoin, valproic acid, or baclofen can be tried
  - Surgical exploration of posterior fossa successful in selected patients
  - Radiofrequency ablation useful in some

- **Pearl**

The diagnosis can sometimes be made before the patient says a word: a man unshaven unilaterally in the V_2 distribution has tic douloureux until proved otherwise.

Reference

Kumar GK et al: When is facial pain trigeminal neuralgia? Postgrad Med 1998;104:149. [PMID: 9793561]

12

Normal Pressure Hydrocephalus

- **Essentials of Diagnosis**
  - Subacute loss of higher cognitive function
  - Urinary incontinence
  - Gait apraxia
  - In some, history of head trauma or meningitis
  - Normal opening pressure on lumbar puncture
  - Enlarged ventricles without atrophy by CT or MRI

- **Differential Diagnosis**
  - Dementia or incontinence due to other cause
  - Parkinson's disease
  - Alcoholic cerebellar degeneration
  - Wernicke-Korsakoff syndrome
  - Encephalitis

- **Treatment**
  - Lumbar puncture provides temporary amelioration of symptoms
  - Ventriculoperitoneal shunting, most effective when precipitating event is identified and recent

- **Pearl**

An apraxic gait differs from an ataxic gait—-the former is magnetic, as though the floor were a magnet and the patient had shoes with metal soles.

12

Reference

Vanneste JA: Diagnosis and management of normal-pressure hydrocephalus. J Neurol 2000;247:5. [PMID: 10701891]

13

Geriatric Disorders

Dementia

- **Essentials of Diagnosis**
  - Persistent and progressive impairment in intellectual function, including loss of short-term memory, word-finding difficulties, apraxia (inability to perform previously learned tasks), agnosia (inability to recognize objects), and visuospatial problems (becoming lost in familiar surroundings)
  - Behavioral disturbances, psychiatric symptoms common
  - Alzheimer's disease accounts for roughly two-thirds of cases; vascular dementia causes most others

- **Differential Diagnosis**
  - Normal age-related cognitive changes or drug effects
  - Delirium, depression, or other psychiatric disorder
  - Metabolic disorder (eg, hypercalcemia, hyper- and hypothyroidism, or vitamin B_{12} deficiency)
  - Tertiary syphilis
  - Normal-pressure hydrocephalus, subdural hematoma
  - Parkinson's disease
  - Dementia associated with less common disorders, such as Pick's disease, Creutzfeldt-Jakob disease, or AIDS

- **Treatment**
  - Correct sensory deficits, treat underlying disease, remove offending medications, and treat depression, when present
  - Caregiver education, referral to Alzheimer Association, advance care planning early
  - Consider anticholinesterase inhibitor, such as donepezil
  - Treat behavioral problems (eg, agitation) with behavioral interventions or medications directed against target symptom

- **Pearl**

Vitamin B_{12} deficiency can cause reversible dementia without hematologic abnormalities.

Reference

Patterson CJ et al: The recognition, assessment and management of dementing disorders: conclusions from the Canadian Consensus Conference on Dementia. CMAJ 1999;160(12 Suppl):S1. [PMID: 10410645]

Delirium

- **Essentials of Diagnosis**
  - Rapid onset of acute confusional state, usually lasting less than 1 week
  - Fluctuating mental status with marked deficit of short-term memory
  - Inability to concentrate, maintain attention, or sustain purposeful behavior
  - Increased anxiety and irritability
  - Risk factors include dementia, organic brain lesion, alcohol dependence, medications, and various medical problems
  - Mild to moderate delirium at night, often precipitated by hospitalization, drugs, or sensory deprivation ("sundowning")

- **Differential Diagnosis**
  - Depression or other psychiatric disorder
  - Medical condition, such as hypoxemia, hypercalcemia, hyponatremia, infection, thiamin deficiency
  - Subarachnoid hemorrhage
  - Medication side effect
  - Subclinical status epilepticus
  - Pain

- **Treatment**
  - Identify and treat underlying cause
  - Promote restful sleep; keep patient up and interactive during day
  - Frequent reorientation by staff, family, clocks, calendars
  - When medication needed, low-dose haloperidol or atypical antipsychotic, avoid benzodiazepines except in alcohol and benzodiazepine withdrawal
  - Avoid potentially offending medications, particularly anticholinergic and psychoactive medications
  - Avoid restraints, lines, and tubes

- **Pearl**

Delirium tremens is the most flagrant example but also the least common.

Reference

Chan D et al: Delirium: making the diagnosis, improving the prognosis. Geriatrics 1999;54:28. [PMID: 10086025]

Constipation

- **Essentials of Diagnosis**
  - Infrequent stools (less than three times a week)
  - Straining with defecation more than 25% of the time

- **Differential Diagnosis**
  - Normal bowel function that does not match patient expectations of bowel function
  - Anorectal dysfunction
  - Slow bowel transit
  - Dietary factors, including low-calorie diet
  - Obstructing cancer
  - Metabolic disorder, such as hypercalcemia
  - Medications (opioids, iron, calcium channel blockers)

- **Treatment**
  - In absence of pathology, increase fiber and liquid intake
  - In presence of slow transit constipation, stool softeners such as docusate, osmotically active agents such as sorbitol and lactulose
  - In refractory cases or with opioid use, stimulant laxatives (eg, senna) may be necessary
  - In presence of anorectal dysfunction, suppositories often necessary

- **Pearl**

One patient's constipation is another's diarrhea.

13

Reference

Schaefer DC et al: Constipation in the elderly. Am Fam Physician 1998; 58:907. [PMID: 9767726]

Hearing Impairment

■ **Essentials of Diagnosis**

  • Difficulty understanding speech, difficulty listening to television or talking on the telephone, tinnitus, hearing loss limiting personal or social life

  • "Whisper test": patient is unable to repeat numbers whispered in each ear

  • Hearing loss on formal audiologic evaluation (pure tone audiometry, speech reception threshold, bone conduction testing, acoustic reflexes, and tympanometry); hearing loss of >40 dB will cause difficulty understanding normal speech

■ **Differential Diagnosis**

  • Sensorineural hearing loss (presbycusis, ototoxicity due to medications, tumors or infections of cranial nerve VIII, injury by vascular events)

  • Conductive hearing loss (cerumen impaction, otosclerosis, chronic otitis media, Meniere's disease, trauma, tumors)

■ **Treatment**

  • Cerumen removal if impaction present (Debrox, gentle irrigation with warm water)

  • Consider assistive listening devices (telephone amplifiers, low-frequency doorbells, closed-captioned television decoders) and hearing aids

  • Educate family to speak slowly and to face the patient directly when speaking

■ **Pearl**

Impaired hearing and vision may result in pseudodementia due to contraction of the older patient's environment.

Reference

Fook L et al: Hearing impairment in older people: a review. Postgrad Med J 2000;76:537. [PMID: 10964114]

Decubitus Ulcers (Pressure Sores)

- ■ **Essentials of Diagnosis**
    - Ulcers over bony or cartilaginous prominences (sacrum, hips, heels)
    - Stage I (nonblanchable erythema of intact skin); stage II (partial thickness skin loss involving the epidermis or dermis); stage III (full-thickness skin loss extending to the deep fascia); stage IV (full-thickness skin loss involving muscle or bone)
    - Risk factors: immobility, incontinence, malnutrition, cognitive impairment, older age

- ■ **Differential Diagnosis**
    - Herpes simplex virus ulcers
    - Venous insufficiency ulcers
    - Underlying osteomyelitis
    - Ulcerated skin cancer
    - Pyoderma gangrenosum

- ■ **Treatment**
    - Reduce pressure (reposition patient every 2 hours, use specialized mattress)
    - Treat underlying conditions that may prevent wound healing (infection, malnutrition, poor functional status, incontinence, comorbid illnesses)
    - Control pain
    - Select dressing to keep the wound moist and the surrounding tissue intact (hydrocolloids, silver sulfadiazine, or, if heavy exudate, calcium alginate or foams)
    - Perform debridement if necrotic tissue present (wet-to-dry dressings, sharp debridement with scalpel, collagenase, or moisture-retentive dressings)
    - Surgical procedures may be necessary to treat extensive pressure ulcers

- ■ **Pearl**

There is no "early" decubitus; pathogenesis begins from within, and skin loss is the last part of the process.

Reference

Cervo FA et al: Pressure ulcers. Analysis of guidelines for treatment and management. Geriatrics 2000;55:55. [PMID: 10732005]

Weight Loss (Involuntary)

- **Essentials of Diagnosis**
  - Weight loss exceeding 5% in 1 month or 10% in 6 months
  - Weight should be measured regularly and compared with previous measures and normative data for age and gender
  - The cause of weight loss is usually diagnosed by history and physical examination
  - Most useful tests for further evaluation: chest x-ray, complete blood count, serum chemistries (including glucose, thyroid-stimulating hormone, creatinine, calcium, liver function tests, albumin), urinalysis, and fecal occult blood testing

- **Differential Diagnosis**
  - Medical disorders (congestive heart failure, chronic lung disease, chronic renal failure, peptic ulcers, dementia, ill-fitting dentures, dysphagia, malignancy, diabetes mellitus, hyperthyroidism, malabsorption, systemic infections, hospitalization)
  - Social problems (poverty, isolation, inability to shop or prepare food, alcoholism, abuse and neglect, poor knowledge of nutrition, food restrictions)
  - Psychiatric disorders (depression, schizophrenia, bereavement, anorexia nervosa, bulimia)
  - Drug effects (serotonin reuptake inhibitors, NSAIDs, digoxin, antibiotics)

- **Treatment**
  - Directed at underlying cause of weight loss, which is usually multifactorial
  - Frequent meals, hand-feed, protein-calorie supplements
  - Among patients with psychosocial causes of malnutrition, referral to community services such as senior centers
  - "Watchful waiting" when cause is unknown after basic evaluation (25% of cases)
  - Consider enteral tube feedings if treatment would improve quality of life, remembering the importance of identifying goals of care before instituting feedings

- **Pearl**

Pay attention to the definition: gradual weight loss over many years is the rule in older patients, and aggressive evaluation may be harmful.

Reference

Gazewood JD et al: Diagnosis and management of weight loss in the elderly. J Fam Pract 1998;47:19. [PMID: 9673603]

Falls

- ■ Essentials of Diagnosis
  - Frequently not mentioned to physicians
  - Evidence of trauma or fractures, but this may be subtle, especially in the hip
  - Decreased activity, social isolation, or functional decline due to fear of falling or as a result of it

- ■ Differential Diagnosis
  - Visual impairment
  - Gait impairment due to muscular weakness, podiatric disorder, or neurologic dysfunction
  - Environmental hazards such as poor lighting, stairways, rugs, warped floors
  - Polypharmacy (especially with use of sedative-hypnotics)
  - Postural hypotension
  - Presyncope, vertigo, dysequilibrium, and syncope

- ■ Treatment
  - Review need for and encourage proper use of assistive devices (eg, cane, walker)
  - Evaluate and treat for osteoporosis
  - Evaluate vision
  - Review medications
  - Assess home and environmental safety and prescribe modifications as indicated

- ■ Pearl

The occasional older person crawls into bed after a fall causing a hip fracture and stays there, and presents with altered mental status only; look for shortening and external rotation of the hips in all older patients with new-onset dementia.

Reference

Fuller GF: Falls in the elderly. Am Fam Physician 2000;61:2159. [PMID: 10779256]

Polypharmacy

- **Essentials of Diagnosis**
  - Risk factors: older age, cognitive impairment, taking five or more medications, multiple prescribing physicians, and recent discharge from a hospital
  - A medical regimen that includes at least one unnecessary or inappropriate medication, such that the likelihood of adverse effects (from the number or type of medications) exceeds the likelihood of benefit
  - Medications used to prevent illness without improving symptoms have increasingly marginal risk-benefit profiles in patients with limited life expectancies
  - Over-the-counter drugs and vitamin supplements often added on by patient without physician's awareness

- **Differential Diagnosis**
  - Appropriate use of multiple medications to treat older adults for multiple comorbid conditions

- **Treatment**
  - Regularly review all medications, instructions, and indications
  - Keep dosing regimens as simple as possible
  - Avoid managing an adverse drug reaction with another drug
  - Select medications that can treat more than one problem

- **Pearl**

For any new symptom in an older patient, consider medications first.

Reference

Monane M et al: Optimal medication use in elders. Key to successful aging. West J Med 1997;167:233. [PMID: 9348752]

Insomnia

- **Essentials of Diagnosis**
  - Difficulty in initiating or maintaining sleep, or nonrestorative sleep that causes impairment of social or occupational functioning
  - For acute insomnia (< 3 weeks), presence of recent life stress or new medications
  - May be related to a psychiatric disorder, such as major depression or posttraumatic stress disorder

- **Differential Diagnosis**
  - Psychiatric illness (depression, anxiety, mania, psychoses, stress, panic attacks)
  - Drug effect (caffeine, theophylline, serotonin reuptake inhibitors, diuretics, others); withdrawal from sedative-hypnotic medications or alcohol
  - Comorbid disease causing chronic pain, dyspnea, urinary frequency, reflux esophagitis, or delirium
  - Akathisia
  - Noisy environment, excessive daytime napping
  - Disordered circadian rhythms (jet lag, shift work, dementia)

- **Treatment**
  - Treat underlying cause of insomnia by removing or modifying mitigating factors
  - Maintain good sleep hygiene (avoid stimulants, minimize noise, keep regular sleep schedule, avoid daytime naps, exercise regularly)
  - Refer for polysomnography if primary sleep disorder is suspected
  - Consider short-term (< 4 weeks) intermittent use of trazodone or a sedative-hypnotic (eg, zolpidem or a benzodiazepine with short-half-life)
  - Diphenhydramine best avoided because of its anticholinergic side effects

- **Pearl**

The need for sleep diminishes with age, though patients may perceive a need for 8 hours of sleep throughout life.

Reference

Insomnia: assessment and management in primary care. National Heart, Lung, and Blood Institute Working Group on Insomnia. Am Fam Physician 1999;59:3029. [PMID: 10392587]

14

Psychiatric Disorders

Panic Disorder

- **Essentials of Diagnosis**
  - Sudden, recurrent, unexpected panic attacks
  - Characterized by palpitations, tachycardia, sensation of dyspnea or choking, chest pain or discomfort, nausea, dizziness, diaphoresis, numbness, depersonalization
  - Sense of doom; fear of losing control or of dying
  - Persistent worry about future attacks
  - Change in behavior due to anxiety about being in places where an attack might occur (agoraphobia)

- **Differential Diagnosis**
  - Endocrinopathies (eg, hyperthyroidism)
  - Cardiac illness (eg, supraventricular tachycardia, myocardial infarction)
  - Pulmonary illness (eg, chronic obstructive pulmonary disease, asthma)
  - Pheochromocytoma
  - Medication or substance use or withdrawal
  - Other anxiety disorders (eg, generalized anxiety disorder, posttraumatic stress disorder)
  - Major depressive disorder
  - Somatoform disorders

- **Treatment**
  - Cognitive-behavioral therapy
  - Antidepressant medication (selective serotonin reuptake inhibitors, tricyclic antidepressants, monoamine oxidase inhibitors)
  - Benzodiazepines as adjunctive treatment
  - May have only a single attack; reassurance, education thus important early

- **Pearl**

In younger patients with multiple emergency room visits for cardiac complaints and negative evaluations, panic attack is the most common diagnosis.

Reference

Saeed SA et al: Panic disorder: effective treatment options. Am Fam Physician 1998;57:2405. [PMID: 9614411]

Generalized Anxiety Disorder

- ■ Essentials of Diagnosis
  - Excessive, persistent worry
  - Worry is difficult to control
  - Physiologic symptoms of restlessness, fatigue, irritability, muscle tension, sleep disturbance

- ■ Differential Diagnosis
  - Endocrinopathies (eg, hyperthyroidism)
  - Pheochromocytoma
  - Medication or substance use (eg, caffeine, nicotine, amphetamine, pseudoephedrine)
  - Medication or substance withdrawal (eg, alcohol, benzodiazepines)
  - Major depressive disorder
  - Adjustment disorder
  - Other anxiety disorders (eg, obsessive-compulsive disorder)
  - Somatoform disorders
  - Personality disorders (eg, avoidant, dependent, obsessive-compulsive)

- ■ Treatment
  - Psychotherapy, especially cognitive-behavioral
  - Relaxation techniques (eg, biofeedback)
  - Buspirone, extended-release venlafaxine, benzodiazepines

- ■ Pearl

In patients with anxiety and depression, treat the depression first.

Reference

Rickels K et al: The clinical presentation of generalized anxiety in primary-care settings: practical concepts of classification and management. J Clin Pathol 1997;58(Suppl 11):4. [PMID: 9363042]

Stress Disorders

- **Essentials of Diagnosis**
  - Includes acute stress disorder and posttraumatic stress disorder
  - Exposure to a traumatic event
  - Intrusive thoughts, nightmares, flashbacks
  - Mental distress or physiologic symptoms (eg, tachycardia, diaphoresis) when exposed to stimuli that cue the trauma
  - Avoidance of thoughts, feelings, or situations associated with the trauma
  - Isolation, detachment from others, emotional numbness
  - Sleep disturbance, irritability, hypervigilance, startle response, poor concentration
  - High comorbidity with depression and substance abuse

- **Differential Diagnosis**
  - Other anxiety disorders (eg, panic disorder, generalized anxiety disorder)
  - Major depressive disorder
  - Adjustment disorder
  - Psychotic disorders
  - Substance use or withdrawal
  - Neurologic syndrome secondary to head trauma

- **Treatment**
  - Individual and group psychotherapy
  - Cognitive-behavioral therapy
  - Antidepressant medication (selective serotonin reuptake inhibitors, tricyclic antidepressants, phenelzine)

- **Pearl**

Consider this diagnosis in any patient with mood symptoms and a history of trauma such as rape, combat, or physical or sexual abuse.

14

Reference

Peebles-Kleiger MJ et al: Office management of posttraumatic stress disorder. A clinician's guide to a pervasive problem. Postgrad Med 1998;103(5):181-3, 187-8, 194-6. (UI: 98253219)

Phobic Disorders

- **Essentials of Diagnosis**
  - Includes specific and social phobias
  - Persistent, irrational fear due to the presence or anticipation of an object or situation
  - Exposure to the phobic object or situation results in excessive anxiety
  - Avoidance of phobic object or situation
  - Social phobia: fear of humiliation or embarrassment in a performance or social situation (eg, speaking or eating in public)

- **Differential Diagnosis**
  - Other anxiety disorders (eg, generalized anxiety disorder, panic disorder, posttraumatic stress disorder)
  - Psychotic disorders

- **Treatment**
  - Behavioral therapy (eg, exposure)
  - Hypnosis
  - Benzodiazepines as necessary for anticipated situations that cannot be avoided (eg, flying)
  - Beta-blockers for anticipated, circumscribed social phobia (performance anxiety)
  - Paroxetine for social phobia

- **Pearl**

The most common anxiety disorder, especially for public speaking.

14

Reference

den Boer JA: Social phobia: epidemiology, recognition, and treatment. BMJ 1997;315:796. [PMID: 9345175]

Obsessive-Compulsive Disorder

- ■ Essentials of Diagnosis
  - Obsessions: recurrent, distressing, intrusive thoughts
  - Compulsions: repetitive behaviors (eg, hand washing, checking) that patient cannot resist performing
  - Patient recognizes obsessions and compulsions as excessive
  - Obsessions and compulsions cause distress and interfere with functioning

- ■ Differential Diagnosis
  - Psychotic disorders
  - Other anxiety disorders
  - Major depressive disorder
  - Somatoform disorders
  - Obsessive-compulsive personality disorder: lifelong pattern of preoccupation with orderliness and perfectionism but without presence of true obsessions or compulsions
  - Substance intoxication
  - Tic disorder (eg, Tourette's syndrome)

- ■ Treatment
  - Behavioral therapy (eg, exposure, response prevention)
  - Selective serotonin reuptake inhibitors or clomipramine

- ■ Pearl

Lack of insight makes a diagnosis of psychotic disorder more likely.

Reference

Khouzam HR: Obsessive-compulsive disorder. What to do if you recognize baffling behavior. Postgrad Med 1999;106:133. [PMID: 10608970]

Somatoform Disorders (Psychosomatic Disorders)

- **Essentials of Diagnosis**
  - Includes conversion, somatization, pain disorder with psychologic factors, hypochondriasis, and body dysmorphic disorder
  - Symptoms may involve one or more organ systems and are unintentional
  - Subjective complaints exceed objective findings
  - Symptom development may correlate with psychosocial stress, and symptoms are real to the patient

- **Differential Diagnosis**
  - Major depressive disorder
  - Anxiety disorders (eg, generalized anxiety disorder)
  - Factitious disorder
  - Malingering
  - Organic disease producing symptoms

- **Treatment**
  - Attention to building therapeutic relationship between patient and a single primary provider
  - Acknowledgment that patient's distress is real
  - Avoidance of confrontation regarding reality of the symptoms
  - Follow-up visits at regular intervals
  - Focus on functioning and empathy regarding patient's psychosocial difficulties
  - Continued vigilance about organic disease
  - Psychotherapy, especially group cognitive-behavioral
  - Biofeedback; hypnosis

- **Pearl**

Table 14-1. Somatoform disorders

| | | Symptom production | |
		Unconscious	**Conscious**
Motivation	**Unconscious**	Somatoform disorders	Factitious disorders
	Conscious	(Not applicable)	Malingering

Reference

Righter EL et al: Managing somatic preoccupation. Am Fam Physician 1999; 59:3113. [PMID: 10392593]

Factitious Disorder

- **Essentials of Diagnosis**
  - Also known as Munchausen syndrome
  - Intentional production or feigning of symptoms
  - Motivation for symptoms is unconscious, to assume the sick role
  - External incentives for symptom production are absent
  - Patient may produce symptoms in another person in order to indirectly assume the sick role (Munchausen by proxy)
  - High correlation with personality disorders

- **Differential Diagnosis**
  - Somatoform disorders
  - Malingering
  - Organic disease producing symptoms

- **Treatment**
  - Gentle confrontation regarding diagnosis
  - Emphasis on patient's strengths
  - Empathy with patient's long history of suffering
  - Attention to building therapeutic relationship between patient and a single primary provider
  - Psychotherapy
  - Many with less severe forms eventually stop or decrease self-destructive behaviors upon confrontation

- **Pearl**

When an obscure disorder eluding diagnosis develops in a patient recently enrolled in studies in the medical field, a factitious etiology is high on the list—if not at the top.

14

Reference

Wise MG et al: Factitious disorders. Prim Care 1999;26:315. [PMID: 10318750]

Personality Disorders

- **Three Clusters**
    1. Odd, eccentric: paranoid, schizoid; schizotypal personality disorders
    2. Dramatic: borderline, histrionic, narcissistic; antisocial personality disorders
    3. Anxious, fearful: avoidant, dependent; obsessive-compulsive personality disorders

- **Essentials of Diagnosis**
    - History dating from childhood or adolescence of recurrent maladaptive behavior
    - Minimal introspective ability
    - Major recurrent difficulties with interpersonal relationships
    - Enduring pattern of behavior stable over time, deviating markedly from cultural expectations
    - Increased risk of major depressive disorder

- **Differential Diagnosis**
    - Anxiety disorders
    - Dissociative disorders
    - Major depressive disorder
    - Bipolar disorder
    - Psychotic disorders
    - Substance use or withdrawal
    - Personality change due to medical illness (eg, central nervous system neoplasm, stroke)

- **Treatment**
    - Maintenance of a highly structured environment and clear, consistent interactions with the patient
    - Individual or group therapy (eg, cognitive-behavioral, interpersonal)
    - Antipsychotic medications may be required transiently in times of stress or decompensation
    - Serotonergic medications if depression or anxiety is prominent
    - Serotonergic medications or mood stabilizers if emotional lability is prominent

- **Pearl**

One of the most challenging therapeutic problems in all of medicine.

Reference

Dhossche DM et al: Assessment and importance of personality disorders in medical patients: an update. South Med J 1999;92:546. [PMID: 10372846]

Psychotic Disorders

- **Essentials of Diagnosis**
  - Includes schizophrenia, schizoaffective and schizophreniform disorders, delusional disorder, brief psychotic disorder, and shared psychotic disorder
  - Loss of ego boundaries, gross impairment in reality testing
  - Prominent delusions or auditory hallucinations
  - May have flat or inappropriate affect and disorganized speech, thought processes, or behavior
  - Brief psychotic disorder: symptoms last less than 1 month, then resolve completely

- **Differential Diagnosis**
  - Major depressive or manic episode with psychotic features
  - Medication or substance use (eg, steroids, levodopa, cocaine, amphetamines)
  - Heavy metal toxicity
  - Psychotic symptoms associated with dementia
  - Delirium
  - Complex partial seizures
  - Central nervous system neoplasm
  - Multiple sclerosis
  - Systemic lupus erythematosus
  - Endocrinopathies (eg, hypothyroidism, Cushing's syndrome)
  - Infectious disease (eg, neurosyphilis)
  - Nutritional deficiency (eg, thiamin, vitamin B_{12})
  - Acute intermittent porphyria
  - Personality disorders (eg, paranoid, schizoid, schizotypal)

- **Treatment**
  - Antipsychotic medications: atypical agents (risperidone, olanzapine, quetiapine, clozapine) less likely to cause extrapyramidal symptoms
  - Attempt to stabilize living situation and provide structured environment
  - Psychotherapy may be effective for brief psychotic disorder after episode resolves
  - Behavioral therapy (eg, skills training)

- **Pearl**

The presence of hallucinations or delusions means psychosis—whether organic or functional in origin is determined next.

Reference

McGrath J et al: Fortnightly review. Treatment of schizophrenia. BMJ 1999; 319:1045. [PMID: 10521199]

Major Depressive Disorder

- ■ Essentials of Diagnosis
  - Depressed mood or anhedonia (loss of interest or pleasure in usual activities), with hopelessness, intense feelings of sadness
  - Poor concentration, thoughts of suicide, worthlessness, guilt
  - Symptoms include sleep or appetite disturbance (increased or decreased), malaise, psychomotor retardation or agitation
  - Increased isolation and social withdrawal, decreased libido
  - May have psychotic component (eg, self-deprecatory auditory hallucinations), or multiple somatic complaints
  - Symptoms last longer than 2 weeks and impair functioning

- ■ Differential Diagnosis
  - Bipolar disorder; adjustment disorder
  - Dysthymic disorder: presence of some depressive symptoms for at least 2 years
  - Bereavement
  - Substance abuse (eg, alcohol) or withdrawal (eg, cocaine, amphetamine)
  - Medication use (eg, steroids, interferon, reserpine)
  - Medical illness (eg, hypothyroidism, stroke, Parkinson's disease, neoplasm, polymyalgia rheumatica)
  - Delirium or dementia
  - Anxiety disorders (eg, generalized anxiety disorder, posttraumatic stress disorder)
  - Personality disorders

- ■ Treatment
  - Assess suicidal risk in all patients
  - Antidepressant medications: selective serotonin reuptake inhibitors, tricyclic antidepressants, venlafaxine, nefazodone, bupropion, mirtazapine, monoamine oxidase inhibitors
  - Psychotherapy (eg, cognitive-behavioral, interpersonal)
  - Interventions to help with resocialization (eg, supportive groups, day treatment programs)
  - Education of patient and family about depression
  - Electroconvulsive therapy for refractory cases
  - Antipsychotic medication if psychotic component present

- ■ Pearl

Ask about history of mania before starting an antidepressant; bipolar patients may develop a manic episode when treated with an antidepressant.

Reference

Doris A et al: Depressive illness. Lancet 1999;354:1369. [PMID: 10533878]

Bipolar Disorder

- **Essentials of Diagnosis**
  - History of manic episode: grandiosity, decreased need for sleep, pressured speech, racing thoughts, distractibility, increased activity, excessive spending or hypersexuality
  - Depressive episodes may alternate with periods of mania
  - Manic episode may have psychotic component

- **Differential Diagnosis**
  - Substance intoxication (eg, cocaine, amphetamine, alcohol)
  - Medication use (eg, steroids, thyroxine, methylphenidate)
  - Infectious disease (eg, neurosyphilis, complications of HIV infection)
  - Endocrinopathies (eg, hyperthyroidism, Cushing's syndrome)
  - Central nervous system neoplasm
  - Complex partial seizures
  - Personality disorders (eg, borderline, narcissistic)

- **Treatment**
  - Mood stabilizer: lithium, valproic acid, carbamazepine
  - Antipsychotic medication (eg, olanzapine) for acute mania or psychotic component
  - Psychotherapy may be helpful once acute mania is controlled

- **Pearl**

Inexperienced clinicians seeing their first manic patient invariably diagnose hyperthyroidism.

Reference

Griswold KS et al: Management of bipolar disorder. Am Fam Physician 2000;62:1343. [PMID: 11011863]

14

Alcohol Dependence

- **Essentials of Diagnosis**
  - Intoxication: somnolence, slurred speech, ataxia, nystagmus, impaired attention or memory, coma
  - Physiologic dependence with symptoms of withdrawal when intake is interrupted
  - Tolerance to the effects of alcohol
  - Presence of alcohol-associated medical illnesses (eg, liver disease, cerebellar degeneration)
  - Recurrent use resulting in multiple legal problems, hazardous situations, or failure to fulfill role obligations
  - Continued drinking despite strong medical and social contraindications and life disruptions
  - High comorbidity with depression

- **Differential Diagnosis**
  - Alcohol use secondary to underlying major psychiatric illness
  - Other sedative-hypnotic dependence or intoxication (eg, benzodiazepines)
  - Intoxication by other substances or medications (eg, opioids)
  - Withdrawal from other substances (eg, cocaine, amphetamine)
  - Pathophysiologic disturbance such as hypoxia, hypoglycemia, stroke, central nervous system infection, or subdural hematoma

- **Treatment**
  - Total abstinence, not "controlled drinking," should be the goal
  - Substance abuse counseling and groups (eg, Alcoholics Anonymous)
  - Disulfiram in selected patients; naltrexone may also be of benefit, in conjunction with substance abuse counseling
  - Treat underlying depression if present

- **Pearl**

Mood or anxiety disorders are difficult to diagnose when a patient is actively drinking.

Reference

O'Connor PG et al: Patients with alcohol problems. N Engl J Medicine 1998; 338:592. [PMID: 9475768]

Alcohol Withdrawal

- ■ Essentials of Diagnosis
  - • Symptoms when patient with dependence abruptly stops drinking
  - • Autonomic hyperactivity, tremor, wakefulness, psychomotor agitation, anxiety, seizures, hallucinations or delusions
  - • Life-threatening severe withdrawal with disorientation and frightening hallucinations (delirium tremens)

- ■ Differential Diagnosis
  - • Delirium secondary to other medical illness (eg, infection, hypoglycemia, hepatic disease)
  - • Withdrawal from other sedative-hypnotics (eg, benzodiazepines) or opioids
  - • Substance intoxication (eg, cocaine, amphetamine)
  - • Anxiety disorders
  - • Manic episode
  - • Seizure disorder

- ■ Treatment
  - • Benzodiazepines, with target of keeping vital signs normal
  - • Haloperidol if hallucinations are present
  - • Thiamin, folate, and multivitamins
  - • Encourage hydration

- ■ Pearl

The longer the period between discontinuation of alcohol and the appearance of symptoms, the worse the delirium tremens.

Reference

Hall W et al: The alcohol withdrawal syndrome. Lancet 1997;349:1897 [PMID: 971770].

14

Opioid Dependence & Withdrawal

- ■ Essentials of Diagnosis
  - Intoxication: somnolence, slurred speech, ataxia, coma, respiratory depression, miotic pupils
  - Physical dependence with tolerance
  - Continued use despite disruptions in social and occupational functioning
  - Withdrawal: nausea, vomiting, abdominal cramps, lacrimation, rhinorrhea, dilated pupils, dysphoria, irritability, diaphoresis, insomnia, tachycardia, fever
  - Withdrawal uncomfortable but not life-threatening

- ■ Differential Diagnosis
  - Alcohol or other sedative-hypnotic intoxication, dependence, or withdrawal
  - Intoxication by or withdrawal from other substances or medications
  - Medical illness while intoxicated: hypoxia, hypoglycemia, stroke, central nervous system infection or hemorrhage; during withdrawal: other gastrointestinal or infectious disease

- ■ Treatment
  - Naloxone for suspected overdose with close medical observation
  - Methadone maintenance after withdrawal for selected patients
  - Clonidine may be helpful in alleviating the autonomic symptoms of withdrawal
  - Methadone may be used to treat acute withdrawal but only under specific federal guidelines
  - Substance abuse counseling and groups (eg, Narcotics Anonymous)

- ■ Pearl

Many opioids are prescribed in fixed-drug combinations with agents such as acetaminophen, which may have differing or additional toxicities.

Reference

Effective medical treatment of opiate addiction. National Consensus Development Panel on Effective Medical Treatment of Opiate Addiction. JAMA 1998;280:1936. [PMID: 9851480]

14

Sexual Dysfunctions

- **Essentials of Diagnosis**
  - Includes hypoactive sexual arousal disorder, sexual aversion disorder, female sexual arousal disorder, male erectile disorder, orgasmic disorder, premature ejaculation
  - Persistent disturbance in the phases of the sexual response cycle (eg, absence of desire, arousal, or orgasm)
  - Causes significant distress or interpersonal difficulty
  - Conditioning may cause or exacerbate dysfunction

- **Differential Diagnosis**
  - Underlying medical condition (eg, chronic illness, various hormone deficiencies, diabetes mellitus, hypertension, peripheral vascular disease, pelvic pathology)
  - Medication (eg, selective serotonin reuptake inhibitors, numerous antihypertensives) or substance use (eg, alcohol)
  - Depression

- **Treatment**
  - Encourage increased communication with sexual partner
  - Decrease performance anxiety via sensate focus, relaxation exercises
  - Sex or couples therapy, especially if life or relationship stressors are present
  - Estrogen replacement in women or testosterone replacement in men if levels are low
  - Erectile dysfunction in men: consider vacuum device, alprostadil, penile injection or implant, sildenafil
  - Premature ejaculation: selective serotonin reuptake inhibitors may help

- **Pearl**

Sexual dysfunction is often undiagnosed in women; relevant inquiries should be made if there are ill-defined and poorly explained somatic symptoms.

Reference

Morgentaler A: Male impotence. Lancet 1999;354:1713. [PMID: 9551480]

Eating Disorders

- ### Essentials of Diagnosis
  - Includes anorexia nervosa and bulimia nervosa
  - Severe abnormalities in eating behavior
  - Disturbance in perception of body shape or weight
  - Anorexia: refusal to maintain a minimally normal body weight
  - Bulimia: repeated binge eating, followed by compensatory behavior to prevent weight gain (eg, vomiting, use of laxatives, excessive exercise, fasting)
  - Medical sequelae include gastrointestinal disturbances, electrolyte imbalance, cardiovascular abnormalities, amenorrhea or oligomenorrhea, caries or periodontitis

- ### Differential Diagnosis
  - Major depressive disorder
  - Body dysmorphic disorder: excessive preoccupation with an imagined defect in appearance
  - Obsessive-compulsive disorder
  - Weight loss secondary to medical illness (eg, neoplasm, gastrointestinal disease, hyperthyroidism, diabetes)

- ### Treatment
  - Psychotherapy (eg, cognitive-behavioral, interpersonal)
  - Family therapy, particularly for adolescent patients
  - Selective serotonin reuptake inhibitors (eg, fluoxetine) may be of benefit
  - Medical management of associated physical sequelae
  - Consider inpatient or partial hospitalization for severe cases

- ### Pearl

If bulimia is suspected, examine the knuckles, teeth, and perioral skin for signs of self-induced vomiting.

Reference

Becker AE et al: Eating disorders. N Engl J Medicine 1999;340:1092. (PMID: 10194240]

15

Dermatologic Disorders

Atopic Dermatitis (Atopic Eczema)

- **Essentials of Diagnosis**
  - Pruritic, exudative, or lichenified eruption on face, neck, upper trunk, wrists, hands, antecubital and popliteal folds
  - Involves face and extensor surfaces more typically in infants
  - Personal or family history of allergies or asthma
  - Recurring; remission possible in adolescence
  - Peripheral eosinophilia, increased serum IgE—not needed for diagnosis

- **Differential Diagnosis**
  - Seborrheic dermatitis
  - Contact dermatitis
  - Scabies
  - Impetigo
  - Eczema herpeticum may be superimposed on atopic dermatitis.
  - Eczematous dermatitis may be presenting feature of immuno-deficiency syndromes in infants

- **Treatment**
  - Avoidance of anything that dries or irritates skin
  - Frequent emollients
  - Topical corticosteroids
  - Topical tacrolimus (FK506) dramatically beneficial in severe atopic dermatitis
  - Phototherapy sometimes helpful
  - Sedative antihistamines relieve pruritus
  - Atopic patients frequently colonized with staphylococci; systemic antibiotics helpful in flares
  - Systemic steroids or cyclosporine only in highly selected cases
  - Dietary restrictions may be of benefit in limited cases when specific food allergies are implicated

- **Pearl**

While RAST testing is useful to exclude food allergies, positive results correlate poorly with food challenges and are difficult to interpret.

Reference

Rothe MJ et al: Atopic dermatitis: An update. J Am Acad Dermatol 1996;35:1. [PMID: 96272959]

Nummular Eczema

- **Essentials of Diagnosis**
  - Middle-aged and older men most frequently affected
  - Discrete coin-shaped, crusted, erythematous, 1–5 cm plaques that may contain vesicles
  - Usually begins on lower legs, dorsal hands, or extensor surfaces of arms but may spread
  - Pruritus often severe

- **Differential Diagnosis**
  - Tinea corporis
  - Psoriasis
  - Xerotic dermatitis
  - Impetigo
  - Contact dermatitis

- **Treatment**
  - Avoidance of agents capable of drying or irritating skin (hot or frequent baths, extensive soaping, etc)
  - Frequent emollients
  - Topical corticosteroids (potency appropriate to location and severity) applied twice daily and tapered as tolerated
  - Topical tar preparations
  - Phototherapy may be helpful in severe cases
  - Sedative antihistamines to relieve pruritus, given at bedtime
  - Antibiotics when signs of impetiginization are present (fissures, crusts, erosions, or pustules)
  - Systemic steroids in highly selected, refractory cases

- **Pearl**

If it scales, scrape it—KOH preparation should always be examined to rule out tinea corporis.

Reference

Rietschel RL et al: Nonatopic eczemas. J Am Acad Dermatol 1988;18:569. [PMID: 88170171]

Seborrheic Dermatitis & Dandruff

- ■ Essentials of Diagnosis
  - Loose, dry, moist, or greasy scales with or without underlying crusted, pink or yellow-brown plaques
  - Predilection for scalp, eyebrows, eyelids, nasolabial creases, lips, ears, presternal area, axillae, umbilicus, groin, and gluteal crease
  - Infantile form on scalp known as cradle cap

- ■ Differential Diagnosis
  - Psoriasis
  - Impetigo
  - Atopic dermatitis
  - Contact dermatitis
  - Pityriasis rosea
  - Tinea versicolor
  - Pediculosis capitis (head lice)

- ■ Treatment
  - Selenium sulfide, tar, zinc, or ketoconazole shampoos
  - Topical corticosteroids
  - Topical ketoconazole cream
  - Systemic corticosteroids and antibiotics in selected generalized or severe cases
  - Patient should be aware that chronic therapy is required to suppress this condition

- ■ Pearl

New-onset severe seborrheic dermatitis can occur in patients with Parkinson's disease and with HIV infection.

Reference

Hay RJ et al: Dandruff and seborrheic dermatitis: Causes and management. Clin Exp Dermatol 1997;22:3. [PMID: 97471102]

15

Allergic Contact Dermatitis

- **Essentials of Diagnosis**
  - Erythema, edema, and vesicles in an area of contact with suspected agent
  - Weeping, crusting, or secondary infection may follow
  - Intense pruritus
  - Pattern of eruption may be diagnostic (eg, linear streaked vesicles in poison oak or ivy)
  - History of previous reaction to suspected contactant
  - Patch testing usually positive
  - Common allergens include nickel, plants, neomycin, topical anesthetics, fragrances, preservatives, hair dyes, textile dyes, nail care products, adhesives, and constituents of rubber and latex products

- **Differential Diagnosis**
  - Nonallergenic contact dermatitis
  - Scabies
  - Impetigo
  - Dermatophytid reaction
  - Atopic dermatitis
  - Seborrheic dermatitis

- **Treatment**
  - Identify and avoid contactant
  - Topical corticosteroids for localized involvement
  - Wet compresses with aluminum acetate solutions for weeping lesions
  - Oral corticosteroids for acute, severe cases; tapering may require 2–3 weeks to avoid rebound

- **Pearl**

If the agent can be aerosolized, as with Rhus *(poison oak and ivy), noncardiogenic pulmonary edema may result—eg, a campfire burning* Rhus *branches.*

Reference

Belsito DV: The diagnostic evaluation, treatment, and prevention of allergic contact dermatitis in the new millennium. J Allergy Clin Immunol 2000;105:409. [PMID: 10719287]

15

Pityriasis Rosea

- ■ Essentials of Diagnosis
  - Oval, salmon-colored, symmetric papules with long axis following cleavage lines
  - Lesions show "collarette of scale" at periphery
  - Trunk most frequently involved; sun-exposed areas often spared
  - A "herald" patch precedes eruption by 1–2 weeks; some patients report prodrome of constitutional symptoms
  - Pruritus common but usually mild
  - Variations in mode of onset, morphology, distribution, and course are common
  - Attempts to isolate infective agent have been disappointing

- ■ Differential Diagnosis
  - Secondary syphilis
  - Tinea corporis
  - Seborrheic dermatitis
  - Tinea versicolor
  - Viral exanthem
  - Drug eruption
  - Psoriasis

- ■ Treatment
  - Usually none required; most cases resolve spontaneously in 3–10 weeks
  - Topical steroids or oral antihistamines for pruritus
  - UVB phototherapy may expedite involution of lesions
  - Short course of systemic corticosteroids in selected severe cases

- ■ Pearl

As in all similar rashes: RPR.

15

Reference

Allen RA et al: Pityriasis rosea. Cutis 1995;56:198. [PMID: 96127440]

Psoriasis

- **Essentials of Diagnosis**
  - Silvery scales on bright red, well-demarcated plaques on knees, elbows, and scalp
  - Pitted nails or onychodystrophy
  - Pinking of intergluteal folds
  - Pruritus mild or absent
  - Associated with psoriatic arthritis
  - Lesions may be induced at sites of injury (Koebner phenomenon)
  - Many variants

- **Differential Diagnosis**
  - Cutaneous candidiasis
  - Tinea corporis
  - Nummular eczema
  - Seborrheic dermatitis
  - Pityriasis rosea
  - Secondary syphilis
  - Pityriasis rubra pilaris
  - Nail findings may mimic onychomycosis
  - Cutaneous features of reactive arthritis may mimic psoriasis
  - Plaque stage of cutaneous T cell lymphoma may mimic psoriasis

- **Treatment**
  - Topical steroids, calcipotriene, tar preparations, anthralin, salicylic acid, or tazarotene
  - Tar shampoos, topical steroids, calcipotriene, keratolytic agents, or intralesional steroids for scalp lesions
  - Phototherapy (UVB, psoralen plus UVA, or the Goeckerman regimen) for widespread disease
  - Systemic steroids *not* used because of risk of severe rebound or induction of pustular psoriasis
  - In selected severe cases, systemic methotrexate, cyclosporine, or acitretin

- **Pearl**

Look carefully at the nails under magnification. Pitting may be subtle but can clinch the diagnosis.

Reference

Stern RS: Psoriasis. Lancet 1997;350:349. [PMID: 9251649]

Exfoliative Dermatitis (Erythroderma)

- ■ Essentials of Diagnosis
  - Erythema and scaling over most of the body
  - Itching, malaise, fever, chills, lymphadenopathy, weight loss
  - Preexisting dermatosis causes more than half of cases
  - Skin biopsy to identify cause
  - Leukocyte gene rearrangement studies if Sézary syndrome suspected and biopsies nondiagnostic

- ■ Differential Diagnosis
  - Erythrodermic psoriasis
  - Pityriasis rubra pilaris
  - Drug eruption
  - Atopic dermatitis
  - Contact dermatitis
  - Severe seborrheic dermatitis
  - Sézary syndrome of cutaneous T cell lymphoma
  - Hodgkin's disease

- ■ Treatment
  - Soaks and emollients
  - Midpotency topical steroids, possibly under occlusive suit
  - Hospitalization may be required
  - Specific systemic therapies
  - Discontinue offending agent in drug-induced cases
  - Antibiotics for secondary bacterial infections

- ■ Pearl

Unexplained erythroderma in a middle-aged person raises the index of suspicion for a visceral malignancy.

Reference

Rothe MJ et al: Erythroderma. Dermatol Clin 2000;18:405. [PMID: 10943536]

Cutaneous T Cell Lymphoma (Mycosis Fungoides)

- **Essentials of Diagnosis**
  - Early stage: erythematous 1- to 5-cm patches, sometimes pruritic, on lower abdomen, buttocks, upper thighs, and, in women, breasts
  - Middle stages: infiltrated, erythematous, scaly plaques
  - Advanced stages: skin tumors, erythroderma, lymphadenopathy, or visceral involvement
  - Skin biopsy critical; serial biopsies may be required to confirm diagnosis
  - CD4/CD8 ratios, tests to detect clonal rearrangement of the T cell receptor gene

- **Differential Diagnosis**
  - Psoriasis
  - Drug eruption
  - Eczematous dermatoses
  - Leprosy
  - Tinea corporis
  - Other lymphoreticular malignancies

- **Treatment**
  - Treatment depends on stage of disease
  - Early and aggressive therapy may control cutaneous lesions—not shown to prevent progression
  - High-potency corticosteroids, mechlorethamine, or carmustine (BCNU) topically
  - Phototherapy (psoralen plus UVA) in early stages
  - Total skin electron beam radiation, photophoresis, systemic chemotherapy, retinoids, and alpha interferon for advanced disease
  - Denileukin diftitox (DAB389IL-2; diphtheria toxin fused to recombinant IL-2)

- **Pearl**

Early stage disease usually progresses slowly, and many patients die of other causes.

Reference

Lorincz AL: Cutaneous T cell lymphoma (mycosis fungoides). Lancet 1996; 347:871. [PMID: 8622396]

15

Lichen Planus

- **Essentials of Diagnosis**
  - Small pruritic, violaceous, polygonal, flat-topped papules; may show white streaks (Wickham's striae) on surface
  - On flexor wrists, dorsal hands, trunk, thighs, shins, ankles, glans penis
  - Oral mucosa frequently affected with ulcers or reticulated white patches
  - Vulvovaginal and perianal lesions show leukoplakia or erosions
  - Scalp involvement (lichen planopilaris) causes scarring alopecia
  - Nail changes infrequent but can include pterygium
  - Trauma may induce additional lesions (Koebner phenomenon)
  - Linear, annular, and hypertrophic variants
  - Hepatitis C infection more prevalent in lichen planus patients; screening indicated
  - Skin biopsy when diagnosis not clear

- **Differential Diagnosis**
  - Lichenoid drug eruption
  - Pityriasis rosea
  - Psoriasis
  - Secondary syphilis
  - Mucosal lesions: lichen sclerosus, candidiasis, erythema multiforme, leukoplakia, pemphigus vulgaris, bullous pemphigoid
  - Discoid lupus erythematosus

- **Treatment**
  - Topical or intralesional steroids for limited cutaneous or mucosal lesions
  - Systemic corticosteroids, psoralen plus UVA, oral isotretinoin, low-molecular-weight heparin for generalized disease
  - Cyclosporine for severe cases
  - Monitor for malignant transformation to squamous cell carcinoma in erosive mucosal disease
  - Aggressive management to avoid debilitating scarring in vulvar lichen planus

- **Pearl**

To the uninitiated, oral lichen planus may be misdiagnosed as thrush, leading to inappropriate assessment for immunocompromise.

Reference

Cribier B et al: Treatment of lichen planus. An evidence-based medicine analysis of efficacy. Arch Dermatol 1998;134:1521. [PMID: 99092348]

15

Morbilliform Drug Eruption

- **Essentials of Diagnosis**
  - Erythema, small papules
  - Occurs within first 2 weeks of drug treatment; may appear later
  - Pruritus prominent
  - Eruption symmetric, beginning proximally and then generalizing
  - Ampicillin, amoxicillin, allopurinol, and trimethoprim-sulfamethoxazole most common causes
  - Amoxicillin eruptions more frequent in patients with infectious mononucleosis; sulfonamide rashes common in HIV-infected patients

- **Differential Diagnosis**
  - Viral exanthems
  - Early stages of erythema multiforme major or drug hypersensitivity syndrome
  - Scarlet fever
  - Toxic shock syndrome
  - Acute graft-versus-host disease

- **Treatment**
  - Discontinue offending agent unless this represents a greater risk to the patient than the eruption
  - Topical corticosteroids and oral antihistamines
  - Avoid rechallenge in complex exanthems and in some HIV-infected patients

- **Pearl**

No matter how obvious the cause of this or any such eruption, consider syphilis.

15

Reference

Wolverton SE: Update on cutaneous drug reactions. Adv Dermatol 1997;13:65. [PMID: 98212498]

Photosensitive Drug Eruption

■ Essentials of Diagnosis

- Morphology variable; photodistribution critical to diagnosis
- Phototoxic reactions resemble sunburn; related to dose of both medication and UV radiation; tetracyclines, amiodarone, furosemide, thiazides, phenothiazines, sulfonylureas, and NSAIDs common causes
- Photoallergic reactions typically red, scaly, pruritic; immune-related
- Pseudoporphyria caused by naproxen, tetracyclines, furosemide, dapsone, and other medications
- Photodistributed lichenoid reactions most frequently due to thiazides, quinidine, NSAIDs

■ Differential Diagnosis

- Porphyria cutanea tarda or other porphyrias
- Lupus erythematosus or dermatomyositis
- Photoallergic contact dermatitis
- Phototoxic contact dermatitis
- Polymorphous light eruption or other idiopathic photosensitivity disorders
- Pellagra
- Xeroderma pigmentosum or other genetic photosensitivity disorders

■ Treatment

- Avoidance of the causative agent
- Sun avoidance, protection with broad-spectrum sunscreens containing physical blockers
- Soothing local measures or topical corticosteroids

■ Pearl

UVA radiation is the most common trigger, so broad-spectrum sunscreens are essential.

Reference

Gould JW et al: Cutaneous photosensitivity diseases induced by exogenous agents. J Am Acad Dermatol 1995;33:551. [PMID: 95403739]

Fixed Drug Eruption

- **Essentials of Diagnosis**
    - Lesions recur at same site with each repeat exposure to the causative medication
    - From one to six lesions
    - Oral, genital, facial, and acral lesions most common
    - Lesions begin as erythematous, edematous, round, sharply demarcated patches or plaques
    - May evolve to targetoid, bullous, or erosive
    - Postinflammatory hyperpigmentation common
    - Offending agents: NSAIDs, sulfonamides, barbiturates, tetracyclines, erythromycin, and laxatives with phenolphthalein

- **Differential Diagnosis**
    - Bullous pemphigoid
    - Erythema multiforme
    - Sweet's syndrome (acute febrile neutrophilic dermatosis)
    - Residual hyperpigmentation can appear similar to pigmentation left behind by numerous other inflammatory disorders
    - The differential of genital lesions includes psoriasis, lichen planus, and syphilis

- **Treatment**
    - Avoidance of the causative agent
    - Symptomatic care of lesions

- **Pearl**

Fixed drug eruption should always be considered in the differential diagnosis of penile erosions.

15

Reference

Korkij W et al: Fixed drug eruption. A brief review. Arch Dermatol 1984; 120:520. [PMID: 84152903]

Bullous Drug Reactions (Erythema Multiforme Major, Stevens-Johnson Syndrome, and Toxic Epidermal Necrolysis)

- **Essentials of Diagnosis**
  - Flu-like symptoms frequently precede eruption
  - Initial lesions erythematous and macular; may become targetoid, form bullae, or may desquamate
  - Two or more mucosal surfaces (oral, conjunctival, anogenital) usually affected; gastrointestinal tract or respiratory tract involved in severe cases
  - Skin biopsies confirm diagnosis
  - Stevens-Johnson syndrome : < 10% of body surface involvement; toxic epidermal necrolysis: > 30% of body surface involvement
  - Sulfonamide drugs, phenytoin, carbamazepine, phenobarbital, penicillins, allopurinol, and NSAIDs most frequent offenders
  - In anticonvulsant hypersensitivity reactions, hepatitis, nephritis, or pneumonitis may occur

- **Differential Diagnosis**
  - Generalized bullous fixed drug eruption
  - Staphylococcal scalded skin syndrome
  - Infection-induced erythema multiforme major (most frequently associated with *Mycoplasma pneumoniae* infection)
  - Early disease may be confused with morbilliform drug eruptions or erythema multiforme minor
  - Bullous pemphigoid and pemphigus vulgaris
  - Graft-versus-host disease

- **Treatment**
  - Discontinuation of provocative agent
  - Extensive involvement may require transfer to a burn unit for fluid and electrolyte management
  - Antibiotics
  - Systemic corticosteroids is controversial
  - Wet dressings, oral and ophthalmologic care, pain relief
  - Intravenous immunoglobulin may be considered in severe cases of toxic epidermal necrolysis
  - Rechallenge with phenytoin, carbamazepine, or phenobarbital should be avoided because cross-reactivity is common; valproic acid is an alternative

- **Pearl**

Be very wary of spiking fevers and systemic symptoms in patients taking potentially offending drugs; it may take days until the rash appears.

Reference

Roujeau JC et al: Medication use and the risk of Stevens-Johnson syndrome or toxic epidermal necrolysis. N Engl J Med 1995;333:1600. [PMID: 96072888]

15

Diffuse Pruritus

- ■ Essentials of Diagnosis
  - May be idiopathic, but workup needed to rule out the internal causes
  - Excoriations are an objective sign of pruritus but not always present

- ■ Differential Diagnosis
  - Hepatic disease, especially cholestatic
  - Hepatitis C with or without liver failure
  - Uremia
  - Hypothyroidism or hyperthyroidism
  - Intestinal parasites
  - Polycythemia vera
  - Lymphomas, leukemias, myeloma, other malignancies
  - Neuropsychiatric diseases (anorexia nervosa, delusions of parasitosis)
  - Scabies

- ■ Treatment
  - Sedative antihistamines for symptomatic relief
  - Topical menthol lotions
  - Aspirin for pruritus of polycythemia vera
  - Cholestyramine, naloxone, prednisone, and colchicine helpful in some with hepatobiliary pruritus
  - Optimization of dialysis, erythropoietin (epoetin alfa), emollients, cholestyramine, phosphate binders, and phototherapy helpful in some with uremic pruritus

15

- ■ Pearl

Excoriations spare areas out of the patient's reach, such as the "butterfly zone" on the back.

Reference

Kantor GR et al: Generalized pruritus and systemic disease. J Am Acad Dermatol 1983;9:375. [PMID: 84033411]

Lichen Simplex Chronicus & Prurigo Nodularis

- **Essentials of Diagnosis**
    - Chronic, severe, localized itching
    - Lichen simplex chronicus: well-circumscribed, erythematous plaques with accentuated skin markings, often on the extremities and posterior neck
    - Prurigo nodularis: multiple pea-sized firm, erythematous or brownish, dome-shaped, excoriated nodules, typically on the extremities

- **Differential Diagnosis**
    - Lichen simplex chronicus: secondary phenomenon in atopic dermatitis, stasis dermatitis, insect bite reactions, contact dermatitis, or pruritus of other cause
    - Lesions of psoriasis, cutaneous lymphoma, lichen planus, and tinea corporis may resemble lichen simplex chronicus
    - Prurigo nodularis: associated with HIV disease, renal failure, hepatic diseases (especially hepatitis), atopic dermatitis, anemia, emotional stress, pregnancy, and gluten enteropathy
    - Prurigo nodularis: similar to hypertrophic lichen planus and scabietic nodules

- **Treatment**
    - Avoid scratching involved areas—occlusion with steroid tape, semipermeable dressings, or even Unna boots may be of value
    - Intralesional steroids or topical superpotent steroids helpful in treating individual lesions; topical doxepin or capsaicin creams sometimes effective
    - Oral antihistamines of limited benefit
    - Phototherapy, isotretinoin, topical calcipotriene, and oral cyclosporine are alternatives
    - Thalidomide in recalcitrant, severe prurigo nodularis—pregnancy prevention and monitoring for side effects are critical

- **Pearl**

These lesions are a response to chronic rubbing or picking: no specific cause is suggested.

Reference

Jones RO: Lichen simplex chronicus. Clin Podiatr Med Surg 1996;13:47. [PMID: 97002584]

Acne Vulgaris

- **Essentials of Diagnosis**
  - Often occurs at puberty, though onset may be delayed until the third or fourth decade
  - Open and closed comedones the hallmarks
  - Severity varies from comedonal to papular or pustular inflammatory acne to cysts or nodules
  - Face, neck, upper chest, and back may be affected
  - Pigmentary changes and severe scarring can occur

- **Differential Diagnosis**
  - Acne rosacea, perioral dermatitis, gram-negative folliculitis, tinea faciei, and pseudofolliculitis
  - Trunk lesions may be confused with staphylococcal folliculitis, miliaria, or eosinophilic folliculitis
  - May be induced by topical, inhaled, or systemic steroids, oily topical products, and anabolic steroids
  - Foods neither cause nor exacerbate acne
  - In women with resistant acne, hyperandrogenism should be considered; may be accompanied by hirsutism and irregular menses

- **Treatment**
  - Improvement usually requires 4–6 weeks
  - Topical retinoids very effective for comedonal acne but usefulness limited by irritation
  - Topical benzoyl peroxide agents
  - Topical antibiotics (erythromycin combined with benzoyl peroxide, clindamycin) effective against comedones and mild inflammatory acne
  - Oral antibiotics (tetracycline, doxycycline, minocycline) for moderate inflammatory acne; erythromycin is an alternative when tetracyclines contraindicated
  - Low-dose oral contraceptives containing a nonandrogenic progestin can be effective in women
  - Diluted intralesional corticosteroids effective in reducing highly inflammatory papules and cysts
  - Oral isotretinoin useful in some who fail antibiotic therapy; pregnancy prevention and monitoring essential
  - Surgical and laser techniques available to treat scarring

- **Pearl**

Don't waste time continuing failing therapies in scarring acne—treat aggressively if needed to prevent further scars.

Reference

Leyden JJ: Therapy for acne vulgaris. N Engl J Med 1997;336:1156. [PMID: 97238758]

Rosacea

- **Essentials of Diagnosis**
  - A chronic disorder of the mid face in middle-aged and older people
  - History of flushing evoked by hot beverages, alcohol, or sunlight
  - Erythema, sometimes persisting for hours or days after flushing episodes
  - Telangiectases become more prominent over time
  - Many patients have acneiform papules and pustules
  - Some advanced cases show large inflammatory nodules and nasal sebaceous hypertrophy (rhinophyma)

- **Differential Diagnosis**
  - Acne vulgaris
  - Seborrheic dermatitis
  - Lupus erythematosus
  - Dermatomyositis
  - Carcinoid syndrome
  - Topical steroid-induced rosacea
  - Polymorphous light eruption
  - Demodex (mite) folliculitis in HIV-infected patients
  - Perioral dermatitis

- **Treatment**
  - Treatment is suppressive and chronic
  - Topical metronidazole and oral tetracyclines effective against papulopustular disease
  - Daily sunscreen use and avoidance of flushing triggers helpful in slowing progression
  - Oral isotretinoin can produce dramatic improvement in resistant cases, but relapse common
  - Laser therapy may obliterate telangiectases
  - Surgery in severe rhinophyma

- **Pearl**

Watch for ocular symptoms—blepharitis, conjunctivitis, or even keratitis may occur in up to 58% of patients.

Reference

Wilkin JK: Rosacea. Arch Dermatol 1994;130:359. [PMID: 94175563]

Erysipelas & Cellulitis

- ■ Essentials of Diagnosis
    - • Cellulitis: an acute infection of the subcutaneous tissue, most frequently caused by *Streptococcus pyogenes* or *Staphylococcus aureus*
    - • Erythema, edema, tenderness are the hallmarks of cellulitis; vesicles, exudation, purpura, necrosis may follow
    - • Lymphangitic streaking may be seen
    - • Demarcation from uninvolved skin indistinct
    - • Erysipelas: involves superficial dermal lymphatics
    - • Erysipelas characterized by a warm, red, tender, edematous plaque with a sharply demarcated, raised, indurated border; classically occurs on the face
    - • Both erysipelas and cellulitis require a portal of entry
    - • Recurrence seen in lymphatic damage or venous insufficiency
    - • A prodrome of malaise, fever, and chills may accompany either entity

- ■ Differential Diagnosis
    - • Acute contact dermatitis
    - • Scarlet fever
    - • Lupus erythematosus
    - • Erythema nodosum
    - • Early necrotizing fasciitis or clostridial gangrene
    - • Underlying osteomyelitis
    - • Evolving herpes zoster
    - • Fixed drug eruption
    - • Venous thrombosis
    - • Beriberi

15

- ■ Treatment
    - • Appropriate systemic antibiotics
    - • Local wound care and elevation

- ■ Pearl
Look for tinea pedis as a portal of entry in patients with leg cellulitis.

Reference

Danik SB et al: Cellulitis. Cutis 1999;64:157. [PMID: 10590915]

Folliculitis, Furuncles, & Carbuncles

- **Essentials of Diagnosis**
  - Folliculitis: thin-walled pustules at follicular orifices, particularly extremities, scalp, face, and buttocks; develop in crops and heal in a few days
  - Furuncle: acute, round, tender, circumscribed, perifollicular abscess; most undergo central necrosis and rupture with purulent discharge
  - Carbuncle: two or more confluent furuncles with multiple sites of drainage
  - Classic folliculitis caused by *S aureus*
  - Staphylococcal infections increased in HIV-infected patients, diabetics, alcoholics, and dialysis patients

- **Differential Diagnosis**
  - Pseudofolliculitis barbae
  - Acne vulgaris and acneiform drug eruptions
  - Pustular miliaria (heat rash)
  - Fungal folliculitis
  - Herpes folliculitis
  - Hot tub folliculitis caused by pseudomonas
  - Gram-negative folliculitis (in acne patients on long-term antibiotic therapy)
  - Eosinophilic folliculitis (AIDS patients)
  - Nonbacterial folliculitis (occlusion or oil-induced)
  - Hidradenitis suppurativa of axillae or groin
  - Dissecting cellulitis of scalp

- **Treatment**
  - Thorough cleansing with antibacterial soaps
  - Mupirocin ointment in limited disease
  - Oral antibiotics (dicloxacillin or cephalexin) for more extensive involvement
  - Warm compresses and systemic antibiotics for furuncles and carbuncles
  - Culture for methicillin-resistant strains in unresponsive lesions
  - Avoid incision and drainage with acutely inflamed lesions; may be helpful when furuncle becomes localized and fluctuant
  - Culture anterior nares in recurrent cases to rule out *S aureus*
  - Mupirocin, oral rifampin to anterior nares for *S aureus*

- **Pearl**

When these lesions occur without obvious cause, a glycosylated hemoglobin may reveal diabetes.

Reference

Rhody C: Bacterial infections of the skin. Prim Care 2000;27:459. [PMID: 10815055]

Tinea Corporis (Ringworm)

- ■ Essentials of Diagnosis
  - Single or multiple circular, sharply circumscribed, erythematous, scaly plaques with elevated borders and central clearing
  - Frequently involves neck, extremities, and trunk
  - A deep, pustular form affecting the follicles (Majocchi's granuloma) may occur
  - Other types affect face (tinea faciei), hands (tinea manuum), feet (tinea pedis), and groin (tinea cruris)
  - Skin scrapings for microscopic examination or culture establish diagnosis
  - Widespread tinea may be presenting sign of HIV infection

- ■ Differential Diagnosis
  - Pityriasis rosea
  - Impetigo
  - Nummular dermatitis
  - Seborrheic dermatitis
  - Psoriasis
  - Granuloma annulare
  - Secondary syphilis
  - Subacute cutaneous lupus erythematosus

- ■ Treatment
  - One or two uncomplicated lesions usually respond to topical antifungals (allylamines or azoles)
  - A low-potency steroid cream during initial days of therapy may decrease inflammation
  - Oral griseofulvin standard therapy in extensive disease, follicular involvement, or in the immunocompromised host—itraconazole and terbinafine also effective
  - Infected household pets (especially cats and dogs) may transmit and should be treated

- ■ Pearl

Be wary of combination products containing antifungals and potent steroids: skin atrophy and reduced efficacy may result.

Reference

Drake LA et al: Guidelines of care for superficial mycotic infections of the skin. J Am Acad Dermatol 1996;34:282. [PMID: 08642094]

Onychomycosis (Tinea Unguium)

- ■ Essentials of Diagnosis
  - Yellowish discoloration, piling up of subungual keratin, friability, and separation of the nail plate
  - May show only overlying white scale if superficial
  - Nail shavings for immediate microscopic examination, culture, or histologic examination with periodic acid-Schiff stain to establish diagnosis; repeated sampling may be required

- ■ Differential Diagnosis
  - Candidal onychomycosis shows erythema, tenderness, swelling of the nail fold (paronychia)
  - Psoriasis
  - Lichen planus
  - Allergic contact dermatitis from nail polish
  - Contact urticaria from foods or other sensitizers
  - Nail changes associated with reactive arthritis, Darier's disease, crusted scabies

- ■ Treatment
  - Antifungal creams not effective
  - Oral terbinafine and itraconazole effective in many
  - Establish diagnosis before initiating therapy
  - Adequate informed consent critical; patients must decide if benefits of oral therapy outweigh risks
  - Weekly prophylactic topical antifungals to suppress tinea pedis may prevent tinea unguium recurrences

- ■ Pearl

There is a significant recurrence rate after oral therapy.

15

Reference

Epstein E: How often does oral treatment of toenail onychomycosis produce a disease-free nail? An analysis of published data. Arch Dermatol 1998; 134:1551. [PMID: 9875192]

Tinea Versicolor (Pityriasis Versicolor)

- **Essentials of Diagnosis**
  - Finely scaling patches on upper trunk and upper arms, usually asymptomatic
  - Lesions yellowish or brownish on pale skin, or hypopigmented on dark skin
  - Caused by yeast of the malassezia species
  - Short, thick hyphae and large numbers of spores on microscopic examination
  - Wood's light helpful in defining extent of lesions

- **Differential Diagnosis**
  - Seborrheic dermatitis
  - Pityriasis rosea
  - Pityriasis alba
  - Hansen's disease (leprosy)
  - Secondary syphilis (macular syphilid)
  - Vitiligo
  - Postinflammatory pigmentary alteration from another inflammatory dermatosis

- **Treatment**
  - Topical agents in limited disease (selenium sulfide shampoos or lotions, zinc pyrithione shampoos, imidazole shampoos, topical allylamines)
  - Oral agents in more diffuse involvement (single-dose ketoconazole repeated after 1 week, or 5–7 days of itraconazole)
  - Oral terbinafine not effective
  - Dyspigmentation may persist for months after effective treatment
  - Relapse likely if prophylactic measures not taken; a single monthly application of topical agent may be effective

- **Pearl**

Scrapings look like "spaghetti and meatballs"—the only entity in medicine best described as an Italian dinner entree.

Reference

Drake LA et al: Guidelines of care for superficial mycotic infections of the skin: Pityriasis (tinea) versicolor. J Am Acad Dermatol 1996;34:287. [PMID: 08642095]

15

Cutaneous Candidiasis

- **Essentials of Diagnosis**
  - Candidal intertrigo causes superficial denuded, pink to beefy-red patches that may be surrounded by tiny satellite pustules in genitocrural, subaxillary, gluteal, interdigital, and submammary areas
  - Oral candidiasis shows grayish white plaques that scrape off to reveal a raw, erythematous base
  - Oral candidiasis more common in elderly, debilitated, malnourished, diabetic, or HIV-infected patients as well as those taking antibiotics, systemic steroids, or chemotherapy
  - Angular cheilitis (perlèche) sometimes due to candida
  - Perianal candidiasis may cause pruritus ani
  - Candidal paronychia causes thickening and erythema of the nail fold and occasional discharge of thin pus

- **Differential Diagnosis**
  - Candidal intertrigo: dermatophytosis, bacterial skin infections, seborrheic dermatitis, contact dermatitis, deep fungal infection, inverse psoriasis, erythrasma, eczema
  - Oral candidiasis: lichen planus, leukoplakia, geographic tongue, herpes simplex infection, erythema multiforme, pemphigus
  - Candidal paronychia: acute bacterial paronychia, paronychia associated with hypoparathyroidism, celiac disease, acrodermatitis enteropathica, or reactive arthritis
  - Chronic mucocutaneous candidiasis

- **Treatment**
  - Control exacerbating factors (eg, hyperglycemia in diabetics, chronic antibiotic use, estrogen-dominant oral contraceptives, systemic steroids, ill-fitting dentures, malnutrition)
  - Treat localized skin disease with topical azoles or polyenes
  - Soaks with aluminum acetate solutions for raw, denuded lesions
  - Fluconazole and itraconazole for systemic therapy
  - Nystatin suspension or clotrimazole troches for oral disease
  - Treat chronic paronychia with topical imidazoles or 4% thymol in chloroform
  - Avoid chronic water exposure

- **Pearl**

  The key in cutaneous candidiasis: is it local, systemic, or due to immunosuppression? The history gives the answer.

Reference

Hay RJ: The management of superficial candidiasis. J Am Acad Dermatol 1999;40(6 Part 2):S35. [PMID: 10367915]

15

Herpes Simplex

- **Essentials of Diagnosis**
  - Orolabial herpes: initial infection usually asymptomatic; gingivo-stomatitis may occur
  - Recurrent grouped blisters on erythematous base (cold sore or fever blister); lips most frequently involved
  - UV exposure a common trigger
  - Genital herpes: primary infection presents as systemic illness with grouped blisters and erosions on penis, rectum, or vagina
  - Recurrences common, present with painful grouped vesicles; active lesions infectious; asymptomatic shedding also occurs
  - A prodrome of tingling, itching, or burning
  - More severe and persistent in immunocompromised patients
  - Eczema herpeticum is diffuse, superimposed upon a preexisting inflammatory dermatosis
  - Herpetic whitlow; infection of fingers or hands
  - Tzanck smears, fluorescent antibody tests, viral cultures, and skin biopsies diagnostic

- **Differential Diagnosis**
  - Impetigo
  - Zoster
  - Syphilis, chancroid, lymphogranuloma venereum, or granuloma inguinale
  - Oral aphthosis, coxsackievirus infection (herpangina), erythema multiforme, pemphigus, or primary HIV infection

- **Treatment**
  - Sunblock to prevent orolabial recurrences
  - Early acute intermittent therapy with acyclovir, famciclovir, or valacyclovir
  - Prophylactic suppressive therapy for patients with frequent recurrences
  - Short-term prophylaxis before intense sun exposure, dental procedures, and laser resurfacing for patients with recurrent orolabial disease
  - Suppressive therapy for immunosuppressed patients
  - Intravenous foscarnet for resistance

- **Pearl**

Think of genital herpes in chronic heel pain—the virus lives in the sacral ganglion and refers pain to that site.

Reference

Conant MA et al: Genital herpes. J Am Acad Dermatol 1996;35:601. [PMID: 97012475]

Zoster (Herpes Zoster, Shingles)

- ■ Essentials of Diagnosis
  - Occurs unilaterally within the distribution of a sensory nerve with some spillover into neighboring dermatomes
  - Prodrome of pain and paresthesia followed by papules and plaques of erythema which quickly develop vesicles
  - Vesicles become pustular, crust over, and heal
  - May disseminate (20 or more lesions outside the primary dermatome) in the elderly, debilitated, or immunosuppressed; visceral involvement (lungs, liver, or brain) may follow
  - Involvement of the nasal tip (Hutchinson's sign) a harbinger of ophthalmic zoster
  - Ramsay Hunt syndrome (ipsilateral facial paralysis, zoster of the ear, and auditory symptoms) from facial and auditory nerve involvement
  - Postherpetic neuralgia more common in older patients
  - Tzanck smears useful but cannot differentiate zoster from zosteriform herpes simplex
  - Direct fluorescent antibody test rapid and specific

- ■ Differential Diagnosis
  - Herpes simplex infection
  - Prodromal pain can mimic the pain of angina, duodenal ulcer, appendicitis, and biliary or renal colic
  - Zoster 30 times more common in the HIV-infected; ascertain HIV risk factors

- ■ Treatment
  - Heat or topical anesthetics locally
  - Antiviral therapy
  - Intravenous acyclovir for disseminated or ocular zoster
  - Bed rest to reduce risk of neuralgia in the elderly
  - Prednisone does not prevent neuralgia
  - Topical capsaicin, local anesthetics, nerve blocks, analgesics, tricyclic antidepressants, and gabapentin for postherpetic neuralgia
  - Patients with active lesions should avoid contact with neonates and immunosuppressed individuals

- ■ Pearl

"Shingles"—the word—is a linguistic corruption from Latin cingulum *("girdle"), reflecting the common thoracic presentation of this disorder.*

Reference

Cohen JI et al: Recent advances in varicella-zoster virus infection. Ann Intern Med 1999;130:922. [PMID: 99296103]

15

Molluscum Contagiosum

- ### Essentials of Diagnosis
  - Patients with AIDS, particularly those with a CD4 count of less than 100/μL, are at highest risk; large lesions on face and genitalia
  - Patients with malignancies, sarcoidosis, extensive atopic dermatitis, or history of diffuse topical steroid use are also predisposed
  - Smooth, firm, dome-shaped, pearly papules; characteristic central umbilication and white core
  - Frequently generalized in young children
  - Sexually transmitted in immunocompetent adults; usually with less than 20 lesions; on lower abdomen, upper thighs, and penile shaft

- ### Differential Diagnosis
  - Warts
  - Varicella
  - Bacterial infection
  - Basal cell carcinoma
  - Lichen planus
  - Cutaneous cryptococcal infection may mimic molluscum lesions in patients with AIDS

- ### Treatment
  - Avoid aggressive treatment in young children; possible therapies for children include topical tretinoin or imiquimod, or continuous application of occlusive tape
  - Cryotherapy, curettage, or a topical agent (eg, podophyllotoxin) for adults with genital disease
  - Antiretroviral therapies resulting in increasing CD4 counts are most effective for HIV-infected patients

- ### Pearl

As in so many other cases, this once trivial disease was made prominent by the HIV epidemic.

Reference

Lewis EJ et al: An update on molluscum contagiosum. Cutis 1997;60:29. [PMID: 9252731]

15

Common Warts (Verrucae Vulgares)

- **Essentials of Diagnosis**
  - Scaly, rough, spiny papules or plaques
  - Most frequently seen on hands, may occur anywhere on skin
  - Caused by human papillomavirus

- **Differential Diagnosis**
  - Actinic keratosis
  - Squamous cell carcinoma
  - Seborrheic keratosis
  - Acrochordon (skin tag)
  - Nevus
  - Molluscum contagiosum
  - Verrucous zoster in HIV-infected patients
  - Extensive warts suggest epidermodysplasia verruciformis, HIV infection, or lymphoproliferative disorders

- **Treatment**
  - Avoid aggressive treatment in young children; spontaneous resolution is common
  - Cryotherapy
  - Patient-applied salicylic acid products
  - Office-applied cantharidin
  - Curettage and electrodesiccation
  - Pulsed dye laser therapy
  - Sensitization with squaric acid in resistant cases
  - Intralesional bleomycin
  - Oral cimetidine has low efficacy but may be a useful adjunct
  - Topical imiquimod less effective in common warts than genital warts

- **Pearl**

The first tumor of Homo sapiens *proved to be caused by a virus.*

Reference

Benton EC: Therapy of cutaneous warts. Clin Dermatol 1997;15:449. [PMID: 97399323]

15

Genital Warts (Condylomata Acuminata)

- ■ **Essentials of Diagnosis**
  - Gray, yellow, or pink lobulated multifocal papules
  - Occur on the penis, vulva, cervix, perineum, crural folds, or perianal area; also may be intraurethral or intra-anal
  - Caused by human papillomavirus; sexually transmitted
  - Increased risk of progression to cervical cancer, anal cancer, or bowenoid papulosis in certain HPV subtypes
  - Children with genital warts should be evaluated for sexual abuse, but childhood infection can also be acquired via perinatal vertical transmission or digital autoinoculation

- ■ **Differential Diagnosis**
  - Psoriasis
  - Lichen planus
  - Bowenoid papulosis and squamous cell carcinoma
  - Seborrheic keratosis
  - Pearly penile papules
  - Acrochordon (skin tag)
  - Secondary syphilis (condyloma latum)

- ■ **Treatment**
  - Treatment may remove lesions but has not been shown to reduce transmission or prevent progression to cancer
  - Cryotherapy, topical podophyllum resin, topical trichloroacetic acid, electrofulguration, and carbon dioxide laser; plume generated by lasers or electrofulguration is potentially infectious to health care personnel
  - Imiquimod is as effective as cryotherapy; women have a higher response rate than men
  - Pap smear for women with genital warts and female sexual partners of men with genital warts
  - Biopsy suspicious lesions; HIV-infected patients with genital warts are at increased risk of HPV-induced carcinomas

- ■ **Pearl**

Subclinical disease, common and impossible to eradicate, is neither investigated nor treated.

Reference

Beutner KR et al: Genital warts and their treatment. Clin Infect Dis 1999; 28(Suppl 1):S37. [PMID: 99152435]

15

Pediculosis

- **Essentials of Diagnosis**

  - Three types of lice *(Pediculus humanus),* each with a predilection for certain body parts
  - Dermatitis caused by inflammatory response to louse saliva
  - Pediculosis capitis (head lice): intense scalp pruritus, presence of nits, possible secondary impetigo and cervical lymphadenopathy; most common in children, rare in blacks
  - Pediculosis corporis (body lice): rarely found on skin, causes generalized pruritus, erythematous macules or urticarial wheals, excoriations and lichenification; homeless and those living in crowded conditions most frequently affected
  - Pediculosis pubis (crabs): usually sexually transmitted; generally limited to pubic area, axillae, and eyelashes; lice may be observed on skin and nits on hairs; maculae ceruleae (blue macules) may be seen
  - Body lice can transmit trench fever, relapsing fever, and epidemic typhus

- **Differential Diagnosis**

  - Head lice: impetigo, hair casts, seborrheic dermatitis
  - Body lice: scabies, urticaria, impetigo, dermatitis herpetiformis
  - Pubic lice: scabies, anogenital pruritus, eczema

- **Treatment**

  - Head lice: topical permethrins with interval removal of nits and re-treatment in 1 week.
  - Pyrethrins available over the counter; resistance common
  - Treat household contacts
  - Body lice: launder clothing and bedding (at least 30 minutes at 150 °F in dryer, or iron pressing of wool garments); patient should then bathe; no pesticides required
  - Pubic lice: treatment is same as for head lice; eyelash lesions treated with thick coating of petrolatum maintained for 1 week; recurrence is more common in HIV-infected patients

- **Pearl**

Body lice infestation is an underappreciated cause of iron deficiency in the homeless population.

Reference

Chosidow O: Scabies and pediculosis. Lancet 2000;355:819. [PMID: 10711939]

Scabies

- ■ Essentials of Diagnosis
    - • Caused by *Sarcoptes scabiei* mite
    - • Pruritogenic papular eruption favoring finger webs, wrists, antecubital fossae, axillae, lower abdomen, genitals, buttocks, and nipples
    - • Itching usually worse at night
    - • Face and scalp are spared (except in children and the immunosuppressed)
    - • Burrows appear as short, slightly raised, wavy lines in skin, sometimes with vesicles
    - • Secondary eczematization, impetigo, and lichenification in longstanding infestation
    - • Red nodules on penis or scrotum
    - • A crusted form in institutionalized, HIV-infected, or malnourished individuals
    - • Burrow scrapings permit microscopic confirmation of mites, ova, or feces; many cases diagnosed on clinical grounds

- ■ Differential Diagnosis
    - • Atopic dermatitis
    - • Papular urticaria
    - • Insect bites
    - • Dermatitis herpetiformis
    - • Pediculosis corporis
    - • Pityriasis rosea

- ■ Treatment
    - • Permethrin 5% cream applied from the neck down for 8 hours; clothing and bed linens laundered thoroughly; repeat therapy in 1 week
    - • Lindane used infrequently because of potential toxicity
    - • Oral ivermectin in refractory cases, institutional epidemics, or immunosuppressed patients
    - • Treat all household and sexual contacts
    - • Persistent postscabietic pruritic papules may require topical or intralesional corticosteroids

- ■ Pearl

A condition occurring in all walks of life, not only in the underserved.

Reference

Chosidow O: Scabies and pediculosis. Lancet 2000;355:819. [PMID: 10711939]

Erythema Multiforme Minor

- ■ Essentials of Diagnosis
  - Uniformly associated with herpes simplex infection (orolabial more than genital)
  - Episodes follow orolabial herpes by 1–3 weeks and may recur with succeeding outbreaks
  - Early sharply demarcated erythematous papules which become edematous
  - Later "target" lesions with three zones: central duskiness that may vesiculate; edematous, pale ring; and surrounding erythema
  - Dorsal hands, dorsal feet, palms, soles, and extensor surfaces most frequently affected, with few to hundreds of lesions
  - Mucosal involvement (usually oral) in 25%
  - Biopsies often diagnostic

- ■ Differential Diagnosis
  - Stevens-Johnson in evolution
  - Pemphigus vulgaris
  - Bullous pemphigoid
  - Urticaria
  - Acute febrile neutrophilic dermatosis (Sweet's syndrome)

- ■ Treatment
  - Chronic suppressive antiherpetic therapy prevents 90% of recurrences
  - Facial and lip sunscreens may also decrease recurrences by limiting herpes outbreaks
  - Episodes usually self-limited (resolving in 1–4 weeks) and do not require therapy
  - Systemic corticosteroids discouraged

- ■ Pearl

Even when a history of herpes cannot be elicited, empiric antivirals may prevent recurring target lesions.

Reference

Singla R et al: Erythema multiforme due to herpes simplex virus. Recurring target lesions are the clue to diagnosis. Postgrad Med 1999;106:151. [PMID: 20024264]

Cutaneous Kaposi's Sarcoma

- **Essentials of Diagnosis**
  - Disease limited to the lower extremities, spreads slowly
  - Classic form occurs in elderly men of Mediterranean, East European, or Jewish descent
  - Vascular neoplasm presenting with one or several red to purple macules which progress to papules or nodules
  - African endemic form cutaneous and locally aggressive in young adults or lymphadenopathic and fatal in children
  - AIDS-associated form shows cutaneous lesions on head, neck, trunk, and mucous membranes; may progress to nodal, pulmonary, and gastrointestinal involvement
  - The form associated with iatrogenic immunosuppression can mimic either classic or AIDS-associated type
  - Human herpesvirus 8 the causative agent in all types
  - Skin biopsy for diagnosis

- **Differential Diagnosis**
  - Dermatofibroma
  - Bacillary angiomatosis
  - Pyogenic granuloma
  - Prurigo nodularis
  - Blue nevus
  - Melanoma
  - Cutaneous lymphoma

- **Treatment**
  - In AIDS-associated cases, combination antiretroviral therapy—increasing CD4 counts—is the treatment of choice
  - Intralesional vincristine or interferon, radiation therapy, cryotherapy, alitretinoin gel, laser ablation, or excision
  - Systemic therapy with liposomal doxorubicin or other cytotoxic drugs in certain cases with rapid progression or visceral involvement

- **Pearl**

The first alert to the HIV epidemic was a New York dermatologist reporting two cases of atypical Kaposi's sarcoma to the Centers for Disease Control—a single physician giving thought to a patient's problem can still make a difference.

Reference

Antman K et al: Kaposi's sarcoma. N Engl J Medicine 2000;342:1027. [PMID: 10749966]

Seborrheic Keratosis

- **Essentials of Diagnosis**
  - Age at onset generally fourth to fifth decades
  - Oval, raised, brown to black, warty, "stuck on"-appearing, well-demarcated papules or plaques; greasy hyperkeratotic scale may be present
  - Usually multiple; some patients have hundreds
  - Chest and back most frequent sites; scalp, face, neck, and extremities also involved
  - Rapid eruptive appearance of numerous lesions (Leser-Trélat sign) may signify internal malignancy

- **Differential Diagnosis**
  - Melanoma
  - Actinic keratosis
  - Nevus
  - Verruca vulgaris
  - Solar lentigo
  - Basal cell carcinoma, pigmented type
  - Squamous cell carcinoma
  - Dermatosis papulosa nigra in dark-skinned patients; numerous small papules on face, neck, and upper chest
  - Stucco keratosis shows hyperkeratotic, gray, verrucous, exophytic papules on the extremities, can be easily scraped off

- **Treatment**
  - Seborrheic keratoses do not require therapy
  - Cryotherapy or curettage effective in removal, may leave dyspigmentation
  - Electrodesiccation and laser therapy

- **Pearl**

A public health menace this is not, but look closely at all such lesions to exclude cutaneous malignancies.

Reference

Pariser RJ: Benign neoplasms of the skin. Med Clin North Am 1998;82:1285. [PMID: 9889749]

15

Actinic Keratosis (Solar Keratosis)

- **Essentials of Diagnosis**
  - Most common in fair-skinned individuals and in organ transplant recipients and other immunocompromised patients
  - Discrete keratotic, scaly papules; red, pigmented, or skin-colored
  - Found on the face, ears, scalp, dorsal hands, and forearms
  - Induced by chronic sun exposure
  - Lesions may become hypertrophic and develop a cutaneous horn
  - Lower lip actinic keratosis (actinic cheilitis) presents as diffuse, slight scaling of the entire lip
  - Some develop into squamous cell carcinoma

- **Differential Diagnosis**
  - Squamous cell carcinoma
  - Bowen's disease (squamous cell carcinoma in-situ)
  - Seborrheic keratosis
  - Discoid lupus erythematosus

- **Treatment**
  - Cryotherapy standard when limited number of sites present
  - Topical fluorouracil effective for extensive disease; usually causes a severe inflammatory reaction
  - Laser therapy for severe actinic cheilitis
  - Biopsy atypical lesions or those that do not respond to therapy
  - Sun protection, sunscreen use

- **Pearl**

In patients with facial pain, check for a history of actinic keratosis; when these lesions become carcinomas, they can invade the local sheath of the fifth cranial nerve and produce this symptom.

15

Reference

Salasche SJ: Epidemiology of actinic keratoses and squamous cell carcinoma. J Am Acad Dermatol 2000;42(1 Part 2):4. [PMID: 10607349]

Basal Cell Carcinoma

- ■ Essentials of Diagnosis
  - Dome-shaped semitranslucent papule with overlying telangiectases, or a plaque of such nodules around a central depression; central area may crust or ulcerate
  - Most occur on head and neck, but the trunk and extremities also affected
  - Pigmented, cystic, sclerotic, and superficial clinical variants
  - Immunosuppressive medications increase frequency and aggressiveness; patients with albinism or xeroderma pigmentosum or exposed to radiation therapy or arsenic also at increased risk
  - Chronic, local spread typical, metastasis rare
  - Biopsy critical for diagnosis

- ■ Differential Diagnosis
  - Squamous cell carcinoma
  - Actinic keratosis
  - Seborrheic keratosis
  - Paget's disease
  - Melanoma
  - Nevus
  - Psoriasis
  - Nevoid basal cell carcinoma syndrome

- ■ Treatment
  - Simple excision with histologic examination of margins
  - Curettage with electrodesiccation in superficial lesions of trunk or small nodular tumors in select locations
  - Mohs' microsurgery with immediate mapping of margins for lesions with aggressive histology, recurrences, or in areas where tissue conservation is important
  - Ionizing radiation is an alternative
  - Sun protection, regular sunscreen use, regular skin screening

- ■ Pearl

An extremely common malignancy—with millions of cases annually worldwide.

Reference

Goldberg LH: Basal cell carcinoma. Lancet 1996;347:663. [PMID: 96175905]

15

Squamous Cell Carcinoma

- ■ Essentials of Diagnosis
  - Chronic UV exposure, certain HPV infections, radiation exposure, long-standing scars, certain HIV infections, and chronic immunosuppression predispose
  - Immunosuppressed renal transplant patients may have 250 times the baseline risk
  - Patients with albinism, xeroderma pigmentosum, and epidermodysplasia verruciformis at increased risk
  - Hyperkeratotic, firm, indurated, red or skin-colored papule, plaque, or nodule, most commonly in sun-damaged skin
  - May ulcerate and form crust; many arise in actinic keratoses
  - Lesions confined to the epidermis are squamous cell carcinoma in-situ or Bowen's disease; all others are considered invasive
  - Metastasis infrequent but devastating; lesions on lip or in scars and those with subcutaneous or perineural involvement are at higher risk
  - Regional lymphatics primary route of spread
  - Skin biopsies usually diagnostic

- ■ Differential Diagnosis
  - Keratoacanthoma (a rapidly growing and sometimes self-involuting variant of squamous cell carcinoma)
  - Actinic keratosis, hypertrophic form
  - Basal cell carcinoma
  - Verruca vulgaris
  - Chronic nonhealing ulcers due to other causes (venous stasis, infection, etc)

- ■ Treatment
  - Simple excision with histologic examination of margins
  - Mohs' microsurgery with immediate mapping of margins for high-risk lesions or in areas where tissue conservation is important
  - Curettage and electrodesiccation in small in-situ lesions
  - Ionizing radiation
  - Evaluate patients with aggressive lesions or perineural involvement on histologic examination for metastatic disease
  - Prophylactic radiotherapy in high-risk lesions
  - Regular screening examinations and sun protection

- ■ Pearl

The main reason to treat all actinic keratoses: preventing this.

Reference

Goldman GD: Squamous cell cancer: a practical approach. Semin Cutan Med Surg 1998;17:80. [PMID: 98332265]

Malignant Melanoma

- ■ Essentials of Diagnosis
  - • Higher incidence in those with fair skin, blue eyes, blond or red hair, blistering sunburns, chronic sun exposure, family history, immunodeficiency, many nevi, dysplastic nevi, giant congenital nevus, and certain genetic diseases such as xeroderma pigmentosum
  - • ABCD warning signs: Asymmetry, Border irregularity, Color variegation, and Diameter over 6 mm
  - • Clinical characteristics vary depending on subtype and location
  - • Early detection is critical; advanced-stage disease has high mortality
  - • Epiluminescence microscopy to identify high-risk lesions
  - • Biopsies for diagnosis must be deep enough to permit measurement of thickness; partial biopsies should be avoided

- ■ Differential Diagnosis
  - • Seborrheic keratosis
  - • Basal cell carcinoma, pigmented type
  - • Nevus (ordinary melanocytic nevus, dysplastic nevus)
  - • Solar lentigo
  - • Pyogenic granuloma
  - • Kaposi's sarcoma
  - • Pregnancy-associated darkening of nevi

- ■ Treatment
  - • Prognosis for localized disease determined by histologic features
  - • Appropriate staging workup including history, physical examination, laboratory tests, and scans to evaluate for metastatic spread
  - • Sentinel lymph node biopsy; lymph node dissection if evidence of lymphatic disease
  - • Reexcision with appropriate margins determined by histologic characteristics of the tumor
  - • Adjuvant therapy for high risk
  - • Close follow-up

15

- ■ Pearl

When a mole is suspicious or changing, it belongs in formalin.

Reference

Lang PG Jr: Malignant melanoma. Med Clin North Am 1998;82:1325.
  [PMID: 9889751]

Nevi (Congenital Nevi, Acquired Nevi)

- **Essentials of Diagnosis**
  - Common acquired nevi have homogeneous surfaces and color patterns, smooth and sharp borders, and are round or oval in shape
  - Color may vary from flesh-colored to brown
  - Flat or raised depending on the subtype or stage of evolution
  - Excisional biopsy to rule out melanoma in changing nevi or those with ABCD warning signs (see Malignant Melanoma)
  - Congenital nevi darkly pigmented; sometimes hairy papules or plaques that may be present at birth
  - Large congenital nevi (those whose longest diameter will be greater than 20 cm in adulthood) are at increased risk for melanoma; when found on head, neck, or posterior midline, associated with underlying leptomeningeal melanocytosis

- **Differential Diagnosis**
  - Dysplastic nevus
  - Melanoma
  - Lentigo simplex
  - Solar lentigo
  - Dermatofibroma
  - Basal cell carcinoma
  - Molluscum contagiosum
  - Blue nevus
  - Café au lait spot
  - Epidermal nevus
  - Becker's nevus

- **Treatment**
  - Excision of cosmetically bothersome nevi, and for those at high risk of developing melanoma
  - Biopsy suspicious lesions
  - Partial biopsies should be avoided when excisional biopsies feasible
  - Head or spinal scans in children with large congenital nevi occurring on the head, neck, or posterior midline

- **Pearl**

Any nevus with suspicious features should be considered melanoma until proved otherwise.

Reference

Schleicher SM et al: Congenital nevi. Int J Dermatol 1995;34:8259. [PMID: 8647657]

Bullous Pemphigoid

- **Essentials of Diagnosis**
  - Age at onset seventh or eighth decade, though also occurs in young children
  - Caused by autoantibodies to two specific components of the hemidesmosome
  - Occasionally drug-induced (penicillamine, furosemide, captopril, enalapril, penicillin, sulfasalazine, nalidixic acid)
  - Large, tense blisters that rupture, leaving denuded areas which heal without scarring
  - Erythematous patches and urticarial plaques even in the absence of bullae
  - Predilection for groin, axillae, flexor forearms, thighs, and shins; may occur anywhere; some have oral involvement
  - Frequently pruritic
  - Diagnosis by lesional biopsy, perilesional direct immunofluorescence, and indirect immunofluorescence

- **Differential Diagnosis**
  - Epidermolysis bullosa acquisita
  - Cicatricial pemphigoid
  - Herpes gestationis
  - Linear IgA dermatosis
  - Dermatitis herpetiformis

- **Treatment**
  - Prednisone initially
  - Nicotinamide plus tetracycline
  - Aggressive immunosuppression may be required (azathioprine, low-dose methotrexate, or mycophenolate mofetil); monitor patients for side effects and infections
  - Topical steroids for localized mild disease that breaks through medical treatment
  - Pemphigoid usually self-limited, lasting months to years

- **Pearl**

With adequate therapy, most patients achieve lasting remission.

Reference

Nousari HC et al: Pemphigus and bullous pemphigoid. Lancet 1999;354:667. [PMID: 10466686]

15

Pemphigus Vulgaris

- ■ Essentials of Diagnosis
  - Presents in fifth or sixth decade
  - Caused by autoantibodies to desmogleins; occasionally drug-induced (penicillamine, captopril)
  - Thin-walled, fragile blisters; rupture to form painful erosions that crust and heal slowly without scarring
  - Most initially present with oral involvement
  - Scalp, face, neck, axillae, and groin common sites; esophagus, trachea, conjunctiva, and other mucosal surfaces may also be involved
  - Lateral pressure applied to perilesional skin induces more blistering (Nikolsky's sign)
  - Diagnosis by lesional biopsy of intact blisters, perilesional direct immunofluorescence, indirect immunofluorescence

- ■ Differential Diagnosis
  - Paraneoplastic pemphigus (usually associated with lymphomas and leukemias)
  - Pemphigus foliaceus
  - Fogo selvagem (endemic Brazilian pemphigus)
  - Bullous pemphigoid
  - Erythema multiforme, Stevens-Johnson syndrome, toxic epidermal necrolysis
  - Linear IgA dermatosis
  - Epidermolysis bullosa acquisita
  - Patients presenting with only oral lesions may be misdiagnosed with aphthous stomatitis, erythema multiforme, herpes simplex, lichen planus, or cicatricial pemphigoid

- ■ Treatment
  - Viscous lidocaine and antibiotic rinses for oral erosions
  - Early and aggressive systemic therapy required; mortality high in untreated patients
  - High doses of oral prednisone combined with another immunosuppressive (azathioprine or mycophenolate mofetil)
  - Monitor for side effects and infections
  - Plasmapheresis, intravenous immune globulin, and intramuscular gold are alternatives

- ■ Pearl

Before the advent of corticosteroids, this disease was often fatal.

Reference

Nousari HC et al: Pemphigus and bullous pemphigoid. Lancet 1999;354:667. [PMID: 10466686]

Urticaria (Hives) & Angioedema

- **Essentials of Diagnosis**
  - Pale or red, evanescent, edematous papules or plaques surrounded by red halo (flare) with severe itching or stinging; appear suddenly and resolve in hours
  - Acute (complete remission within 6 weeks) or chronic
  - Subcutaneous swelling (angioedema) occurs alone or with urticaria; eyelids and lips often affected; respiratory tract involvement may produce airway obstruction, and gastrointestinal involvement may cause abdominal pain; anaphylaxis possible
  - Can be induced by drugs (penicillins, aspirin, other NSAIDs, opioids, radiocontrast dyes, ACE inhibitors)
  - Foods a frequent cause of acute urticaria (nuts, strawberries, shellfish, chocolate, tomatoes, melons, pork, garlic, onions, eggs, milk, azo dye additives)
  - Infections also a cause (streptococcal upper respiratory infections, viral hepatitis, helminthic infections, or infections of the tonsils, a tooth, sinuses, gallbladder, prostate)

- **Differential Diagnosis**
  - Hereditary or acquired complement-mediated angioedema
  - Physical urticarias (pressure, cold, heat, solar, vibratory, cholinergic, aquagenic)
  - Urticarial hypersensitivity reactions to insect bites
  - Urticarial vasculitis
  - Bullous pemphigoid
  - Erythema multiforme
  - Granuloma annulare
  - Lyme borreliosis (erythema migrans)

- **Treatment**
  - Treat acute urticaria with antihistamines and avoid identified triggers; short course of prednisone in some cases
  - Chronic urticaria treated with antihistamines on a regular rather than as-needed basis; chronic prednisone discouraged
  - Second-generation nonsedating antihistamines during waking hours
  - Workup to rule out usual triggers

- **Pearl**

Angiotensin-converting enzyme (ACE) inhibitor-induced angioedema may occur at any time—even years—after beginning the medicine.

Reference

Greaves MW: Chronic urticaria. N Engl J Med 1995; 332:1767. [PMID: 95281009]

Granuloma Annulare

- ■ Essentials of Diagnosis
  - • White or red flat-topped, asymptomatic papules that spread with central clearing to form annular plaques; cause unknown
  - • May coalesce, then involute spontaneously
  - • Predilection for dorsum of fingers, hands, or feet; elbows or ankles also favored sites
  - • Generalized form sometimes associated with diabetes; subcutaneous form most common in children
  - • Skin biopsy secures diagnosis

- ■ Differential Diagnosis
  - • Necrobiosis lipoidica
  - • Tinea corporis
  - • Erythema migrans (Lyme disease)
  - • Sarcoidosis
  - • Secondary syphilis
  - • Erythema multiforme
  - • Subacute cutaneous lupus erythematosus
  - • Annular lichen planus
  - • Leprosy (Hansen's disease)
  - • Rheumatoid nodules (subcutaneous form)

- ■ Treatment
  - • None required in mild cases; 75% of patients with localized disease clear in 2 years
  - • Intralesional or potent topical corticosteroids effective for single lesions
  - • Prednisone contraindicated in generalized disease due to relapse upon withdrawal
  - • Anecdotal success with dapsone, nicotinamide, potassium iodide, systemic retinoids, antimalarials, and psoralen plus UVA (PUVA)

- ■ Pearl

Suspect HIV infection in generalized granuloma annulare in non-diabetics.

Reference

Smith MD et al: Granuloma annulare. Int J Dermatol 1997;36:326. [PMID: 97343421]

15

Discoid (Chronic Cutaneous) Lupus Erythematosus

- **Essentials of Diagnosis**
  - Dull red macules or papules developing into sharply demarcated hyperkeratotic plaques with follicular plugs
  - Lesions heal from the center with atrophy, dyspigmentation, and telangiectasias
  - Localized lesions most common on scalp, nose, cheeks, ears, lower lip, and neck
  - Scalp lesions cause scarring alopecia
  - Generalized disease involves trunk and upper extremities
  - Cutaneous involvement only rarely progresses to systemic lupus erythematosus, but one-fourth of SLE patients develop DLE
  - Abnormal serologies, leukopenia, and albuminuria identify DLE patients likely to progress; children with DLE more likely to progress
  - Skin biopsy for diagnosis; direct immunofluorescence

- **Differential Diagnosis**
  - Seborrheic dermatitis
  - Rosacea
  - Lupus vulgaris (cutaneous tuberculosis)
  - Sarcoidosis
  - Bowen's disease (squamous cell carcinoma in-situ)
  - Polymorphous light eruption
  - Tertiary syphilis
  - Lichen planopilaris of the scalp

- **Treatment**
  - Screen for systemic disease with history, physical, and laboratory tests
  - Aggressive sun protection, including a high-SPF sunscreen
  - Potent topical corticosteroids or intralesional steroids for localized lesions
  - Systemic therapy with antimalarials
  - Monitor laboratory studies; ophthalmologic consultation every 6 months
  - Thalidomide in resistant cases; pregnancy prevention and monitoring for side effects critical

15

- **Pearl**

Relapses are common, and long-term therapy is often required.

Reference

Donnelly AM et al: Discoid lupus erythematosus. Australas J Dermatol 1995;36:3. [PMID: 7763220]

Androgenetic Alopecia (Common Baldness)

- **Essentials of Diagnosis**
  - Genetic predisposition plus excessive androgen response
  - Men in third and fourth decades: gradual loss of hair, chiefly from vertex and frontotemporal regions; rate variable
  - Women: diffuse hair loss throughout the mid scalp, sparing frontal hairline
  - Appropriate laboratory workup for women with signs of hyperandrogenism (hirsutism, acne, abnormal menses)
  - Hair pull test may show a normal or increased number of telogen hairs; hair shafts narrow but not fragile

- **Differential Diagnosis**
  - Telogen effluvium
  - Alopecia induced by hypothyroidism
  - Alopecia induced by iron deficiency
  - Secondary syphilis
  - Trichotillomania
  - Tinea capitis
  - Alopecia areata in evolution

- **Treatment**
  - Early topical minoxidil effective in about one-third with limited disease
  - Oral finasteride prevents further loss and increases hair counts (except on the temples); contraindicated in women of childbearing potential; lacks efficacy in postmenopausal women
  - Wigs or interwoven hair for cosmetic purposes
  - Hair transplantation with minigrafts
  - Women with hyperandrogenism may respond to antiandrogen therapies

- **Pearl**

Anxious patients with this condition support an enormous market for uninvestigated products.

Reference

Drake LA et al: Guidelines for care of androgenetic alopecia. J Am Acad Dermatol 1996;35:465. [PMID: 96378724]

15

Alopecia Areata

- ■ Essentials of Diagnosis
  - Usually occurs without associated disease, but patients with alopecia areata have an increased incidence of atopic dermatitis, Down's syndrome, lichen planus, vitiligo, autoimmune thyroiditis, and systemic lupus erythematosus
  - Rapid and complete hair loss in one or several round or oval patches
  - Occurs on the scalp or in the beard, eyebrows, or eyelashes; other hair-bearing areas less frequently affected
  - Short broken hairs on patch periphery
  - During active disease, telogen hairs near the patches easily pulled; gray hairs spared
  - The patches show preservation of follicles and normal scalp
  - Some patients have nail pitting
  - Some progress to total loss of scalp hair (alopecia totalis); a few lose all body hair (alopecia universalis)
  - Biopsy with horizontal sectioning if diagnosis unclear

- ■ Differential Diagnosis
  - Tinea capitis
  - Discoid lupus erythematosus, early lesions
  - Lichen planopilaris, early lesions
  - Secondary syphilis
  - Trichotillomania
  - Metastatic or cutaneous malignancy
  - Loose anagen syndrome
  - Androgenic alopecia

- ■ Treatment
  - Course is variable: some patches regrow spontaneously, others resist therapy
  - Intralesional steroid injections for regrowth
  - Topical anthralin, corticosteroids, or minoxidil, contact sensitization with squaric acid, and psoralens plus UVA
  - Psychologic stress can be devastating; emotional support, patient education essential

- ■ Pearl

Spontaneous recovery is common in patients with limited disease who are postpubertal at onset.

Reference

Price VH: Treatment of hair loss. N Engl J Med 1999;341:964. [PMID: 99412080]

Vitiligo

- **Essentials of Diagnosis**
  - Depigmented white patches surrounded by a normal, hyperpigmented, or occasionally inflamed border
  - Hairs in affected area usually turn white
  - Localized form may affect one nondermatomal site or may be segmental
  - Usually treatment-resistant
  - Generalized form most common; involvement symmetric and tends to affect skin around orifices
  - Universal form depigments entire body surface
  - Acrofacial form affects the distal fingers and facial orifices
  - Ocular abnormalities (iritis, uveitis, and retinal pigmentary abnormalities) increased in vitiligo patients
  - Associated with insulin-dependent diabetes, pernicious anemia, autoimmune thyroiditis, alopecia areata, and Addison's disease

- **Differential Diagnosis**
  - Leukoderma associated with metastatic melanoma
  - Occupational vitiligo from phenols or other chemicals
  - Morphea
  - Lichen sclerosis
  - Tinea versicolor
  - Pityriasis alba
  - Postinflammatory hypopigmentation
  - Hansen's disease (leprosy)
  - Cutaneous T cell lymphoma
  - Lupus erythematosus
  - Piebaldism
  - Tuberous sclerosis

15

- **Treatment**
  - Spontaneous repigmentation infrequently occurs
  - Cosmetic camouflage
  - Sun protection to avoid severe burns in affected areas
  - Potent topical steroids in focal lesions may help repigment
  - Psoralen plus UVA may help in generalized disease, but inadvertent burns are common
  - Total permanent depigmentation with monobenzone an option in extensive disease
  - Patient education, emotional support

- **Pearl**

An under-appreciated part of the endocrine immunopathies: its presence should call for thyroid, adrenal, and gastric antibody studies.

Reference

Kovacs SO: Vitiligo. J Am Acad Dermatol 1998;38(5 Part 1):647. [PMID: 9591808]

Melasma (Chloasma Faciei)

- ■ Essentials of Diagnosis
  - • Most frequently seen in women during pregnancy or menopause—also associated with oral contraceptives and phenytoin use
  - • Well-demarcated symmetric brown patches with irregular borders
  - • Typically on cheeks and forehead but may also involve nipples, genitals, or forearms
  - • Exacerbated by sun exposure

- ■ Differential Diagnosis
  - • Postinflammatory hyperpigmentation
  - • Contact photodermatitis from perfumes
  - • Exogenous ochronosis (from hydroquinones, phenol, or resorcinol)
  - • Drug-induced hyperpigmentation (minocycline, gold, etc)

- ■ Treatment
  - • Sun protection, including broad-spectrum sunscreen with UVA coverage
  - • Bleaching creams with hydroquinone moderately effective, sometimes combined with topical retinoids and mild topical steroid (contraindicated during pregnancy or lactation)

- ■ Pearl

Pregnancy-induced melasma clears within months; medication-induced disease persists for years.

Reference

Grimes PE: Melasma. Etiologic and therapeutic considerations. Arch Dermatol 1995;131:1453. [PMID: 96094883]

15

Acanthosis Nigricans

- **Essentials of Diagnosis**
    - Symmetric velvety hyperpigmented plaques on axillae, groin, and neck; the face, umbilicus, inner thighs, anus, flexor surfaces of elbows and knees, and mucosal surfaces may also be affected
    - Associated with insulin-resistant states such as obesity
    - Laboratory evaluation of testosterone and DHEAS levels in women with the type A syndrome of insulin resistance
    - Patients with the type B syndrome have acanthosis nigricans and insulin resistance secondary to anti-insulin receptor autoantibodies generated by autoimmune diseases
    - Associated with some drugs (testosterone, nicotinic acid, oral contraceptives, corticosteroids)
    - Widespread lesions or disease occurring in a nonobese patient arouse suspicion of malignant acanthosis nigricans associated with adenocarcinomas of the stomach, lung, and breast
    - Workup for malignancy if palmar involvement present

- **Differential Diagnosis**
    - Confluent and reticulated papillomatosis of Gougerot and Carteaud
    - Epidermal nevus
    - Dowling-Degos disease

- **Treatment**
    - Weight loss for obese patients
    - Malignant form often responds to treatment of the causal tumor

- **Pearl**

May be a harbinger of impending diabetes even before fasting glucose levels are elevated.

15

Reference

Schwartz RA: Acanthosis nigricans. J Am Acad Dermatol 1994;31:1. [PMID: 94292614]

Erythema Nodosum

- ■ Essentials of Diagnosis
  - A reactive inflammation of the subcutis associated with infections (streptococcal, tuberculous, yersinia, salmonella, shigella, systemic fungal infections), drugs (oral contraceptives, sulfonamides, bromides), sarcoidosis, and inflammatory bowel disease
  - Symmetric, erythematous, tender plaques or nodules 1–10 cm in diameter on anterior shins
  - Lesions also seen on upper legs, neck, and arms
  - Onset accompanied by malaise, leg edema, and arthralgias
  - Lesions flatten over a few days leaving a violaceous patch, then heal without atrophy or scarring
  - All lesions generally resolve within 6 weeks
  - Chronic form with prolonged course not associated with underlying diseases
  - Deep skin biopsy for diagnosis

- ■ Differential Diagnosis
  - Erythema induratum (secondary to tuberculosis)
  - Nodular vasculitis
  - Poststeroid panniculitis
  - Lupus panniculitis
  - Erythema multiforme
  - Syphilis
  - Subcutaneous fat necrosis associated with pancreatitis

- ■ Treatment
  - Treat underlying causes
  - Bed rest, gentle support hose; avoid vigorous exercise
  - NSAIDs
  - Potassium iodide
  - Intralesional steroids in persistent cases
  - Systemic steroids in severe cases; contraindicated when the underlying cause is infectious

15

- ■ Pearl

Chronic lesions unresponsive to therapy should prompt a workup for subclinical tuberculosis infection.

Reference

Cribier B et al: Erythema nodosum and associated diseases. Int J Dermatol 1998;37:667. [PMID 98433780]

Pyoderma Gangrenosum

- **Essentials of Diagnosis**
  - Often chronic and recurrent; may be accompanied by a poly-articular arthritis
  - Associated with inflammatory bowel disease and lymphoprolif-erative disorders; also seen with hepatitis B or C, HIV infection, systemic lupus erythematosus, pregnancy, and other conditions
  - Up to half of cases idiopathic
  - Lesions begin as inflammatory pustules, sometimes at a trauma site
  - Erythematous halo enlarges, then ulcerates
  - Ulcers painful with ragged, undermined, violaceous borders; bases appear purulent
  - Ulcers heal slowly, form atrophic scars
  - Diagnosis of exclusion; biopsies with special stains and cultures to rule out infections (mycobacterial, fungal, tertiary syphilis, gangrene, amebiasis)

- **Differential Diagnosis**
  - Folliculitis, insect bites, or Sweet's syndrome (acute febrile neutro-philic dermatosis)
  - Ulcers secondary to underlying infection
  - Ulcers secondary to underlying neoplasm
  - Factitious ulcerations from injected substances
  - Vasculitis (especially Wegener's granulomatosis)
  - Coumarin necrosis

- **Treatment**
  - Treat inflammatory bowel disease when present
  - Local compresses, occlusive dressings, potent topical steroids, intralesional steroids, or topical tacrolimus
  - High-dose systemic steroids in widespread disease; if control is not established or if a steroid taper is unsuccessful, a steroid-sparing agent (cyclosporine, mycophenolate mofetil, etc) is added
  - Dapsone, sulfasalazine, and clofazimine also steroid-sparing

- **Pearl**

Often confused with factitious ulcerations as the clinical presentations are quite similar.

Reference

Powell FC et al: Pyoderma gangrenosum. Clin Dermatol 2000;18:283. [PMID: 10856660]

15

Leg Ulcers From Venous Insufficiency

- ### Essentials of Diagnosis
  - Occurs in patients with signs of venous insufficiency
  - Irregular ulcerations, often on medial aspect of lower legs; fibrinous eschar at the base
  - Light rheography to assess venous insufficiency
  - Measurement of the ankle/brachial index to eliminate arterial component
  - Atypical or persistent ulcers should be biopsied to rule out other causes

- ### Differential Diagnosis
  - Arterial insufficiency
  - Pyoderma gangrenosum
  - Diabetic neuropathy and microangiopathy
  - Vasculitis
  - Cryoglobulins
  - Infection (mycobacteria, fungi)
  - Trauma
  - Sickle cell anemia or thalassemia
  - Neoplasm (eg, basal cell or squamous cell carcinoma, melanoma, lymphoma)

- ### Treatment
  - Clean ulcer base, remove eschar regularly
  - Topical antibiotics (metronidazole) reduce bacterial growth and odor; topical steroids when inflammation present
  - Cover ulcer with occlusive permeable biosynthetic dressing
  - Compression therapy with Unna's boot or elastic bandage essential
  - Becaplermin (recombinant platelet-derived growth factor) in diabetics with refractory ulcers
  - Cultured epidermal cell grafts or bilayered skin substitutes in highly refractory ulcers
  - Compression stockings to reduce edema and risk of further ulcerations

- ### Pearl

Venous stasis ulcers disappear as arterial insufficiency develops—no preload, no ulcer.

Reference

Alguire PC et al: Chronic venous insufficiency and venous ulceration. J Gen Intern Med 1997;12:374. [PMID: 9192256]

15

Gynecologic, Obstetric, & Breast Disorders

Abnormal Uterine Bleeding

- **Essentials of Diagnosis**
  - Excessive menses, intermenstrual bleeding, or both; postmenopausal bleeding
  - Common soon post-menarche, 4–6 years pre-menopause

- **Differential Diagnosis**
  - Pregnancy (especially ectopic), spontaneous abortion
  - Anovulation (eg, polycystic ovaries, hypothyroidism)
  - Uterine myoma or carcinoma, polyp, trauma
  - Cervicitis, carcinoma of the cervix
  - Adenomyosis
  - Exogenous hormones (eg, unopposed estrogen, medroxyprogesterone acetate, levonorgestrel, oral contraceptives)
  - Coagulation disorders (eg, von Willebrand's disease)

- **Treatment**
  - Exclude pregnancy
  - Transfusion, oral iron when deficiency proved
  - Papanicolaou smear (all ages) and endometrial biopsy (all postmenopausal women and those over age 35 with chronic anovulation or more than 6 months of bleeding)
  - Active bleeding with significant anemia: high-dose estrogen (25 mg intravenously or oral contraceptive taper: two pills twice daily for 3 days tapering over 2 weeks to one daily); high-dose progestin when high-dose estrogen contraindicated
  - Chronic bleeding: oral contraceptives or cyclic progestin; NSAIDs can reduce blood loss
  - Hysterectomy or endometrial ablation for bleeding refractory to hormonal therapy
  - Hysterectomy if endometrial cancer, hyperplasia with atypia

- **Pearl**

Ectopic pregnancy is considered first and promptly as the most serious cause of acute uterine (and intraperitoneal) blood loss.

Reference

Munro MG: Medical management of abnormal uterine bleeding. Obstet Gynecol Clin North Am 2000;27:287. [PMID: 10857120]

Dysmenorrhea

- ■ Essentials of Diagnosis
  - Occurs in 50% of menstruating women
  - Low, midline, cramping pelvic pain radiating to back or legs; pain starting before or with menses, peaking after 24 hours, and subsiding after 2 days, often associated with nausea, diarrhea, headache, and flushing
  - Primary dysmenorrhea: pain without pelvic pathology and beginning 1–2 years after menarche
  - Secondary dysmenorrhea: pain with underlying pathology such as endometriosis or adenomyosis, developing years after menarche

- ■ Differential Diagnosis
  - Endometriosis
  - Adenomyosis
  - Uterine myoma
  - Cervical stenosis, uterine anomalies
  - Chronic endometritis or pelvic inflammatory disease
  - Intrauterine device

- ■ Treatment
  - NSAIDs prior to the onset of bleeding, continued for 2–3 days
  - Suppression of ovulation with oral contraceptives or medroxyprogesterone acetate
  - In secondary dysmenorrhea, laparoscopy may be needed diagnostically

- ■ Pearl

Endometriosis is the most important cause; pregnancy is the treatment.

Reference

Coco AS: Primary dysmenorrhea. Am Fam Physician 1999;60:489. [PMID: 10465224]

16

Mucopurulent Cervicitis

- **Essentials of Diagnosis**
  - A sexually transmitted infection most commonly caused by *Neisseria gonorrhoeae* or chlamydia; endocervical inflammation can result from herpesvirus, trichomonas, or candida
  - Usually asymptomatic but may have abnormal vaginal discharge, postcoital bleeding, or dysuria
  - Red, friable cervix with purulent, often blood-streaked endocervical discharge
  - Must be distinguished from physiologic ectopy of columnar epithelium common in young women

- **Differential Diagnosis**
  - Pelvic inflammatory disease
  - Cervical carcinoma or dysplasia
  - Cervical ulcer secondary to syphilis, chancroid, or granuloma inguinale
  - Normal epithelial ectopy
  - Cervical inflammation due to vaginal infection

- **Treatment**
  - In general, treat only if tests are positive for *N gonorrhoeae* or chlamydia; empirically in a high risk or noncompliant patient
  - Ceftriaxone for gonorrhea, erythromycin or doxycycline (once pregnancy excluded) for chlamydiosis
  - Sexual abstinence until treatment completed, with therapy for partner

- **Pearl**

Any patient with cervicitis, irrespective of the cause, should be tested for HIV, syphilis, and hepatitis C.

16

Reference

Miller KE et al: Update on the prevention and treatment of sexually transmitted diseases. Am Fam Physician 2000;61:379. [PMID: (UI: 10670504]

Vaginitis

- **Essentials of Diagnosis**
  - Vaginal burning, pain, pruritus, discharge
  - Results from atrophy, infection, or allergic reaction
  - Common infectious causes include *Candida albicans, Trichomonas vaginalis,* bacterial vaginosis (gardnerella and other anaerobes)
  - Trichomonas is sexually transmitted and causes profuse, malodorous discharge and vaginal irritation
  - Bacterial vaginosis may be asymptomatic or associated with a thin, gray, "fishy" discharge
  - *C albicans* associated with pruritus, burning, and a thick, white, nonmalodorous discharge
  - KOH and pH are usually diagnostic: Trichomonads are motile, pH > 4.5; bacterial vaginosis reveals clue cells, pH > 4.5; hyphae and spores with a normal pH (< 4.5) mean candida

- **Differential Diagnosis**
  - Physiologic discharge, ovulation
  - Atrophic vaginitis, vulvar dystrophies (lichen sclerosis), and vulvar neoplasia in older women
  - Cervicitis, syphilis, herpesvirus outbreak
  - Cervical carcinoma
  - Foreign body (retained tampon)
  - Contact dermatitis (eg, condoms, perfumed products, soap)
  - Pubic lice, scabies

- **Treatment**
  - Limit vaginal irritants
  - Culture cervix for *Neisseria gonorrhoeae* and chlamydia if no other cause for symptoms
  - For *T vaginalis:* metronidazole (2 g as a single dose) for both patient and partner
  - For *C albicans:* antifungal (eg, clotrimazole) vaginal cream or suppository or single-dose oral fluconazole (150 mg)
  - For bacterial vaginosis: metronidazole (500 mg twice daily for 7 days or vaginal gel twice daily for 5 days)

16

- **Pearl**

Pubic lice may simulate vaginitis and may be seen in all walks of life despite the contrary bias.

Reference

Egan ME et al: Diagnosis of vaginitis. Am Fam Physician 2000;62:1095. [PMID: 10997533]

Myoma of the Uterus
(Fibroid Tumor, Leiomyoma, Fibromyoma)

- **Essentials of Diagnosis**
  - Irregular enlargement of uterus caused by benign smooth muscle tumors
  - Occurs in 40–50% of women over age 40
  - May be asymptomatic or cause heavy or irregular vaginal bleeding, anemia, urinary frequency, pelvic pressure, dysmenorrhea
  - Acute pelvic pain rare
  - May be intramural, submucosal, subserosal, intraligamentous, cervical, or parasitic (ie, deriving its blood supply from an adjacent organ)
  - Pelvic ultrasound confirms diagnosis

- **Differential Diagnosis**
  - Pregnancy
  - Adenomyosis
  - Ovarian or adnexal mass
  - Abnormal uterine bleeding due to other causes
  - Leiomyosarcoma
  - Renal infarct
  - Tamoxifen therapy

- **Treatment**
  - Exclude pregnancy
  - Papanicolaou smear and endometrial biopsy
  - Pelvic examinations regularly for small asymptomatic myomas
  - Hormonal therapy for menometrorrhagia
  - GnRH agonists for 3–6 months for women planning surgery or nearing menopause
  - Medical therapies often ineffective for large or submucosal myomas; resection may be necessary

16

- **Pearl**

Infarction of a myoma may cause a spectacular elevation in serum LDH, simulating hemolysis if the hematocrit is also falling from associated bleeding.

Reference

Nowak RA: Fibroids: pathophysiology and current medical treatment. Baillieres Best Pract Res Clin Obstet Gynaecol 1999;13:223. [PMID: 10755039]

Endometriosis

- ■ Essentials of Diagnosis
  - Seen in 10% of all menstruating women, 25% of infertile women
  - Progressive, recurrent, characterized by aberrant growth of endometrium outside the uterus
  - Classic triad: cyclic pelvic pain, dysmenorrhea, and dyspareunia
  - May be associated with infertility or pelvic mass
  - Pelvic examination may or may not be normal
  - Hematochezia, painful defecation, or hematuria if bowel or bladder invaded
  - Ultrasound often normal
  - Laparoscopy confirms diagnosis

- ■ Differential Diagnosis
  - Other causes of chronic pelvic pain
  - Primary dysmenorrhea
  - Adenomyosis

- ■ Treatment
  - NSAIDs
  - Ovulation suppression until fertility is desired
  - GnRH analogs (eg, leuprolide) for no longer than 6 months
  - Laparoscopy with ablation of lesions for refractory pain helpful in up to two-thirds of patients; 50% recur
  - Hysterectomy with bilateral salpingo-oophorectomy for those who have completed childbearing

- ■ Pearl

The only benign disease in medicine which behaves like metastatic carcinoma; endometriosis occurs anywhere in the body, including fingers, lungs, and other organs.

16

Reference

Wellbery C: Diagnosis and treatment of endometriosis. Am Fam Physician 1999;60:1753. [PMID: 10537390]

Pelvic Inflammatory Disease
(PID, Salpingitis, Endometritis, Tubo-ovarian Abscess)

- **Essentials of Diagnosis**
  - Most common in young, sexually active women with multiple partners
  - Upper genital tract associated with *Neisseria gonorrhoeae* and *Chlamydia trachomatis,* anaerobes, *Haemophilus influenzae,* enteric gram-negative rods, and streptococci
  - A major cause of chronic pelvic pain, infertility and pelvic adhesions
  - Symptoms and severity vary
  - Lower abdominal, adnexal, cervical motion tenderness; fever, abnormal cervical discharge, leukocytosis
  - Absence of competing diagnosis
  - Right upper quadrant pain (Fitz-Hugh and Curtis syndrome) from associated perihepatitis
  - Pelvic ultrasound may reveal a tubo-ovarian abscess.
  - Laparoscopy for cases with uncertain diagnosis or no improvement despite antibiotic therapy

- **Differential Diagnosis**
  - Any cause of acute abdominal-pelvic pain or peritonitis
  - Appendicitis, diverticulitis
  - Ruptured ovarian cyst, ovarian torsion
  - Ectopic pregnancy
  - Acute cystitis, urinary calculi

- **Treatment**
  - Oral antibiotics for mild cases (14-day course) covering *N gonorrhoeae* and chlamydia
  - Hospitalization and intravenous antibiotics for toxic, adolescent, HIV-infected, or pregnant patients
  - Surgical drainage of tubo-ovarian abscess
  - Screen for HIV, hepatitis, syphilis
  - Sexual abstinence until treatment completed; partner should be treated

16

- **Pearl**

PID is occasionally if irreverently referred to as "Hollywood appendicitis" in the entertainment industry.

Reference

Munday PE: Pelvic inflammatory disease—an evidence-based approach to diagnosis. J Infect 2000;40:31. [PMID: 10762109]

Pelvic Organ Prolapse

- ■ Essentials of Diagnosis
  - Common in older multiparous women as a delayed result of child-birth injury to pelvic floor
  - Includes prolapse of the uterus, bladder, rectum, small bowel or vaginal cuff
  - Often asymptomatic; may have pelvic pressure or pulling, vaginal bulge, low back pain, difficulties with defecation or voiding
  - Pelvic examination confirms the diagnosis
  - Prolapse may be slight, moderate, or marked
  - Attenuation of pelvic structures with aging can accelerate development

- ■ Differential Diagnosis
  - Vaginal or cervical neoplasm
  - Rectal prolapse
  - Rectal carcinoma

- ■ Treatment
  - Supportive measures (eg, Kegel exercises), high-fiber diet, weight reduction, and limit straining and lifting
  - Conjugated estrogen creams to decrease vaginal irritation
  - Pessaries may reduce prolapse and its symptoms; ineffective for very large prolapse
  - Corrective surgery for symptomatic prolapse that significantly affects quality of life

- ■ Pearl

Lack of awareness of this entity may result in misdiagnosis of a pelvic tumor or abscess; the history should provide the answer.

Reference

Shull BL: Pelvic organ prolapse: anterior, superior, and posterior vaginal segment defects. Am J Obstet Gynecol 1999;181:6. [PMID: 10411783]

16

Spontaneous Abortion

- **Essentials of Diagnosis**
  - Vaginal bleeding and pelvic pain and cramping before the 20th week of pregnancy
  - Occurs in up to 20% of pregnancies
  - Threatened abortion: pregnancy may continue or abortion may ensue; cervix closed, bleeding and cramping mild, intrauterine pregnancy confirmed
  - Inevitable or incomplete abortion: cervix dilated and products of conception may or may not be partially expelled; brisk uterine bleeding
  - Complete abortion: products of conception completely expelled; cervix closed, cramping and bleeding decreased
  - Missed abortion (blighted ovum): failed pregnancy detected by ultrasound; cervix closed, bleeding and cramping mild
  - Serum β-hCG low or falling except in threatened abortion
  - Pelvic ultrasonography contraindicated when bleeding heavy or cervix open

- **Differential Diagnosis**
  - Ectopic pregnancy
  - Menorrhagia, menses, prolapsed uterine myoma
  - Gestational trophoblastic neoplasia
  - Cervical neoplasm or lesion

- **Treatment**
  - Follow hematocrit closely
  - Threatened abortion: β-hCG in 2–3 days; immediate follow-up if brisk bleeding develops
  - Limiting activity ineffective
  - Inevitable or incomplete abortion: immediate suction curettage
  - Missed abortion: suction curettage or wait for spontaneous abortion
  - Rh_o immune globulin to Rh-negative mothers
  - Follow-up to ensure patient is no longer pregnant

- **Pearl**

Over-the-counter diagnostic kits resulting in early diagnosis of pregnancy have demonstrated a high incidence of this disorder—in truth a normal phenomenon in up to one-third of conceptions.

Reference

Ansari AH et al: Recurrent pregnancy loss. An update. J Reprod Med 1998; 43:806. [PMID: 9777621]

16

Menopausal Syndrome

- ■ Essentials of Diagnosis
  - Cessation of menses without other cause, usually due to aging or bilateral oophorectomy
  - Average age is 51; earlier in women who smoke
  - Perimenopause: declining ovarian function over 4–6 years
  - Menstrual irregularity, hot flushes, night sweats, vaginal dryness
  - Elevated serum FSH and LH

- ■ Differential Diagnosis
  - Other causes of amenorrhea, especially pregnancy
  - Hyperthyroidism or hypothyroidism
  - Pheochromocytoma
  - Uterine neoplasm
  - Sjögren's syndrome
  - Depression
  - Anorexia

- ■ Treatment
  - Short-term hormonal therapy
  - Hot flushes often resolve by 2–4 years after menopause
  - For irregular bleeding, oral contraceptives, cyclic or combined continuous estrogen plus progestin, or progestins alone
  - Long-term hormone replacement therapy to decrease risk of osteoporosis
  - Estrogen cream and nonhormonal lubricants for vaginal dryness

- ■ Pearl

Menopause may on occasion be premature, a devastating event for a nulliparous young woman; psychologic support is crucial in the early care of such patients.

16

Reference

Cutson TM et al: Managing menopause. Am Fam Physician 2000;61:1391. [PMID: 10735345]

Preeclampsia-Eclampsia

- **Essentials of Diagnosis**
  - Progressive condition affecting 5–10% of pregnant women
  - Preeclampsia is hypertension plus proteinuria; addition of seizures means eclampsia
  - Headache, blurred vision or scotomas, abdominal pain, altered mental status
  - Funduscopic evidence of acute hypertension, hyperreflexia; encephalopathy
  - Thrombocytopenia, elevated AST or ALT, hemoconcentration or hemolysis
  - Pulmonary edema can occur
  - HELLP syndrome: hemolysis, elevated liver enzymes and low platelets
  - Increased in primiparas and patients with history of preeclampsia, hypertension, diabetes, chronic renal disease, autoimmune disorders

- **Differential Diagnosis**
  - Chronic hypertension due to other cause
  - Chronic renal disease due to other cause
  - Primary seizure disorder
  - Hemolytic uremic syndrome
  - Thrombotic thrombocytopenic purpura

- **Treatment**
  - The only treatment is delivery of the fetus
  - Induce labor at or near term or for severe disease regardless of gestational age
  - Remote from term, mild cases can be observed in the hospital with induction of labor for worsening disease
  - Antihypertensives if blood pressure > 180/110 mm Hg; goal is 150/90 mm Hg
  - For eclampsia, intravenous magnesium sulfate or diazepam

- **Pearl**

Deliver the baby, cure the disease.

Reference

Visser W et al: Prediction and prevention of pregnancy-induced hypertensive disorders. Baillieres Best Pract Res Clin Obstet Gynaecol 1999;13:131. [PMID: 10746098]

16

Mammary Dysplasia (Fibrocystic Disease)

- ■ Essentials of Diagnosis
  - Common age 30–50
  - Painful, often multiple, usually bilateral masses in the breasts
  - Rapid fluctuation in size of masses
  - Pain, increase in size during premenstrual phase of cycle
  - Rare in postmenopausal women not on hormonal therapy
  - Eighty percent of women have histologic fibrocystic changes

- ■ Differential Diagnosis
  - Breast carcinoma
  - Fibroadenoma
  - Fat necrosis
  - Intraductal papilloma

- ■ Treatment
  - Biopsy to exclude carcinoma
  - Ultrasound to differentiate cystic from solid masses
  - Aspiration both diagnostic and therapeutic
  - Regular breast self-examination
  - Supportive brassiere (night and day), NSAIDs, oral contraceptives
  - Danazol (100–200 mg twice daily) for severe pain

- ■ Pearl

Recognize that all women are appropriately fearful of breast cancer in this condition and that medical management is only one part of the picture.

Reference

Zylstra S: Office management of benign breast disease. Clin Obstet Gynecol 1999;42:234. [PMID: 10370844]

Puerperal Mastitis

- **Essentials of Diagnosis**
  - Occurs in nursing mothers within 3 months after delivery
  - Unilateral inflammation of breast or one quadrant of breast
  - Sore or fissured nipple with surrounding redness, tenderness, induration, warmth, fever, malaise
  - Increased incidence in first-time mothers
  - *Staphylococcus aureus* and streptococci are usual causative agents
  - May progress to breast abscess
  - Ultrasound can confirm abscess diagnosis

- **Differential Diagnosis**
  - Local irritation or trauma
  - Benign or malignant tumors (inflammatory carcinoma)
  - Subareolar abscess (occurs in nonlactating women)
  - Fat necrosis

- **Treatment**
  - For very mild cases, warm compresses and increased frequency of breast feeding
  - Oral dicloxacillin or first-generation cephalosporin
  - Hospitalize for intravenous antibiotics if no improvement in 48 hours in toxic patients
  - Increase frequency of breast feeding with expression of any remaining milk
  - Incision and drainage for abscess; stop breast feeding from affected breast (may pump milk and discard)

- **Pearl**

Women with this disorder may appear surprisingly toxic systemically, diverting attention from this diagnosis.

16

Reference

Scott-Conner CE et al: The diagnosis and management of breast problems during pregnancy and lactation. Am J Surg 1995;170:401. [PMID: 7573738]

Chronic Pelvic Pain

- **Essentials of Diagnosis**
  - Subacute pelvic pain of more than 6 months' duration
  - Etiology often multifactorial
  - Up to 40% have been physically or sexually abused
  - Pain that resolves with ovulation suppression suggests gynecologic cause; some nongynecologic conditions also improve with ovulation suppression
  - Concomitant depression very common
  - Ultrasound is usually not diagnostic, nor is physical examination
  - Half of women who undergo laparoscopy have no visible pathology

- **Differential Diagnosis**
  - Gynecologic: endometriosis, adenomyosis, pelvic adhesions, prior PID or chronic PID, leiomyomas
  - Gastrointestinal: irritable bowel syndrome, inflammatory bowel disease, diverticular disease, constipation, neoplasia, hernia
  - Urologic: detrusor overactivity, interstitial cystitis, urinary calculi, urethral syndrome, bladder carcinoma
  - Musculoskeletal: myofascial pain, low back pain, disk problems, nerve entrapment, muscle strain or spasm
  - Psychiatric: somatization, depression, physical or sexual abuse, anxiety

- **Treatment**
  - Evaluate for and treat the above causes, including psychiatric
  - NSAIDs; avoid opioids
  - Ovulation suppression with oral contraceptives, medroxyprogesterone acetate, or a short course of leuprolide acetate can be both diagnostic and therapeutic
  - Diagnostic laparoscopy if medical management fails or diagnosis remains in question
  - Hysterectomy with bilateral oophorectomy for refractory gynecologic pain in women who have completed child-bearing

- **Pearl**

The most difficult management problem in primary care gynecology, medically and psychologically.

Reference

Scialli AR: Evaluating chronic pelvic pain. A consensus recommendation. Pelvic Pain Expert Working Group. J Reprod Med 1999;44:945. [PMID: 10589405]

16

Cervical Dysplasia

- ■ Essentials of Diagnosis
    - Risk factors: early intercourse, multiple sexual partners, smoking, HIV infection
    - Includes low- and high-grade squamous intraepithelial lesions or cervical intraepithelial neoplasia (CIN 1–3)
    - Seventy-five percent of low-grade (CIN 1) regress spontaneously; only 35% of high-grade (CIN 2–3) regress
    - Atypical squamous cells of undetermined significance (ASCUS) associated with underlying dysplasia in 10%; other causes are benign reparative changes, inflammation
    - Atypical glandular cells of undetermined significance (AGUS, AGCUS) associated with significant abnormality (eg, endometrial hyperplasia, adenocarcinoma, or high-grade dysplasia) in 40%
    - Over 90% of squamous dysplasia and cancer due to sexually transmitted infection with human papillomavirus (HPV)
    - Colposcopy to confirm cytologic diagnosis and exclude invasive cancer

- ■ Differential Diagnosis
    - Inflammation due to vaginitis, cervicitis or atrophy
    - Inadequate specimen
    - Inaccurate interpretation of cytology or histology

- ■ Treatment
    - Excision (loop electrosurgical excision procedure, cone biopsy) or ablation (cryotherapy, laser)
    - Atypical cells: treat vaginitis or atrophy if present; colposcopy for recurrence
    - Repeat Pap smear every 4–6 months until three consecutive normal results are reported; routine screening thereafter
    - Low-grade lesions: colposcopy with biopsy confirms diagnosis; expectant management versus ablation or excision
    - High-grade lesions: colposcopy with biopsy to confirm diagnosis; treat with ablation or excision
    - Atypical squamous or glandular cells: colposcopy, endocervical curettage, and, if abnormal bleeding is present, endometrial biopsy

- ■ Pearl

Know your cytopathologist; staging is crucial in this condition.

Reference

Cox JT: Evaluation of abnormal cervical cytology. Clin Lab Med 2000; 20:303. [PMID: 10863643]

Amenorrhea

- ### Essentials of Diagnosis
  - Absence of menses for over 3 months in women with past menses (secondary amenorrhea); absence of menarche by age 16 (primary amenorrhea)
  - May be anatomic, ovarian, or hypothalamic-pituitary-ovarian
  - Anatomic causes: congenital anomalies of the uterus, imperforate hymen, cervical stenosis
  - Ovarian failure: causes include autoimmune diseases, Turner's, ovarian dysgenesis, radiation or chemotherapy
  - Hypothalamic-pituitary-ovarian causes most common; include hyperandrogenic disorders, hypothalamic anovulation, hyperpro-lactinemia, hypothyroidism, and hypothalamic or pituitary lesions
  - Exclusion of pregnancy and measurement of TSH and prolactin secures diagnosis
  - FSH and LH to evaluate for premature ovarian failure or poly-cystic ovarian syndrome
  - Dehydroepiandrosterone sulfate and testosterone to exclude androgen-secreting tumors
  - Withdrawal bleeding in response to progestin (10 mg medrox-yprogesterone acetate for 10 days) indicates that the ovary produces estrogen and that the uterus and outflow tract are intact

- ### Differential Diagnosis
  - Pregnancy
  - Physiologic (adolescence, perimenopause)
  - Causes as outlined above

- ### Treatment
  - Polycystic ovarian syndrome: oral contraceptives offer cycle regularity, decrease the risk of endometrial cancer caused by unopposed estrogen, and treat associated acne and hirsutism
  - Hypo-estrogenic causes: treat underlying disorder, estrogen treatment to prevent osteoporosis
  - Hyperprolactinemia: surgery for macroadenoma, otherwise treat with bromocriptine or expectant management

- ### Pearl
  Though the differential is broad and the evaluation extensive, three processes top the list in all women with amenorrhea: pregnancy, pregnancy, and pregnancy.

Reference
Pletcher JR et al: Menstrual disorders. Amenorrhea. Pediatr Clin North Am 1999;46:505. [PMID: 1-384804]

16

Urinary Incontinence

- ■ Essentials of Diagnosis
  - Uncontrolled loss of urine; classified as stress, urge, or overflow
  - Stress incontinence: urine loss during coughing or exercising; leakage observed on examination during cough or with Valsalva's maneuver
  - Urge incontinence due to spontaneous bladder contractions; accompanied by urgency, associated with frequency and nocturia, normal examination
  - Overflow incontinence caused by overdistention of bladder; uncommon in women, caused by neurologic lesion or outflow obstruction; postvoid residual markedly elevated
  - Evaluation indicated when diagnosis is uncertain or prior to surgical correction
  - Urinary tract infections commonly cause transient incontinence or worsening of preexisting incontinence

- ■ Differential Diagnosis
  - Urinary tract infection
  - Mobility disorders affecting ability to get to the toilet
  - Neurologic causes as outlined above
  - Urinary fistula, urethral diverticulum
  - Medications: diuretics, anticholinergics, antihistamines, alpha-adrenergic blockers

- ■ Treatment
  - Exclude urinary tract infection
  - A voiding diary aids in diagnosis and guiding therapy
  - Kegel exercises, formal training of the pelvic muscles
  - For urge incontinence: timed voids, limit fluid intake and caffeine, anticholinergic medications
  - Surgical treatment is effective in up to 85% for stress incontinence refractory to conservative management

- ■ Pearl

In older patients, be sure rectal sphincter tone is normal; this can be a clue to a spinal cord lesion.

Reference

Keane DP et al: Urinary incontinence: anatomy, physiology and pathophysiology. Baillieres Best Pract Res Clin Obstet Gynaecol 2000;14:207. [PMID: 10897320]

16

17

Common Surgical Disorders

Abdominal Aortic Aneurysm

- ■ Essentials of Diagnosis
  - Overall incidence in patients over age 60 years is 2–6.5%
  - More than 90% originate below the renal arteries
  - Most asymptomatic, discovered incidentally at physical examination or sonography
  - Abdominal ultrasound has sensitivity approaching 100%
  - Back or abdominal pain often precedes rupture
  - Abdominal aortic aneurysm diameter is the most important predictor of aneurysm rupture
  - Most rupture leftward and posteriorly; left knee jerk may thus be lost
  - Generalized arteriomegaly in many patients

- ■ Differential Diagnosis
  - Pancreatic pseudocyst, pancreatitis
  - Multiple myeloma
  - Musculoskeletal causes of back pain
  - Renal colic
  - Bleeding peptic ulcer

- ■ Treatment
  - In asymptomatic patients, depending on age and presence of other medical conditions, surgery is recommended when the aneurysm is >5 cm
  - Resection may be beneficial even for aneurysms as small as 4 cm
  - In symptomatic patients, immediate repair irrespective of size
  - Endovascular repair (transfemoral insertion of a prosthetic graft) considered if the anatomy of aneurysm is suitable (ie, graft can be secured infrarenally); long-term durability of endovascular grafts is unknown

- ■ Pearl

In upper gastrointestinal hemorrhage in patients over age 60 with a normal upper endoscopy, consider aortoenteric fistula.

Reference

Santilli JD et al: Diagnosis and treatment of abdominal aortic aneurysms. Am Fam Physician 1997;56:1081. [PMID: 9310060]

Pharyngoesophageal Diverticulum
(Zenker's Diverticulum)

- ■ Essentials of Diagnosis
  - • Most prevalent in the fifth to eighth decades of life
  - • Results from herniation of the mucosa through a weak point in the muscle layer proximal to the cricopharyngeal muscle
  - • Dysphagia worsening as more is eaten; regurgitation of undigested food, halitosis
  - • Gurgling sounds in the neck on auscultation
  - • Barium swallow confirms diagnosis by demonstrating the sac

- ■ Differential Diagnosis
  - • Esophageal, mediastinal, or neck tumor
  - • Cricopharyngeal achalasia (occasionally associated)
  - • Esophageal web
  - • Achalasia or lower esophageal stricture
  - • Epiphrenic diverticulum (lower esophagus)

- ■ Treatment
  - • There is no medical therapy; all patients should be considered candidates for surgical treatment

- ■ Pearl

Unsuspected Zenker's diverticulum may be inadvertently perforated at upper endoscopy, a reason to perform contrast radiography prior to esophagoduodenoscopy.

Reference

Sideris L et al: The treatment of Zenker's diverticula: a review. Semin Thorac Cardiovasc Surg 1999;11:337. [PMID: 10535375]

17

Malignant Tumors of the Esophagus

- **Essentials of Diagnosis**
  - Progressive dysphagia—initially during ingestion of solid foods, later with liquids; progressive weight loss ominous
  - Smoking, alcohol, asbestos, gastroesophageal reflux disease are risk factors
  - Classic radiographic appearance with irregular mucosal pattern and narrowing, with shelf-like upper border or concentrically narrowed esophageal lumen
  - CT scan delineates extent of disease
  - Adenocarcinoma (often associated with reflux-induced Barrett's esophagus) now has incidence similar to that of squamous cell

- **Differential Diagnosis**
  - Benign tumors of the esophagus (< 1%)
  - Benign esophageal stricture
  - Esophageal diverticulum
  - Esophageal webs
  - Achalasia (may be associated)
  - Globus hystericus

- **Treatment**
  - In 75–80% of patients, local tumor invasion or distant metastasis at the time of presentation precludes cure
  - For patients with localized primary, resection (when feasible) provides the best palliation
  - Adjuvant chemotherapy with radiation therapy or surgical resection results in cure for only 10–15%
  - Expandable metallic stent placement, laser fulguration, feeding tube placement with or without radiation therapy for additional palliation

- **Pearl**

17

True dysphagia—food sticking upon swallowing—has nearly 100% association with anatomic lesions.

Reference

Fox JR et al: Today's approach to esophageal cancer. What is the role of the primary care physician? Postgrad Med 2000;107:109. [PMID: 108444946]

Obstruction of the Small Intestine

- ■ Essentials of Diagnosis
  - • Defined as partial or complete obstruction of the intestinal lumen by an intrinsic or extrinsic lesion
  - • Etiology: adhesions (eg, from prior surgery or pelvic inflammatory disease) 60%, malignancy 20%, hernia 10%, inflammatory bowel disease 5%, volvulus 3%, other 2%.
  - • Crampy abdominal pain, vomiting (often feculent in complete obstruction), abdominal distention, constipation or obstipation
  - • Distended, tender abdomen with or without peritoneal signs; high-pitched tinkling or peristaltic rushes audible
  - • Patients often intravascularly depleted secondary to emesis, decreased oral intake, and sequestration of fluid in the bowel wall and lumen and the peritoneal cavity
  - • Plain films of the abdomen show dilated small bowel with more than three air-fluid levels

- ■ Differential Diagnosis
  - • Adynamic ileus due to any cause (eg, hypokalemia, pancreatitis, nephrolithiasis, recent operation or trauma)
  - • Colonic obstruction
  - • Intestinal pseudo-obstruction

- ■ Treatment
  - • Nasogastric suction
  - • Fluid and electrolyte (especially potassium) replacement with isotonic crystalloid
  - • Most management decisions are based on the distinction between partial and complete obstruction
  - • Surgical exploration for suspected hernia strangulation, or obstruction not responsive to conservative therapy

- ■ Pearl

Although Osler referred to adhesions as "the refuge of the diagnostically destitute," they remain the most common cause of small bowel obstruction.

17

Reference

Wilson MS et al: A review of the management of small bowel obstruction. Members of the Surgical and Clinical Adhesions Research Study (SCAR). Ann R Coll Surg Engl 1999;81:320. [PMID: 10645174]

Functional Obstruction
(Adynamic Ileus, Paralytic Ileus)

- **Essentials of Diagnosis**
  - History of precipitating factor (eg, recent surgery, peritonitis, other serious medical illness, anticholinergic drugs, hypokalemia)
  - Continuous abdominal pain, distention, vomiting, and obstipation
  - Minimal abdominal tenderness; decreased to absent bowel sounds
  - Radiographic images show diffuse gastrointestinal organ distention

- **Differential Diagnosis**
  - Mechanical obstruction due to any cause
  - Specific diseases associated with functional obstruction (ie, perforated viscus, pancreatitis, cholecystitis, appendicitis, nephrolithiasis)
  - Colonic pseudo-obstruction (Ogilvie's syndrome)

- **Treatment**
  - Restriction of oral intake; nasogastric suction in severe cases
  - Attention to electrolyte and fluid imbalance (ie, hypokalemia, dehydration)
  - Prokinetic drugs (metoclopramide, erythromycin) may be tried
  - Laparotomy should be avoided if at all possible to avert the subsequent risk of mechanical obstruction from adhesions

- **Pearl**

Lower lobe pneumonia may on occasion cause adynamic ileus.

Reference

Dorudi S et al: Acute colonic pseudo-obstruction. Br J Surg 1992;79:99. [PMID: 1555081]

17

Acute Appendicitis

- **Essentials of Diagnosis**
  - Consider in all patients with unexplained abdominal pain; 6% of the population will have appendicitis in their lifetime
  - Anorexia invariable
  - Abdominal pain, initially poorly localized or periumbilical, then localizing to the right lower quadrant over 4–48 hours in two-thirds of patients
  - Abdominal plain films and pattern of bowel function are of little diagnostic value
  - Low-grade fever, right lower quadrant tenderness at McBurney's point with or without peritoneal signs
  - Pelvic and rectal examinations are critically important
  - Mild leukocytosis (10,000–18,000/μL) with PMN predominance; microscopic hematuria or pyuria is common
  - Consider pelvic ultrasound (in women) and CT scan to differentiate surgical from nonsurgical pathologic conditions

- **Differential Diagnosis**
  - Gynecologic pathology (eg, ectopic pregnancy, pelvic inflammatory disease, endometriosis, mittelschmerz, twisted ovarian cyst)
  - Urologic pathology (eg, testicular torsion, acute epididymitis)
  - Nephrolithiasis
  - Urinary tract infection or pyelonephritis
  - Perforated peptic ulcer
  - Inflammatory bowel disease
  - Meckel's diverticulitis
  - Mesenteric adenitis
  - Acute cholecystitis
  - Right lower lobe pneumonia

- **Treatment**
  - Open or laparoscopic appendectomy
  - Certainty in diagnosis remains elusive (10–30% of patients are found to have a normal appendix at operation)
  - When diagnosis unclear, observe for several hours with serial examinations, or (if the patient is reliable) schedule return in 8–12 hours for reevaluation

- **Pearl**

The most common cause of the acute abdomen in every decade of life.

Reference

Hardin DM Jr: Acute appendicitis: review and update. Am Fam Physician 1999;60:2027. [PMID: 10569505]

17

Diverticulitis

- **Essentials of Diagnosis**
  - Acute, intermittent cramping left lower abdominal pain; constipation in some cases alternating with diarrhea
  - Fever, tenderness in left lower quadrant, with palpable abdominal mass in some patients
  - Leukocytosis
  - Radiographic evidence of diverticula, thickened interhaustral folds, narrowed lumen
  - CT scan is the safest and most cost-effective diagnostic method

- **Differential Diagnosis**
  - Colorectal carcinoma
  - Appendicitis
  - Strangulating colonic obstruction
  - Colitis due to any cause
  - Pelvic inflammatory disease
  - Ruptured ectopic pregnancy or ovarian cyst
  - Inflammatory bowel disease

- **Treatment**
  - Liquid diet (10 days) and oral antibiotics (metronidazole plus ciprofloxacin or trimethoprim-sulfamethoxazole) for mild first attack
  - Nasogastric suction and broad-spectrum intravenous antibiotics for patients requiring hospitalization (eg, failed outpatient management, inadequate analgesia)
  - Percutaneous catheter drainage for intra-abdominal abscess
  - Emergent laparotomy with colonic resection and diversion for generalized peritonitis, uncontrolled sepsis, visceral perforation, and acute clinical deterioration
  - High-residue diet, stool softener, psyllium mucilloid for chronic therapy

17

- **Pearl**

Left-sided diverticula are more common and more likely to become inflamed; right-sided diverticula are less common and more likely to bleed.

Reference

Ferzoco LB et al: Acute diverticulitis. N Engl J Med 1998;338:1521. [PMID: 9593792]

Pancreatic Pseudocyst

- **Essentials of Diagnosis**
  - Collection of pancreatic fluid in or around the pancreas; may occur as a complication of acute or chronic pancreatitis
  - Characterized by epigastric pain, tenderness, fever, and occasionally a palpable mass
  - Leukocytosis, persistent serum amylase elevation
  - Pancreatic cyst demonstrated by CT scan
  - Complications include hemorrhage, infection, rupture, fistula formation, pancreatic ascites, and obstruction of surrounding organs

- **Differential Diagnosis**
  - Pancreatic phlegmon or abscess
  - Resolving pancreatitis
  - Pancreatic carcinoma
  - Abdominal aortic aneurysm

- **Treatment**
  - Up to two-thirds spontaneously resolve
  - Avoidance of alcohol
  - Percutaneous catheter drainage with nutritional support while avoiding oral feedings effective in many cases
  - Decompression into an adjacent hollow viscus (cystojejunostomy or cystogastrostomy) may be necessary
  - Octreotide to inhibit pancreatic secretion

- **Pearl**

There are only two causes of pulsatile abdominal masses: pancreatic pseudocyst and aneurysm.

Reference

Lillemoe KD et al: Management of complications of pancreatitis. Curr Probl Surg 1998;35:1. [PMID: 9452408]

17

Hernia

- **Essentials of Diagnosis**
    - Protrusion of a viscus through an opening in the wall of the cavity in which it is contained (sac is an outpouching of peritoneum)
    - Lump or swelling in the groin, sometimes associated with sudden pain and bulging during heavy lifting or straining
    - Discomfort is worse at the end of the day, relieved when patient reclines and hernia reduces
    - Clinically distinguishing an indirect from a direct hernia is unimportant, since their operative repair is the same
    - Early symptoms of incarceration are those of partial bowel obstruction; the early discomfort will be periumbilical
    - A femoral hernia is an acquired protrusion of a peritoneal sac through the femoral ring; smaller, more difficult to palpate and to diagnose

- **Differential Diagnosis**
    - Hydrocele
    - Varicocele
    - Inguinal lymphadenopathy
    - Lipoma of the spermatic cord
    - Testicular torsion
    - Femoral artery aneurysm

- **Treatment**
    - In general, all hernias should be repaired unless local or systemic conditions preclude a safe outcome
    - Elective outpatient surgical repair for reducible hernias
    - Attempt reduction of incarcerated (irreducible) hernias (when peritoneal signs are absent) with conscious sedation, Trendelenburg position, and steady, gentle pressure
    - Emergent repair for nonreducible, incarcerated, or strangulated

17

- **Pearl**

The patient tells you he has an inguinal hernia; you tell him he has a femoral hernia.

Reference

Avisse C et al: The inguinal rings. Surg Clin North Am 2000;80:49. [PMID: 10685144]

Intestinal Ischemia

- **Essentials of Diagnosis**

  Acute:
  - Causes are emboli (eg, in atrial fibrillation); thrombosis (eg, in patients with atherosclerosis), or nonocclusive insufficiency (eg, in congestive heart failure)
  - With occlusion, diffuse abdominal pain but minimal physical findings
  - Lactic acidosis suggests bowel infarction rather than ischemia

  Chronic:
  - Results from atherosclerotic plaques of superior mesenteric, celiac axis, and inferior mesenteric; more than one of the above major arteries must be involved because of collateral circulation
  - Epigastric or periumbilical postprandial pain; patients limit intake to avoid pain, resulting in weight loss and less prominent pain

  Ischemic colitis:
  - Occurs primarily with inferior mesenteric artery ischemia; episodic bouts of crampy lower abdominal pain and mild, often bloody diarrhea; lactic acidosis or colonic infarction rare

- **Differential Diagnosis**
  - Diverticulitis and appendicitis
  - Myocardial infarction
  - Pancreatitis
  - Inflammatory bowel disease and colitis due to other causes
  - Visceral malignancy
  - Polyarteritis nodosa
  - Renal colic
  - Cholecystitis

- **Treatment**
  - Decision to operate is challenging given comorbidities
  - Laparotomy with removal of necrotic bowel
  - Pre- and postoperative intra-arterial infusion of papaverine if occlusion is embolic

- **Pearl**

  Abdominal pain in a patient with heart failure receiving digitalis and diuretics is nonocclusive mesenteric ischemia until proved to be otherwise.

17

Reference

Brandt LJ et al: AGA technical review on intestinal ischemia. American Gastrointestinal Association. Gastroenterology 2000;118:954. [PMID: 10784596]

Acute Cholecystitis

- ■ Essentials of Diagnosis
  - Acute, steady right upper quadrant or midabdominal pain; nausea, food intolerance common
  - Classic finding is Murphy's sign, which refers to inspiratory arrest with palpation in the right upper quadrant
  - Fever, leukocytosis, slight elevation in liver function studies, amylase, and lipase
  - Biliary colic and acute cholecystitis often overlap; clinical distinction may be difficult
  - Abdominal ultrasound is the diagnostic procedure of choice, showing stones, ductal anatomy, and inflammation (thickened gallbladder wall and pericholecystic fluid); may be acalculous
  - Radionuclide (HIDA) scan shows a nonopacified gallbladder and diagnoses acute cholecystitis accurately in 97% of cases

- ■ Differential Diagnosis
  - Acute appendicitis
  - Acute pancreatitis
  - Peptic ulcer disease
  - Acute hepatitis
  - Right lower lobe pneumonia
  - Myocardial infarction
  - Radicular pain in thoracic dermatome, eg, preeruptive zoster

- ■ Treatment
  - Bowel rest, intravenous fluids, and analgesics; give parenteral antibiotics to cover coliform organisms
  - Early laparoscopic cholecystectomy leads to reduced morbidity and mortality
  - Immediate cholecystectomy for gallbladder ischemia, perforation, emphysematous cholecystitis; percutaneously placed cholecystostomy catheters used initially in severely ill or elderly patients with high surgical risk
  - Endoscopic retrograde cholangiopancreatography (ERCP) with sphincterotomy should be performed when there are associated common bile duct stones, pancreatitis, or cholangitis

17

- ■ Pearl

In cholecystitis, the patient precisely identifies the time of onset of symptoms—not so in appendicitis.

Reference

Hashizume M et al: The clinical management and results of surgery for acute cholecystitis. Semin Laparosc Surg 1998;5:69. [PMID: 8259091]

Carotid Artery Disease

- **Essentials of Diagnosis**
  - Most common in patients with standard risk factors for atherosclerosis (eg, hypertension, hypercholesterolemia, diabetes mellitus)
  - Many patients asymptomatic
  - Otherwise, amaurosis fugax; transient hemiparesis with or without aphasia or sensory changes; stroke diagnosed if focal findings persist for more than 24 hours
  - Bruit may be present but correlates poorly with degree of stenosis
  - Duplex ultrasound useful in assessing stenosis; gadolinium angiography demonstrates anatomy

- **Differential Diagnosis**
  - Carotid artery dissection
  - Giant cell arteritis
  - Takayasu's arteritis
  - Lipohyalinosis
  - Radiation fibrosis
  - Cardiac emboli
  - Brain tumor or abscess (in patient with stroke)

- **Treatment**
  - Aspirin
  - Thromboplastic agents in highly selected patients with cerebral ischemia: less than 3 hours of symptoms, no hemorrhage on CT
  - Carotid endarterectomy in stenosis > 70% with or without symptoms
  - Surgery of uncertain benefit when stenosis < 70%

- **Pearl**

Only one in four untreated patients with > 70% stenosis will have a stroke; of patients found to have 100% occlusion, only half have suffered a neurologic event.

Reference

Biller J et al: When to operate in carotid artery disease. Am Fam Physician 2000;61:400. [PMID: 10670506]

17

Acute Lower Extremity Arterial Occlusion

- **Essentials of Diagnosis**
  - Typical patient has valvular hypertensive or ischemic heart disease, often peripheral vascular disease as well
  - Some occur following posterior knee dislocation, iatrogenic catheter injury
  - Abrupt onset of pain, dysesthesia
  - Pulses absent, limb cold; occasional atrial fibrillation on cardiac examination
  - Leukocytosis; elevated CK and LDH

- **Differential Diagnosis**
  - Neuropathic pain
  - Deep venous thrombosis
  - Reflex sympathetic dystrophy
  - Systemic vasculitis
  - Cholesterol atheroembolic syndrome

- **Treatment**
  - Embolectomy, either surgically or by Fogarty catheter
  - Fasciotomy if compartment syndrome complicates
  - Heparin if limb judged not to be threatened; occasionally, vasospasm gives false impression of total occlusion, and heparin may help

- **Pearl**

In a patient with an intra-arterial femoral line in the ICU on a ventilator, there will be no history—check distal pulses frequently.

Reference

Thrombolysis in the management of lower limb peripheral arterial occlusion—a consensus document. Working Party on Thrombolysis in the Management of Limb Ischemia. Am J Cardiol 1998;81:207. [PMID: 9591906]

17

18

Common Pediatric Disorders*

Croup

- **Essentials of Diagnosis**
  - Viral croup, usually due to parainfluenza virus, affects younger children
  - Barking cough, stridor, and hoarseness following upper respiratory infection
  - Usually worse at night
  - Lateral neck films can be useful diagnostically; patients with viral croup have subglottic narrowing (steeple sign) and a normal epiglottis
  - Direct laryngoscopy rules out epiglottitis or laryngomalacia in confusing cases but must be performed cautiously with anticipation of intubation

- **Differential Diagnosis**
  - Angioneurotic edema
  - Foreign body in the esophagus or larynx
  - Retropharyngeal abscess
  - Epiglottitis
  - Laryngomalacia

- **Treatment**
  - Treatment of viral croup is supportive; mist therapy is anecdotal
  - Oral hydration, oxygen, racemic epinephrine, and corticosteroids are accepted therapy
  - Most croup is self-limited and lasts less than 5 days

- **Pearl**

Every mother knows that a walk with a child in the cool night air is the treatment of choice.

Reference

Klassen TP: Croup. A current perspective. Pediatr Clin North Am 1999;46:1167. [PMID: 10629679]

---

* The following common childhood diseases are discussed in other chapters: aspiration of foreign body and cystic fibrosis, Chapter 2; pharyngitis, mumps, poliomyelitis, varicella and zoster, infectious mononucleosis, rabies, and rubella, Chapter 8; appendicitis, Chapter 16; otitis media and otitis externa, Chapter 19.

Pyloric Stenosis

- **Essentials of Diagnosis**
  - Increase in size of the muscular layer of the pylorus of unknown cause; occurs in one or two out of 1000 births, with males and whites affected more commonly
  - Vomiting beginning between 2–8 weeks of age; may become projectile; rarely bilious
  - Infant is hungry and nurses avidly, but weight gain is poor and growth retardation occurs
  - Constipation, dehydration, and hypochloremic alkalosis with hypokalemia are typical
  - Palpable olive-sized mass in the subhepatic region best felt after the child has vomited
  - String sign and retained gastric contents on upper gastrointestinal series; ultrasound shows a hypoechoic mass

- **Differential Diagnosis**
  - Gastroesophageal reflux disease
  - Esophageal stenosis or achalasia
  - Small bowel obstruction due to other causes
  - Antral web
  - Adrenal insufficiency
  - Pylorospasm
  - Other causes of growth retardation

- **Treatment**
  - Pyloromyotomy is the treatment of choice
  - Dehydration and electrolyte abnormalities should be corrected prior to surgery
  - Excellent prognosis after surgery

- **Pearl**

Pyloric stenosis: an epigastric mass in a vomiting baby with a hard metabolic alkalosis? Game, set, and match for this diagnosis.

18

Reference

Dinkevich E et al: Pyloric stenosis. Pediatrics in Rev 2000;21:249. [PMID: 10878190]

Down's Syndrome

- ■ Essentials of Diagnosis
  - Occurs in 1 : 600 newborns, with increasing incidence in children of mothers over 35 years of age
  - Ninety-five percent of patients have 47 chromosomes with trisomy 21
  - Characteristic findings are small, broad head, flat nasal bridge, upward slanting palpebral fissures, transverse palmar crease, short hands, and inner epicanthal folds
  - One-third to one-half have congenital heart disease; atlantoaxial subluxation and sensorineural hearing loss more frequent than in the general population; leukemia is 20 times more common, and there is an increased susceptibility to infections

- ■ Differential Diagnosis
  - The chromosome and phenotypic abnormalities are pathognomonic

- ■ Treatment
  - Goal of therapy is to help affected patients develop full potential
  - No convincing evidence exists to support any of the forms of general therapy that have been advocated (eg, megadoses of vitamins, exercise programs)
  - Therapy directed toward specific problems (eg, cardiac surgery, antibiotics)
  - Electrocardiography and echocardiography in the neonatal period, yearly vision and hearing examinations, yearly thyroid screening, and a cervical spine x-ray once during the preschool years

- ■ Pearl

Chromosome 21 codes the beta-amyloid seen ubiquitously in brains of Down's patients and Alzheimer's in adults.

Reference

Saenz RB: Primary care of infants and young children with Down syndrome. Am Fam Physician 1999;59:381. [PMID: 9930130]

18

Respiratory Syncytial Virus (RSV) Disease

- **Essentials of Diagnosis**
  - The most important cause of lower respiratory tract illness in young children, causing half of all cases of bronchiolitis and many cases of pneumonia
  - Epidemics in late fall to early spring; attack rates are high
  - The classic disease (bronchiolitis) is characterized by diffuse wheezing, difficulty feeding, variable fever, cough, tachypnea, and inspiratory retractions
  - Apnea may be the presenting symptom, especially in premature infants
  - Chest x-ray shows hyperinflation and peribronchiolar thickening, occasionally atelectasis
  - RSV antigen detected in nasal or pulmonary secretions in most

- **Differential Diagnosis**
  - Bronchiolitis due to other viruses or bacteria
  - Asthma
  - Foreign body aspiration
  - Chlamydial pneumonitis
  - Pertussis
  - Laryngomalacia
  - Substernal goiter

- **Treatment**
  - Severely ill children should be hospitalized, given humidified oxygen, and kept in respiratory isolation
  - Bronchodilator therapy usually instituted
  - Corticosteroid use considered in hospitalized patients
  - Ribavirin, by continuous aerosolization; given to selected patients at very high risk.

- **Pearl**

  Consider RSV if croup lasts for days to weeks.

18

Reference

Malhotra A et al: Influenza and respiratory syncytial virus. Update on infection, management, and prevention. Pediatr Clin North Am 2000;47:353. [PMID: 10761508]

Roseola Infantum (Exanthema Subitum)

- **Essentials of Diagnosis**

  - A benign illness typically caused by human herpes virus 6 occurring primarily in children 3 months to 4 years of age; 90% of cases occur before the second year
  - Abrupt onset of fever (as high as 40 °C) lasting up to 5 days in an otherwise mildly ill child; dissociation between systemic symptoms and febrile course
  - Fever ceases abruptly; a characteristic rash develops in 20%, consisting of rose-pink maculopapules beginning on the trunk and spreading outward with disappearance in 1–2 days
  - No conjunctivitis or pharyngeal exudate, but there may be mild cough or coryza
  - Rash may occur without fever

- **Differential Diagnosis**

  - Serious bacterial infections
  - Drug allergy
  - Measles
  - Rubella
  - Enterovirus infection
  - Scarlet fever
  - Toxic shock syndrome
  - Kawasaki disease

- **Treatment**

  - Supportive care only; acetaminophen and sponge baths for fever
  - Reassurance for parents
  - Febrile seizures occur, but no more commonly than with other self-limited infections
  - Children are no longer infectious once they are afebrile

- **Pearl**

No other illness exhibits rash after *defervescence.*

Reference

Leach CT: Human herpesvirus-6 and -7 infections in children: agents of roseola and other syndromes. Curr Opin Pediatr 2000;12:269. [PMID: 10836165]

18

Acute Lymphoblastic Leukemia (ALL)

- **Essentials of Diagnosis**
  - The most common malignancy of childhood; peak age at onset is 4 years; accounts for 75% of childhood leukemias
  - Uncontrolled proliferation of immature lymphocytes
  - Intermittent fever, bone pain, petechiae, purpura, pallor; hepatosplenomegaly and lymphadenopathy unusual
  - Single or multiple cytopenias common; serum uric acid and LDH often elevated
  - Bone marrow shows homogeneous infiltration of more than 25% of leukemic blasts; most have blasts expressing common ALL antigen (CALLA)

- **Differential Diagnosis**
  - EBV of CMV infection
  - Immune thrombocytopenic purpura
  - Autoimmune hemolytic anemia
  - Aplastic anemia
  - Juvenile rheumatoid arthritis
  - Pertussis
  - Other malignancies

- **Treatment**
  - Induction therapy (first month of therapy), usually with three or four drugs, including prednisone, vincristine, asparaginase, daunorubicin, or methotrexate
  - Consolidation phase: intrathecal chemotherapy and sometimes cranial irradiation to treat lymphoblasts that may be present in meninges
  - Delayed intensification to further reduce leukemic cells
  - Maintenance therapy with mercaptopurine, weekly methotrexate, and monthly vincristine or prednisone
  - Bone marrow transplant considered in relapsed patients
  - Children with white counts under 50,000/μL at diagnosis or between 1 year and 10 years of age have better prognosis
  - Those with mediastinal mass or chromosomal translocations have a worse prognosis
  - Over 70% of treated patients are cured

- **Pearl**

"Spontaneous cures" of ALL in older literature are likely cases of severe infectious mononucleosis.

Reference

Pui CH et al: Acute lymphoblastic leukemia. N Engl J Med 1998;339:605.
  [PMID: 9718381]

18

Wilms' Tumor (Nephroblastoma)

- **Essentials of Diagnosis**
  - A renal tumor representing 6% of cancers in patients under age 15; peak age at diagnosis is 3
  - Occurs sporadically or as part of a malformation syndrome or cytogenic abnormality
  - Asymptomatic abdominal mass (80%), fever (25%), and hematuria (20%)
  - Five to 10 percent are bilateral
  - Hypertension, genitourinary abnormalities, aniridia, hemihypertrophy occasionally seen
  - Abdominal ultrasound or CT reveals a solid intrarenal mass; 10% of patients will have metastatic disease (lung or liver) at time of diagnosis; ultrasound and chest x-ray may help show spread of metastases

- **Differential Diagnosis**
  - Neuroblastoma originating from the adrenal
  - Other abdominal tumors
  - Polycystic kidneys
  - Renal abscess
  - Hydronephrosis

- **Treatment**
  - Once the diagnosis is made, almost all patients undergo surgical exploration of the abdomen with attempted excision of the tumor and possible nephrectomy
  - Vincristine and dactinomycin routinely used in all patients; doxorubicin administered in those with advanced disease
  - Flank irradiation effective in some patients, and lung irradiation may be used to treat metastases

- **Pearl**

Along with neuroblastoma, a commonly curable tumor once uniformly fatal.

Reference

Petruzzi MJ et al: Wilms' tumor. Pediatr Clin North Am 1997;44:939. [PMID: 9286293]

18

Juvenile Rheumatoid Arthritis (Still's Disease)

- **Essentials of Diagnosis**

  Three types: pauciarticular, polyarticular, systemic:
  - Pauciarticular: fewer than five joints involved; younger females can have uveitis, knee involvement, ANA-positivity; adolescents, usually male, have both large and small joint disease, rarely ANA-positive
  - Polyarticular: five or more joints, occurs at any age; fever and weight loss common; ANA and rheumatoid factor positive in older children
  - Systemic: any age; fever and rash common, with lymphadenopathy, hepatosplenomegaly, pericarditis, and pleuritis; joint symptoms variable, often follow systemic symptoms by weeks to months; rheumatoid factor and ANA routinely negative

- **Differential Diagnosis**
  - Rheumatic fever
  - Infective arthritis
  - Reactive arthritis due to various causes
  - Lyme disease
  - SLE
  - Dermatomyositis
  - Leukemia
  - Inflammatory bowel disease
  - Bone tumors
  - Osteomyelitis

- **Treatment**
  - Goals of treatment are to restore function, relieve pain, and maintain joint function
  - NSAIDs and physical therapy are the mainstays
  - Methotrexate, hydroxychloroquine, sulfasalazine, gold salts, and local corticosteroid injections for those symptomatic after NSAIDs
  - For the most refractory cases, systemic steroids may be required

18

- **Pearl**

  Systemic Still's disease is one of the few causes of biquotidian fever spikes.

Reference

Woo P et al: Juvenile chronic arthritis. Lancet 1998;351:969. [PMID: 9734957]

Colic

- **Essentials of Diagnosis**
  - A syndrome characterized by severe and paroxysmal crying that usually worsens in the late afternoon and evening
  - Abdomen sometimes distended, the facies can be pained, fists are often clenched, infant is unresponsive to soothing
  - Thought to be due to a disturbance in the gastrointestinal tract, but unproved
  - Begins in the first few weeks of life and peaks at 2–3 months; may last into the fifth month of life

- **Differential Diagnosis**
  - Normal crying in an infant
  - Any illness in the infant causing distress, such as otitis media, intestinal cramping, corneal abrasion
  - Food allergy

- **Treatment**
  - Reassurance of parents
  - Education of the parents regarding the baby's cues
  - Phenobarbital elixir and dicyclomine not recommended
  - Elimination of cow's milk from the formula (or from the mother's diet if she is nursing) in refractory cases to rule out milk protein allergy
  - Hypoallergenic diet, soy formula, reduced stimulation may help in difficult cases

- **Pearl**

Rule of Threes: During the first 3 months, a healthy infant cries more than 3 hours a day, for more than 3 days a week, for more than 3 weeks.

Reference

Balon AJ: Management of infantile colic. Am Fam Physician 1997; 55:235. [PMID: 9012281]

18

Tetralogy of Fallot

- **Essentials of Diagnosis**
  - The most common cyanotic heart disease after 1 week of age
  - Ventricular septal defect, obstruction to right ventricular outflow, right ventricular hypertrophy, and overriding aorta
  - Varying cyanosis after the neonatal period, dyspnea on exertion, easy fatigability, growth retardation
  - Right ventricular lift, systolic ejection murmur (rough) maximal at the left sternal border, single loud S_2
  - Elevated hematocrit, boot-shaped heart on chest x-ray
  - Echocardiography, cardiac catheterization, and angiocardiography all useful in confirming the diagnosis

- **Differential Diagnosis**

  Other cyanotic heart diseases:
  - Pulmonary atresia with intact ventricular septum
  - Tricuspid atresia
  - Hypoplastic left heart syndrome
  - Complete transposition of the great arteries
  - Total anomalous pulmonary venous return
  - Persistent truncus arteriosus

- **Treatment**
  - Acute treatment of cyanotic episodes includes supplemental oxygen, placing the patient in the knee-chest position; consideration of intravenous propanolol, morphine
  - Palliation with oral beta-blockers or surgical anastamosis between a systemic artery and the pulmonary artery (Blalock-Taussig shunt) recommended for very small infants with severe symptoms and in those who are not candidates for complete correction
  - Total surgical correction (ventricular septal defect closure and right ventricular outflow tract reconstruction) is the treatment of choice in selected patients; patients are still at risk for sudden death because of arrhythmias
  - Complete repair in childhood has a 10-year survival rate of more than 90% and a 30-year survival rate of 85%

18

- **Pearl**

  The combination of right ventricular hypertrophy, small pulmonary arteries, and pulmonary oligemia is seen in no other condition.

Reference

Waldman JD et al: Cyanotic congenital heart disease with decreased pulmonary blood flow in children. Pediatr Clin North Am 1999;46:385. [PMID: 10218082]

Kawasaki Disease
(Mucocutaneous Lymph Node Syndrome)

■ Essentials of Diagnosis

- Illness of unknown cause characterized by 5 days of fever, non-exudative conjunctivitis, inflamed oral mucous membranes, cervical lymphadenopathy of at least 1.5 cm, rash over the trunk and extremities, and edema
- Cardiovascular complications include myocarditis, pericarditis, and arteritis predisposing to coronary artery aneurysm formation
- Acute myocardial infarction may occur; 1–2% of patients die from this during the initial phase of the disease
- Arthritis, thrombocytosis, and elevated sedimentation rate commonly seen

■ Differential Diagnosis

- Acute rheumatic fever
- Juvenile rheumatoid arthritis
- Viral exanthems
- Infectious mononucleosis
- Streptococcal pharyngitis
- Measles
- Toxic shock syndrome

■ Treatment

- Patients require an echocardiogram to evaluate for coronary aneurysms
- Intravenous immune globulin and high-dose aspirin are the mainstays of therapy
- Corticosteroids contraindicated

■ Pearl

This and anomalous origin of a coronary artery from the pulmonary artery are the sole causes of Q wave infarction in childhood.

Reference

Taubert KA et al: Kawasaki disease. Am Fam Physician 1999;59:3093. [PMID: 10392592]

18

Bacterial Meningitis

- **Essentials of Diagnosis**
  - Signs of systemic illness (fever, malaise), headache, stiff neck, and altered mental status
  - In infants under 12 months of age, such signs of meningeal irritation may be absent
  - Predisposing factors can include ear infection, sinusitis, recent neurosurgical procedures, and skull fracture
  - No symptom or sign reliably distinguishes bacterial cause from meningitis due to viruses, fungi, or other pathogens
  - Organisms depend upon the age: < 1 month, group B or D streptococci, Enterobacteriaceae, listeria; 1–3 months, above pathogens plus *Haemophilus influenzae,* pneumococci, and meningococci; 3 months to 7 years, *H influenzae,* pneumococci, and meningococci
  - Cerebrospinal fluid typically shows elevated protein, low glucose, elevated WBC (> 1000/μL) with a high proportion of PMNs (> 50%)
  - Gram stain and culture often lead to the definitive diagnosis

- **Differential Diagnosis**
  - Meningitis due to nonbacterial organisms
  - Brain abscess
  - Encephalitis
  - Sepsis without meningitis
  - Intracranial mass or hemorrhage

- **Treatment**
  - Prompt empiric antibiotics can be life-saving
  - Exact antibiotic regimen depends upon age of patient; therapy narrowed once the susceptibilities of the organism known
  - Concomitant dexamethasone decreases morbidity and mortality
  - Patients monitored for acidosis, syndrome of inappropriate secretion of vasopressin, and hypoglycemia
  - Coagulopathies may require platelets and fresh frozen plasma
  - Mortality can be up to 20% in neonates, and neurologic sequelae may occur in up to 25% of affected patients

18

- **Pearl**

When bacteria cannot be seen on Gram stain of cerebrospinal fluid in subsequently proved meningitis, meningococcus is the most likely cause.

Reference

Pong A et al: Bacterial meningitis and the newborn infant. Infect Dis Clin North Am 1999;13 :711. [PMID: 10470563]

Henoch-Schönlein Purpura (Anaphylactoid Purpura)

- ■ Essentials of Diagnosis
  - A small-vessel vasculitis affecting skin, gastrointestinal tract, and kidney
  - Occurs slightly more often in males under 10 years of age; two-thirds have a preceding upper respiratory tract infection; occasionally observed in adults
  - Skin lesions often begin as urticaria and progress to a maculopapular eruption, finally becoming a symmetric purpuric rash
  - Eighty percent develop migratory polyarthralgias or polyarthritis; edema of the hands, feet, scalp, and periorbital areas occurs commonly
  - Colicky abdominal pain occurs in two-thirds; renal involvement in 25–50%
  - Platelet count, prothrombin time, and partial thromboplastin time normal; urinalysis may reveal hematuria and proteinuria; serum IgA often elevated

- ■ Differential Diagnosis
  - Immune thrombocytopenic purpura
  - Meningococcemia
  - Rocky Mountain spotted fever
  - Other hypersensitivity vasculitides
  - Juvenile rheumatoid arthritis
  - Kawasaki disease
  - Leukemia
  - Child abuse

- ■ Treatment
  - Pain medications and NSAIDs to treat joint pain and inflammation
  - Corticosteroid therapy for symptomatic relief; does not alter skin or renal manifestations
  - No satisfactory specific treatment
  - Prognosis is generally good

- ■ Pearl

Remember this diagnosis in adults with abdominal pain and palpable purpura—although it is mostly a pediatric problem.

18

Reference

Saulsbury FT: Henoch-Schönlein purpura in children. Report of 100 patients and review of the literature. Medicine (Baltimore) 1999;78:395. [PMID: 10575422]

Intussusception

- **Essentials of Diagnosis**
  - The telescoping of one part of the bowel into another, leading to edema, hemorrhage, ischemia, and eventually infarction
  - Peak is between 6 months and 1 year of age; intussusception is the most common cause of intestinal obstruction in the first 2 years of life
  - Lead points can include hypertrophied Peyer patches, polyps, lymphoma, or other tumors; in children over 6, lymphoma most common lesion
  - Most (90%) are ileocolic; ileoileal, colocolic also
  - Symptoms include intermittent colicky abdominal pain, vomiting, and (late) bloody stool
  - Plain films may show signs of obstruction, but a barium or air-barium enema is the standard for diagnosis

- **Differential Diagnosis**
  - Volvulus
  - Incarcerated hernia
  - Acute appendicitis
  - Acute gastroenteritis
  - Urinary tract infection
  - Small bowel obstruction due to other cause
  - Renal calculus
  - Pancreatitis
  - Perforated viscus

- **Treatment**
  - Patients stabilized with fluid; decompressed with a nasogastric tube
  - Surgical consultation to exclude perforation
  - Air-barium enema has a reduction rate of up to 90%, but never performed if perforation is suspected
  - Reduction by enema may result in perforation as much as 1% of the time
  - If perforation occurs or if enema fails, surgical decompression may be necessary
  - Recurs in up to 10% of cases, usually in the first day after reduction

- **Pearl**

Recurrent intussusception suggests the diagnosis of Peutz-Jeghers syndrome.

Reference

Winslow BT et al: Intussusception. Am Fam Physician 1996;54:213. [PMID: 8677837]

18

Otitis Media

- **Essentials of Diagnosis**
    - Peak incidence between the ages of 6 months and 3 years
    - History may include fever, ear pain, and other nonspecific systemic symptoms
    - Tympanometry shows an opaque, bulging, hyperemic tympanic membrane with a loss of landmarks; pneumatic otoscopy show loss of mobility
    - Breast feeding probably protective; exposure to tobacco smoke and pacifier use thought to increase incidence
    - Although caused by viruses, most cases are assumed to be bacterial
    - Bacterial causes are (1) *Streptococcus pneumoniae,* 40–50%; (2) *Haemophilus influenzae,* 20–30%; (3) *Moraxella catarrhalis,* 10–15%

- **Differential Diagnosis**
    - Otitis externa
    - Hemotympanum
    - Cholesteatoma
    - Foreign body

- **Treatment**
    - Treatment controversial; most children with otitis media not treated in Europe
    - CDC recommendations: (1) Children > 2 not in day care and not exposed to antibiotics in the last 3 months, give amoxicillin, 40–45 mg/kg/d for 5 days; (2) children < 2 in day care or with recent antibiotic exposure, give high-dose amoxicillin, 80–100 mg/kg/d for 10 days; (3) second-line therapy includes amoxicillin-clavulanate, cefuroxime, or intramuscular ceftriaxone
    - Three or more episodes in 6 months or four episodes in a year warrant prophylactic antibiotics; tympanostomy tubes considered with persistent infection

- **Pearl**

Nasotracheal intubation is an overlooked cause of otitis media.

Reference

O'Neill P: Acute otitis media. BMJ 1999;319:833. [PMID: 10496831]

Febrile Seizures

- **Essentials of Diagnosis**
  - Occur in 2–5% of children
  - Peak age is 2 years old, boys more often affected than girls
  - Last less than 15 minutes, are generalized, and occur in developmentally normal children between 6 months and 5 years of age
  - Those that are longer, focal, or multiple are complex
  - Family history a risk factor
  - One in three will have a recurrent seizure, 75% within a year

- **Differential Diagnosis**
  - Meningitis
  - Encephalitis
  - Intracranial hemorrhage
  - Intracranial tumor
  - Trauma

- **Treatment**
  - No treatment for simple febrile seizures
  - Electroencephalography not recommended in the initial workup
  - Lumbar puncture absolutely in children under 12 months of age, recommended for children 12–18 months of age
  - Prophylactic anticonvulsants may lower the risk of recurrence; significant side effects limit their use

- **Pearl**

An excellent case can be made for brain CT or MRI following any first-time seizure irrespective of age.

Reference

McAbee GN et al: A practical approach to uncomplicated seizures in children. Am Fam Physician 2000;62:1109. [PMID: 10997534]

Enuresis

- **Essentials of Diagnosis**
  - Involuntary urination at an age where control is expected, mostly occurring at night
  - Primary enuresis occurs in children who never have had control; secondary in children with at least 6 months of prior control
  - Family history important; three-quarters of children with enuresis have at least one parent who did
  - Afflicts 20% of 5-year-olds, 10% of 7-year-olds, and 5% of 10-year-olds
  - Secondary enuresis often caused by psychosocial stressors
  - Medical problems, including UTI and diabetes mellitus, must be excluded

- **Differential Diagnosis**
  - Urinary tract infection
  - Diabetes mellitus
  - Congenital genitourinary anomalies
  - Constipation
  - Diuretic ingestion

- **Treatment**
  - Therapy for causative medical problems
  - Support and positive reinforcement for children and families
  - Fluid restriction and bladder emptying prior to bedtime
  - Alarm systems effective but take weeks to work
  - Desmopressin works quickly but does not provide long-term control
  - Imipramine not recommended due to side effects and overdose potential

- **Pearl**

Hypokalemia suggests Munchausen by proxy due to administration of diuretic to the child.

Reference

Gimpel GA et al: Clinical perspectives in primary nocturnal enuresis. Clin Pediatr 1998;37:23. [PMID: 9475696]

18

Urinary Tract Infection

- ■ Essentials of Diagnosis
  - Girls at higher risk than boys
  - Bacterial infection of the urinary tract, defined as $> 10^3$ colony-forming units/mL by suprapubic aspiration, $> 10^4$ CFU/mL by catheter, or $> 10^5$ CFU/mL clean catch
  - Most common pathogens are *E coli, klebsiellae, enterococci*, and *Proteus mirabilis*
  - Urinalysis usually positive for leukocytes and bacteria
  - Difficult to differentiate lower tract infections from pyelonephritis

- ■ Differential Diagnosis
  - Appendicitis
  - Gastroenteritis
  - Pelvic inflammatory disease (adolescents)
  - Diabetes mellitus
  - Urethral irritation

- ■ Treatment
  - Antibiotic choice guided by urine culture
  - Treat children 1–24 months of age with cefixime or initial intravenous cefotaxime followed by oral cefixime
  - Voiding cystourethrogram for infants and children once free of infection to rule out vesicoureteral reflux
  - Prophylactic antibiotics continued until voiding cystourethrogram performed

- ■ Pearl

As in adult men, urinary tract infections in children with few exceptions reflect an anatomic defect somewhere in the collecting system: thus, image all.

Reference

Shaw KN et al: Urinary tract infection in the pediatric patient. Pediatr Clin North Am 1999;46:1111. [PMID: 10629676]

Constipation

- **Essentials of Diagnosis**
  - Defined as infrequent bowel movements, usually hard in consistency
  - Hard stools can lead to painful defecation and later withholding and encopresis
  - Constipation can be caused by anatomic abnormalities, neurologic problems, or endocrine disorders; usually no cause identified
  - A positive family history often elicited
  - Children are capable of withholding stool voluntarily
  - Rectal examination to evaluate fissures and assess rectal tone
  - Abdominal radiograph may confirm the diagnosis

- **Differential Diagnosis**
  - Hirschsprung's disease
  - Hypothyroidism
  - Hyperparathyroidism
  - Congenital gastrointestinal malformation
  - Infantile botulism
  - Lead intoxication

- **Treatment**
  - Impacted children will usually require a clean-out; although enemas are sometimes used, severe impaction may require oral polyethylene glycol-electrolyte solution
  - Dietary changes (increased fiber and lower milk and caffeine intake) usually beneficial
  - Mineral oil titrated to one or two soft stools per day is a recommended first-line agent
  - Lactulose may be useful; Docusate sodium suspension is foul-tasting and often hard for children to take
  - Mainstay of therapy is behavioral; long course of toilet sitting and positive feedback necessary
  - Families need to be told repeatedly that functional constipation is difficult to cure and that months to years of treatment may be necessary

- **Pearl**

As always in constipation, accurate definition and structural causes come first.

Reference

Griffin GC et al: How to resolve stool retention in a child. Underwear soiling is not a behavior problem. Postgrad Med 1999;105:159. [PMID: 9924501]

19

Selected Genetic Disorders*

Neurofibromatosis

- **Essentials of Diagnosis**
  - Occurs either sporadically or on a familial basis with autosomal dominant inheritance
  - Two distinct forms: Type 1 (von Recklinghausen's disease), characterized by multiple hyperpigmented macules in neurofibromas; and type 2, characterized by eighth cranial nerve tumors
  - Often present with symptoms and signs of tumor of the spinal or cranial nerves; superficial cutaneous nerve examination reveals palpable mobile nodules
  - Associated cutaneous lesions include axillary freckling and patches of cutaneous pigmentation (café au lait spots)
  - Malignant degeneration of neurofibromas possible, leading to peripheral sarcoma
  - Also associated with meningioma, bone cysts, pheochromocytomas, or scoliosis

- **Differential Diagnosis**
  - Intracranial or intraspinal tumor due to other causes
  - Albright's syndrome
  - Other neurocutaneous dysplasias

- **Treatment**
  - Genetic counseling important
  - Disfigurement may be corrected by plastic surgery
  - Intraspinal or intracranial tumor and tumors of peripheral nerves treated surgically if symptomatic

- **Pearl**

Up to six café au lait spots are allowed before Recklinghausen's disease is considered.

Reference

Gabriel KR: Neurofibromatosis. Curr Opin Pediatr 1997;9:89. [PMID: 9088761]

---

* The following genetic disorders are discussed in other chapters. Chapter 2: Cystic fibrosis; Chapter 5: sickle cell anemia, thalassemia, Von Willebrand's disease; Chapter 12: Huntington's chorea; Chapter 18: Down's syndrome

Acute Intermittent Porphyria

- ■ Essentials of Diagnosis
  - Autosomal dominant with variable expressivity
  - Symptoms begin in the teens or twenties, usually in young women; clinically silent in most, however
  - Caused by deficiency of porphobilinogen deaminase activity, leading to increased excretion of delta-aminolevulinic acid and porphobilinogen in the urine
  - Abdominal pain, acute peripheral or central nervous system dysfunction, recurrent psychiatric illness; cutaneous photosensitivity absent
  - Attacks precipitated by drugs (eg, barbiturates, sulfonamides, estrogens), intercurrent infections, and alcohol
  - Profound hyponatremia occasionally occurs; diagnosis confirmed by demonstrating increasing porphobilinogen in urine during acute attack
  - Absence of fever and leukocytosis

- ■ Differential Diagnosis
  - Other causes of acute abdominal pain (appendicitis, peptic ulcer disease, cholecystitis, diverticulitis, ruptured ectopic pregnancy, familial Mediterranean fever)
  - Polyneuropathy due to other causes
  - Guillain-Barré syndrome
  - Heavy metal poisoning (eg, lead)
  - Psychosis due to other causes
  - Other causes of hyponatremia

- ■ Treatment
  - High-carbohydrate diet may diminish number of episodes in some
  - Acute flares require analgesics and may require intravenous glucose and hematin

- ■ Pearl

In a young woman with abdominal pain and multiple surgical scars, think acute intermittent porphyria before adding another one.

Reference

Grandchamp B: Acute intermittent porphyria. Semin Liver Dis 1998; 18:17. [PMID: 9516674]

19

Alkaptonuria (Ochronosis)

- ### Essentials of Diagnosis
  - Recessively inherited deficiency of the enzyme homogentisic acid oxidase; leads to accumulation of an oxidation product in cartilage and degenerative joint disease of the spine with purplish joints
  - A slight, darkish blue color below the skin in areas overlying cartilage such as ears; some have more hyperpigmentation in scleras and conjunctivas
  - Aortic or mitral stenosis due to accumulation of metabolites in heart valves; predisposition to coronary artery disease occasionally
  - Back pain in spondylitis
  - Diagnosed by demonstrating homogentisic acid in the urine, which turns black spontaneously on air exposure

- ### Differential Diagnosis
  - Ankylosing spondylitis or other spondyloarthropathies
  - Osteoarthritis
  - Amiodarone toxicity
  - Chrysiasis
  - Argyria
  - Rheumatic heart disease

- ### Treatment
  - Similar to that for other arthropathies.
  - Rigid dietary restriction may be helpful

- ### Pearl

The only disease in medicine with black cartilage.

Reference

Fernández-Cañón JM et al: The molecular basis of alkaptonuria. Nat Genet 1996;14:19. [PMID: 8782815]

Gaucher's Disease

- ■ Essentials of Diagnosis
  - Autosomal recessive
  - Deficiency of beta-glucocerebrosidase causes accumulation of sphingolipid within phagocytic cells throughout body
  - Infiltration primarily involves the liver, spleen, bone marrow, and lymph nodes
  - Anemia, thrombocytopenia, splenomegaly are common; erosion of bones due to local infarction with bone pain
  - Bone marrow aspirates reveal typical Gaucher cells, with eccentric nucleus, PAS-positive inclusions; definitive diagnosis requires demonstration of deficient glucose cerebrosidase activity in leukocytes

- ■ Differential Diagnosis
  - Hepatomegaly, splenomegaly, lymphadenopathy due to other causes
  - Idiopathic avascular necrosis of bone, especially the hip
  - Metastatic malignancy to bone

- ■ Treatment
  - Largely supportive
  - Splenectomy for those with bleeding problems due to platelet sequestration
  - Alglucerase, given intravenously on a regular basis, probably improves orthopedic and hematologic problems; major drawback is exceptional cost

- ■ Pearl

A Jewish patient with a hip fracture and splenomegaly has Gaucher's disease until proved otherwise.

Reference

Mistry PK et al: A practical approach to diagnosis and management of Gaucher's disease. Baillieres Clin Haematol 1997;10:817. [PMID: 9497866]

19

Homocystinuria

- **Essentials of Diagnosis**
  - Autosomal recessive disease resulting in extreme elevations of plasma and urinary homocystine levels, a basis for diagnosis for this disorder
  - Patients often present in second and third decades of life with evidence of arterial or venous thromboses without underlying risk factors for hypercoagulability
  - Ectopia lentis almost always present; mental retardation common
  - Repeated venous and arterial thromboses common; reduced life expectancy from myocardial infarction, stroke, and pulmonary embolism

- **Differential Diagnosis**
  - Marfan's syndrome
  - Other causes of mental retardation
  - Other causes of hypercoagulability

- **Treatment**
  - Treatment in infancy with pyridoxine and folate helps some
  - Pyridoxine nonresponders treated with dietary reduction in methionine and supplementation of cysteine, also from infancy
  - Betaine may also be useful
  - Anticoagulation as appropriate for thrombosis

- **Pearl**

Ninety-five percent of ectopia lentis occurs in Marfan's syndrome, with upward lens displacement; the remaining 5% have this disorder, with downward lens dislocation.

Reference

De Franchis R et al: Clinical aspects of cystathionine beta-synthase deficiency: how wide is the spectrum? The Italian Collaborative Study Group on Homocystinuria. Eur J Pediatr 1998;157(Suppl 2):S67. [PMID: 9587029]

19

Marfan's Syndrome

- **Essentials of Diagnosis**
  - Autosomal dominant; a systemic connective tissue disease
  - Characterized by abnormalities of the skeletal system, eye, and cardiovascular system
  - Spontaneous pneumothorax, ectopia lentis, and myopia are characteristic; patients have disproportionately tall stature with long extremities and arachnodactyly, thoracic deformity, and joint laxity or contractures
  - Aortic dilation and dissection most worrisome complication; mitral regurgitation seen occasionally

- **Differential Diagnosis**
  - Homocystinuria
  - Aortic dissection due to other causes
  - Mitral or aortic regurgitation due to other causes
  - Ehlers-Danlos syndrome

- **Treatment**
  - Children should have periodic vision surveillance and annual orthopedic consultation
  - Patients of all ages require echocardiography—often annually—to monitor aortic diameter and mitral valve function; endocarditis prophylaxis usually required
  - Beta-blockade may retard the rate of aortic dilation; criteria for prophylactic replacement of the aortic root are unsettled

- **Pearl**

One of the few disorders in medicine immediately diagnosable by inspection.

Reference

Pyeritz RE: The Marfan syndrome. Annu Rev Med 2000;51:481. [PMID: 10774478]

19

Hemochromatosis

- ## Essentials of Diagnosis
  - The most common genetic disease among white North Americans
  - Autosomal recessive disease caused by *C282Y* mutation in most, with symptoms of hepatic, pancreatic, cardiac, and gonadal dysfunction
  - Hyperabsorption of iron and its parenchymal storage results in tissue injury
  - Symptoms typically occur after age 50 in men and after age 60 in women and depend on which organs are prominently involved
  - Clinical manifestations variably include cirrhosis and often hepatocellular carcinoma, congestive heart failure, diabetes mellitus, erectile dysfunction, arthropathy, and hypopituitarism
  - Elevated serum iron, normal transferrin, percentage saturation of iron >60%, and increased ferritin; glucose intolerance; mildly elevated AST and alkaline phosphatase
  - Liver biopsy characteristic, with iron stain identifying accumulation in parenchymal cells rather than reticuloendothelial system

- ## Differential Diagnosis
  - Other causes of cirrhosis
  - Other causes of congestive heart failure
  - Diabetes mellitus
  - Other causes of hypopituitarism
  - Other causes of iron overload, especially multiple transfusions (more than 100 units) as in homozygous beta-thalassemia

- ## Treatment
  - Screen first-order relatives with ferritin determinations
  - Early recognition and diagnosis (precirrhotic state) is crucial
  - Low-iron diet
  - Weekly phlebotomy to deplete iron stores, followed by maintenance phlebotomy or intramuscular deferoxamine
  - Treat manifestations of liver disease, congestive heart failure, diabetes, and arthropathy
  - Liver transplantation for decompensated cirrhosis

- ## Pearl

19

Widespread iron fortification of foods is arguably carcinogenic, given that hepatocellular carcinoma is the most common cause of death in this disease.

Reference

Powell LW et al: Haemochromatosis in the new millennium. J Hepatol 2000;32(1 Suppl):48. [PMID: 10718794]

Wilson's Disease (Hepatolenticular Degeneration)

- **Essentials of Diagnosis**

  - Autosomal recessive disorder with onset between first and third decades and symptoms of acute or chronic liver or neuropsychiatric dysfunction
  - Excessive deposition of copper in the liver and brain
  - Symptoms of cirrhosis and basal ganglia dysfunction
  - Kayser-Fleischer rings in the cornea (in all cases of neurologic Wilson's disease), hepatomegaly, parkinsonian tremor and rigidity, psychiatric abnormalities
  - Elevated urinary copper excretion (>100 mg/24 h), elevated hepatic copper (>100 mg/g), decreased serum ceruloplasmin (<20 mg/dL) before cirrhosis develops

- **Differential Diagnosis**

  - Other causes of fulminant hepatic failure
  - Other causes of cirrhosis
  - Other causes of psychiatric and neurologic disturbances, especially Parkinson's disease

- **Treatment**

  - Restrict dietary copper (shellfish, organ foods, legumes)
  - Oral penicillamine facilitates urinary excretion of chelated copper; pyridoxine supplementation necessary
  - Trientine if penicillamine cannot be tolerated
  - Oral zinc acetate promotes fecal copper excretion
  - Liver transplantation for fulminant hepatic failure or decompensated cirrhosis

- **Pearl**

One percent of Wilson's disease patients present with hemolytic anemia: copper is toxic to red cell membranes.

Reference

Cuthbert JA: Wilson's disease. Update of a systemic disorder with protean manifestations. Gastroenterol Clin North Am 1998;27:655. [PMID: 9891702]

19

20

Common Disorders of the Eye

Acute Conjunctivitis

- **Essentials of Diagnosis**
  - Acute onset of red, itchy, burning eyes with tearing, eyelid sticking, foreign body sensation, and discharge
  - Conjunctival injection and edema, mucoid or purulent discharge, lid edema and possible preauricular lymph node enlargement
  - Vision is normal or slightly decreased
  - Causes include bacterial and viral (including herpetic) infections and allergy

- **Differential Diagnosis**
  - Acute uveitis
  - Acute angle-closure glaucoma
  - Corneal abrasion or infection
  - Dacryocystitis
  - Nasolacrimal duct obstruction
  - Chronic conjunctivitis
  - Scleritis in autoimmune disease
  - Reactive arthritis

- **Treatment**
  - Topical broad-spectrum ophthalmologic antibiotics
  - Ophthalmology follow-up for persistent symptoms or presence of decreased visual acuity

- **Pearl**

Be certain the red eye is not uveitis or episcleritis before making the diagnosis.

Reference

Hara JH: The red eye: diagnosis and treatment. Am Fam Physician 1996; 54:2423. [PMID: 8961843]

Corneal Ulceration

- **Essentials of Diagnosis**
  - Acute eye pain, photophobia, redness, tearing, discharge, and blurred vision
  - Upper eyelid edema, conjunctival injection with ciliary flush, mucopurulent discharge, white corneal infiltrate with overlying epithelial defect that stains with fluorescein dye, and, in some cases, hypopyon
  - Causes include trauma, contact lens wear, infection (bacterial, herpetic, fungal, acanthamoeba)

- **Differential Diagnosis**
  - Acute uveitis
  - Acute angle-closure glaucoma
  - Acute conjunctivitis
  - Sterile or immunologic ulcer
  - Corneal abrasion or foreign body

- **Treatment**
  - Frequent topical broad spectrum antibiotics and daily ophthalmologic follow-up
  - Prompt ophthalmologic referral for ulcer > 2 mm in diameter
  - *Do not patch a corneal ulcer!*

- **Pearl**

If the cause of corneal ulceration is not apparent, think bulbar syringomyelia.

Reference

Cohen EJ: Cornea and external disease in the new millennium. Arch Ophthalmol 2000;118:979. [PMID: 10900114]

Acute (Angle-Closure) Glaucoma

- **Essentials of Diagnosis**
  - Less than 5% of all glaucoma
  - Acute onset of eye pain and redness, photophobia, blurred vision with colored halos around lights, headaches, nausea, or abdominal pain
  - Decreased vision, conjunctival injection with ciliary flush, steamy cornea, mid-dilated and nonreactive pupil, and elevated intraocular pressure by tonometry
  - Preexisting narrow anterior chamber angle predisposes; older patients, hyperopes, Asians, and Inuits more susceptible
  - Precipitated by pupillary dilation caused by stress, pharmacologic mydriasis), dark environment (eg, movie theater)

- **Differential Diagnosis**
  - Acute conjunctivitis
  - Acute uveitis
  - Corneal abrasion or infection
  - Other types of glaucoma

- **Treatment**
  - Prompt ophthalmologic referral
  - Pharmacotherapy includes systemic acetazolamide, topical miotic (pilocarpine), beta-blocker (timolol), alpha-agonist (apraclonidine, brimonidine), and systemic hyperosmotic agent (eg, glycerol or mannitol).
  - Laser peripheral iridotomy usually curative

- **Pearl**

Don't avoid a dilated funduscopic examination for fear of precipitating acute glaucoma; you would be doing the patient a favor to identify this treatable disease early.

Reference

Morgan A et al: Acute visual change. Emerg Med Clin North Am 1998; 16:825. [PMID: 9889742]

Open-Angle (Chronic) Glaucoma

- **Essentials of Diagnosis**
  - Ninety-five percent or more of glaucoma
  - Insidious onset resulting in eventual complete loss of vision; asymptomatic early; common in blacks, elderly, and myopic patients
  - Tonometry reveals elevated intraocular pressure (> 21 mm Hg) but highly variable
  - Pathologic cupping of optic disk seen funduscopically, can be asymmetric
  - Loss of peripheral visual fields

- **Differential Diagnosis**
  - Normal diurnal variation of intraocular pressure
  - Other types of glaucoma: congenital optic nerve abnormalities; ischemic, compressive, or toxic optic neuropathy
  - Bilateral retinal disorders (chorioretinitis, retinoschisis, retinitis pigmentosa)

- **Treatment**
  - Beta-blocking agents (timolol)
  - Miotics (pilocarpine)
  - Prostaglandin analog (latanoprost)
  - Alpha-adrenergic agents (brimonidine, apraclonidine)
  - Carbonic anhydrase inhibitors (acetazolamide, dorzolamide)
  - Laser trabeculoplasty, trabeculectomy, and aqueous shunt procedure

- **Pearl**

A patient referred by an ophthalmologist for evaluation of dyspnea has beta-blocker-induced asthma or congestive heart failure until proved otherwise.

Reference

Coleman AL: Glaucoma. Lancet 1999;354:1803. [PMID: 10577657]

20

Uveitis

- **Essentials of Diagnosis**
  - Inflammation of the uveal tract, including the iris (iritis), ciliary body (cyclitis), and choroid (choroiditis); categorized as anterior (iridocyclitis), posterior (chorioretinitis), or panuveitis (diffuse)
  - Acute onset of eye pain and redness, photophobia, tearing, and blurred vision (anterior uveitis); gradual visual loss with floaters, but otherwise asymptomatic (posterior uveitis); recurrent and bilateral
  - Injected conjunctiva or sclera with flare and inflammatory cells by slitlamp examination, white cells on corneal endothelium, and iris nodules (anterior uveitis); white cells and opacities in the vitreous, retinal or choroidal infiltrates, edema, and vascular sheathing (posterior uveitis)
  - Multiple causes: post trauma or surgery, lens-induced, HLA-B27-associated autoimmune diseases (eg, ankylosing spondylitis, reactive arthritis, ulcerative colitis), Behçet's syndrome, infectious (herpes simplex or zoster, syphilis, tuberculosis, toxoplasmosis, toxocariasis, histoplasmosis, leprosy, Lyme disease, CMV, candida), psoriatic arthritis, sarcoidosis, Vogt-Koyanagi-Harada syndrome

- **Differential Diagnosis**
  - Acute conjunctivitis
  - Corneal abrasion or infection
  - Retinal detachment
  - Retinitis pigmentosa
  - Intraocular tumor (eg, retinoblastoma, leukemia, malignant melanoma, lymphoma)
  - Retained intraocular foreign body
  - Scleritis

- **Treatment**
  - Prompt ophthalmologic referral in all cases
  - Anterior disease: frequent topical steroids, periocular steroid injection, dilation of the pupil with cycloplegic agent (eg, cyclopentolate, scopolamine, homatropine)
  - Posterior disease: more commonly requires systemic steroids and immunosuppressive agents

- **Pearl**

The most common ocular reflection of systemic disease.

Reference

Lightman S: New therapeutic options in uveitis. Eye 1997;11(Part 2): 222. [PMID: 9349417]

Cataract

- ■ Essentials of Diagnosis
  - Slowly progressive, painless visual loss or blurring, with glare from oncoming headlights and reduced color perception
  - Lens opacification grossly visible or seen by ophthalmoscopy
  - Causes include aging, trauma, drugs (steroids, anticholinesterases, antipsychotics), uveitis, radiation, tumor, retinitis pigmentosa, systemic diseases (diabetes mellitus, hypoparathyroidism, Wilson's disease, myotonic dystrophy, Down's syndrome, atopic dermatitis)

- ■ Differential Diagnosis
  - Generally unmistakable
  - Ectopia lentis may cause some diagnostic confusion

- ■ Treatment
  - Surgical removal with intraocular lens implant for visual impairment or occupational requirement

- ■ Pearl

When bilateral cataracts are removed in succession, the patient is always most grateful for the first procedure because color vision returns.

Reference

Trudo EW et al: Cataracts. Lifting the clouds on an age-old problem. Postgrad Med 1998;103:114. [PMID: 9590990]

20

Retinal Vein Occlusion
(Branch, Hemiretinal, or Central)

- ### Essentials of Diagnosis
  - Sudden, unilateral, and painless visual loss or field defect
  - Local or diffuse venous dilation and tortuosity, retinal hemorrhages, cotton-wool spots, and edema; optic disk edema and hemorrhages; neovascularization of disk, retina, or iris by funduscopy and slitlamp examination
  - Associated underlying diseases include atherosclerosis and hypertension, glaucoma, hypercoagulable state including factor V Leiden or natural anticoagulant deficiency (AT-III, S, C), lupus anticoagulants; hyperviscosity (polycythemia or Waldenström's coagulopathy), Behçet's syndrome, SLE
  - Retrobulbar external venous compression (thyroid disease, orbital tumor) and migraine also may be responsible

- ### Differential Diagnosis
  - Venous stasis
  - Ocular ischemic syndrome
  - Diabetic retinopathy
  - Papilledema
  - Radiation retinopathy
  - Hypertensive retinopathy
  - Retinopathy of anemia
  - Leukemic retinopathy

- ### Treatment
  - Prompt ophthalmologic referral
  - Laser photocoagulation for retinal ischemia and persistent macular edema
  - Surveillance and treatment of underlying diseases

- ### Pearl

Think of hemoglobin SC disease in a pregnant woman with any retinal venous occlusion.

Reference

Baumal CR et al: Treatment of central retinal vein occlusion. Ophthalmic Surg Lasers 1997;28:590. [PMID: 9243663]

Retinal Artery Occlusion (Branch or Central)

- ■ **Essentials of Diagnosis**
  - Sudden unilateral and painless loss of vision or visual field defect
  - Focal wedge-shaped area of retinal whitening or edema within the distribution of a branch arteriole or diffuse retinal whitening with a cherry-red spot at the fovea; arteriolar constriction with segmentation of blood column; visible emboli
  - Macular vision unaffected because of external carotid collateral
  - Associated underlying diseases include carotid plaque or cardiac-source emboli; vasculitis; less common than vein occlusion in hypercoagulable states

- ■ **Differential Diagnosis**
  - Ophthalmic artery occlusion
  - Inherited metabolic or lysosomal storage disease
  - Ocular migraine

- ■ **Treatment**
  - Medical emergency calling for immediate ophthalmologic referral
  - Digital ocular massage, systemic acetazolamide or topical beta-blocker to lower intraocular pressure, anterior chamber paracentesis, and carbogen treatment
  - Consider thrombolysis

- ■ **Pearl**

The retina is part of the central nervous system, and this disorder is thus treated as one does a stroke.

Reference

Kosmorsky GS: Sudden painless visual loss: optic nerve and circulatory disturbances. Clin Geriatr Med 199915:1. [PMID: 9855655]

Retinal Detachment

- **Essentials of Diagnosis**
  - Acute onset of photopsias (flashes of light), floaters ("shade" or "cobwebs"), a curtain or shadow across the visual field, and peripheral or central visual loss
  - Elevation of the retina with a flap tear or break in the retina, vitreous pigmented cells or hemorrhage seen by ophthalmoscopy
  - Risk factors include lattice vitreoretinal degeneration, posterior vitreous separation (especially with vitreous hemorrhage), high myopia, trauma, and previous ocular surgery (especially with vitreous loss)

- **Differential Diagnosis**
  - Retinoschisis
  - Choroidal detachment
  - Posterior vitreous separation

- **Treatment**
  - Immediate ophthalmologic referral
  - Bed rest with bilateral patching
  - Closure of retinal tear by pneumatic retinopexy, scleral buckling with cryopexy, pars plana vitrectomy with drainage, endolaser, cryopexy, membrane peel, gas or silicone oil injection
  - Repair of small tears by laser photocoagulation or cryopexy

- **Pearl**

Retinal detachment is the most common nonorthopedic injury sustained playing tennis doubles.

Reference

Elfervig LS et al: Retinal detachment. Insight 1998;23:66. [PMID: 9866533]

Diabetic Retinopathy

- ■ Essentials of Diagnosis
  - Asymptomatic; may have decreased or fluctuating vision or floaters
  - Nonproliferative: dot and blot hemorrhages, microaneurysms, hard exudates, cotton-wool spots, venous beading, and intraretinal microvascular abnormalities
  - Proliferative: neovascularization of optic disk, retina, or iris; preretinal or vitreous hemorrhages and tractional retinal detachment

- ■ Differential Diagnosis
  - Hypertensive retinopathy
  - Radiation retinopathy
  - Central or branch retinal vein occlusion
  - Ocular ischemic syndrome
  - Sickle cell retinopathy
  - Retinopathy of severe anemia
  - Embolization from intravenous drug abuse (talc retinopathy)
  - Collagen-vascular disease
  - Sarcoidosis
  - Eales' disease

- ■ Treatment
  - Ophthalmologic referral and regular follow-up in all diabetics
  - Laser photocoagulation for macular edema and proliferative disease
  - Pars plana vitrectomy for nonclearing dense vitreous hemorrhage and tractional retinal detachment involving or threatening the macula

- ■ Pearl

Seventy-five percent of diabetics develop significant retinopathy within 15 years after diagnosis; nearly one-fourth never develop retinopathy.

Reference

Ferris FL 3rd et al: Treatment of diabetic retinopathy. N Engl J Med 1999; 341:667. [PMID: 10460819]

20

Age-Related Macular Degeneration

- **Essentials of Diagnosis**
  - Nonexudative (dry) form: central or paracentral blind spot and gradual loss of central vision; may be asymptomatic
  - Small and hard or large and soft drusen, geographic atrophy of the retinal pigment epithelium, and pigment clumping
  - Exudative (wet) form: distortion of straight lines or edges, central or paracentral blind spot, and rapid loss of central vision
  - Gray-green choroidal neovascular membrane, lipid exudates, subretinal hemorrhage or fluid, pigment epithelial detachment, and fibrovascular disciform scars
  - Risk factors include increasing age, positive family history, cigarette smoking, hyperopia, light iris color, hypertension, and cardiovascular disease

- **Differential Diagnosis**
  - Prominent drusen
  - Choroidal neovascularization from other causes (eg, ocular histoplasmosis, angioid streaks, myopic degeneration, traumatic choroidal rupture, optic disk drusen, choroidal tumors, laser scars, and inflammatory chorioretinal lesions)

- **Treatment**
  - Prompt ophthalmologic referral
  - Laser photocoagulation, photodynamic therapy, submacular surgery, and macular translocation for choroidal neovascularization

- **Pearl**

Age-related macular degeneration is the third leading cause of blindness in America (after glaucoma and diabetic retinopathy).

Reference

Fine SL et al: Age-related macular degeneration. N Engl J Med 2000;342:483. [PMID: 10675430]

Hypertensive Retinopathy

- **Essentials of Diagnosis**
  - Usually asymptomatic; may have decreased vision
  - Generalized or localized retinal arteriolar narrowing, almost always bilateral
  - Arteriovenous crossing changes (A-V nicking), retinal arteriolar sclerosis (copper or silver wiring), cotton-wool spots, hard exudates, flame-shaped hemorrhages, retinal edema, arterial macroaneurysms, chorioretinal atrophy
  - Optic disk edema in malignant hypertension

- **Differential Diagnosis**
  - Diabetic retinopathy
  - Radiation retinopathy
  - Central or branch retinal vein occlusion
  - Sickle cell retinopathy
  - Retinopathy of severe anemia
  - Embolization from intravenous drug abuse (talc retinopathy)
  - Autoimmune disease
  - Sarcoidosis
  - Eales' disease

- **Treatment**
  - Treat the hypertension
  - Ophthalmologic referral

- **Pearl**

The only pathognomonic funduscopic change of hypertension is focal arteriolar narrowing—and that is typically seen in hypertensive crisis.

Reference

Schubert HD: Ocular manifestations of systemic hypertension. Curr Opin Ophthalmol 1998;9:69. [PMID: 10387339]

20

Pingueculum & Pterygium

- **Essentials of Diagnosis**
  - Pingueculum: yellow-white flat or slightly raised conjunctival lesion in the interpalpebral fissure adjacent to the limbus but not involving the cornea
  - Pterygium: wing-shaped fold of fibrovascular tissue arising from the interpalpebral conjunctiva and extending onto the cornea
  - Irritation, redness, decreased vision; may be asymptomatic
  - Both lesions can be highly vascularized and injected; their growth associated with sunlight and chronic irritation

- **Differential Diagnosis**
  - Conjunctival intraepithelial neoplasia
  - Dermoid
  - Pannus

- **Treatment**
  - Protect the eyes from sun, dust, and wind with sunglasses or goggles
  - Reduce ocular irritation with artificial tears or mild topical steroid
  - Surgical removal with extreme irritation not relieved with above treatment, extension of pterygium to the pupillary margin, or irregular astigmatism

- **Pearl**

Xanthomas always, xanthelasma sometimes, and pterygium and pingueculum are never associated with hyperlipidemia—except coincidentally.

Reference

Hoffman RS et al: Current options in pterygium management. Int Ophthalmol Clin 1999;39:15. [PMID: 10083903]

Hordeolum & Chalazion

- **Essentials of Diagnosis**
  - Eyelid lump, swelling, pain, and redness
  - Visible or palpable, well-defined subcutaneous nodule within the eyelid; eyelid edema, erythema, and tenderness with or without preauricular node
  - Hordeolum: acute obstruction and infection of eyelid gland (meibomian gland—internal hordeolum, gland of Zeis or Moll—external hordeolum), associated with *Staphylococcus aureus*
  - Chalazion: chronic obstruction and inflammation of meibomian gland with leakage of sebum into surrounding tissue with resultant lipogranuloma; rosacea may be associated

- **Differential Diagnosis**
  - Preseptal cellulitis
  - Sebaceous cell carcinoma
  - Pyogenic granuloma

- **Treatment:**
  - Warm compresses for 15–20 minutes at least 4 times daily
  - Topical antibiotic ointment twice daily
  - Incision and curettage for persistent chalazion (> 6–8weeks)
  - Intralesional steroid injection for chalazion near the nasolacrimal drainage system

- **Pearl**

Hordeolum—this kernel-type abscess gets its name from the Latin word for barleycorn.

Reference

Lederman C et al: Hordeola and chalazia. Pediatr Rev 1999;20:283. [PMID: 10429150]

20

Blepharitis & Meibomianitis

- ■ Essentials of Diagnosis
  - Chronic itching, burning, mild pain, foreign body sensation, tearing, and crusting around the eyes on awakening
  - Crusty, red, thickened eyelids with prominent blood vessels or inspissated oil glands in the eyelid margins, conjunctival injection, mild mucoid discharge, and acne rosacea

- ■ Differential Diagnosis
  - Sebaceous gland carcinoma

- ■ Treatment
  - Warm compresses for 15 minutes, followed by scrubbing the eyelid margins with baby shampoo at least twice daily
  - Artificial tears for irritation
  - Topical antibiotic ointment at bedtime
  - Recurrent or persistent meibomitis treated with doxycycline for 6–8 weeks, followed by slow taper; in women, negative pregnancy test before and contraception during treatment essential

- ■ Pearl

No precaution is too prudent when contemplating treatment of young women with tetracycline.

Reference

Carter SR: Eyelid disorders: diagnosis and management. Am Fam Physician 1998;57:2695. [PMID: 9636333]

21

Common Disorders of the Ear, Nose, & Throat

Chronic Serous Otitis Media

- **Essentials of Diagnosis**
    - Owing to obstruction of the auditory tube, resulting in transudation of fluid
    - Allergic and immune factors probably contribute
    - More common in children but can occur in adults following an upper respiratory tract infection, barotrauma, air travel, or auditory tube obstruction by tumor
    - Painless hearing loss with feeling of fullness or voice reverberation in affected ear
    - Dull, immobile tympanic membrane with loss of landmarks and bubbles seen behind tympanic membrane; intact light reflex
    - Fifteen- to 20-decibel conductive hearing loss by audiometry and Weber tuning fork examination lateralizing to affected ear

- **Differential Diagnosis**
    - Acute otitis media
    - Nasopharyngeal tumor (as causative agent)

- **Treatment**
    - Oral decongestants, antihistamines, and antibiotics
    - Tympanotomy tubes for refractory cases with audiology and otolaryngology referral

- **Pearl**

Unilateral otitis media, especially in a patient of Asian ethnicity, is nasopharyngeal carcinoma until proved otherwise—mirror examination of the nasopharynx is obligatory.

Reference

Osma U et al: The complications of chronic otitis media: report of 93 cases. J Laryngol Otol 2000;114:97. [PMID: 10748823]

Acute Otitis Media

- **Essentials of Diagnosis**
  - Ear pain, with sensation of fullness in ear and hearing loss; fever and chills; onset often following upper respiratory syndrome
  - Dullness and hyperemia of eardrum with loss of landmarks and light reflex
  - Most common organisms in both children and adults include *Streptococcus pneumoniae, Haemophilus influenzae, Moraxella catarrhalis,* and group A streptococcus
  - Complications include mastoiditis, skull base osteomyelitis, sigmoid sinus thromboses, meningitis, brain abscess

- **Differential Diagnosis**
  - Bullous myringitis (associated with mycoplasmal infection)
  - Acute external otitis
  - Otalgia referred from other sources (especially pharynx)
  - Serous otitis

- **Treatment**
  - Antibiotics versus supportive care controversial; oral decongestants
  - Tympanostomy tubes for refractory cases, with audiology and otolaryngology referral
  - Recurrent acute otitis media may be prevented with long-term antibiotic prophylaxis

- **Pearl**

With unexplained fever in a ventilated patient, look in the ears: otitis media can result from auditory tube obstruction by the nasotracheal tube.

Reference

Damoiseaux RA et al: Primary care based randomized, double blind trial of amoxicillin versus placebo for acute otitis media in children aged under 2 years. BMJ 2000;320:350. [PMID: 10657332]

Endolymphatic Hydrops (Meniere's Syndrome)

- ■ Essentials of Diagnosis
  - Etiology is unknown
  - Due to distention of the endolymphatic compartment of the inner ear
  - The four tenets: episodic vertigo and nausea (lasting 1–8 hours), aural pressure, continuous tinnitus, and fluctuating hearing loss
  - Sensorineural hearing loss by audiometry starting in the low frequencies

- ■ Differential Diagnosis
  - Benign positioning vertigo
  - Posterior fossa tumor
  - Vestibular neuronitis
  - Vertebrobasilar insufficiency
  - Psychiatric disorder
  - Multiple sclerosis
  - Syphilis

- ■ Treatment
  - Low-salt diet and diuretic
  - Antihistamines, diazepam, and antiemetics may be given parenterally for acute attacks
  - Aminoglycoside ablation of unilateral vestibular function via middle ear infusion
  - Surgical treatment in refractory cases: decompression of endolymphatic sac, vestibular nerve section, or labyrinthectomy if profound hearing loss present

- ■ Pearl

One of the few unilateral diseases of paired organs.

Reference

Saeed SR: Fortnightly review. Diagnosis and treatment of Meniere's disease. BMJ 1998;316:368. [PMID: 9487176]

Benign Positioning Vertigo

- **Essentials of Diagnosis**
  - Acute onset of vertigo, nausea, tinnitus
  - Provoked by changes in head positioning rather than by maintenance of a particular posture
  - Nystagmus with positive Bárány test (delayed onset of symptoms by movement of head with habituation and fatigue of symptoms)

- **Differential Diagnosis**
  - Endolymphatic hydrops
  - Vestibular neuronitis
  - Posterior fossa tumor
  - Vertebrobasilar insufficiency
  - Migraines

- **Treatment**
  - Intravenous diazepam, antihistamines, and antiemetics for acute attack
  - Reassurance with otolaryngologic referral for persistent symptoms or other neurologic abnormalities
  - Single-session physical therapy protocols may be useful in some patients

- **Pearl**

Learn this well—it's the most common cause of vertigo encountered in primary care settings.

Reference

Furman JM et al: Benign paroxysmal positional vertigo. N Engl J Med 1999; 341:1590. [PMID: 10564690]

Acute Sinusitis

- **Essentials of Diagnosis**
  - Nasal congestion, purulent discharge, facial pain, and headache; teeth may hurt or feel abnormal in maxillary sinusitis; history of allergic rhinitis, acute upper respiratory infection, or dental infection often present
  - Fever, toxicity; tenderness, erythema, and swelling over affected sinus; discolored nasal discharge and poor response to decongestants alone
  - Clouding of sinuses on imaging or by transillumination
  - Coronal CT scans have become the diagnostic study of choice
  - Pain not prominent in chronic sinusitis—a poorly defined entity
  - Typical pathogens include *Streptococcus pneumoniae,* other streptococci, *Haemophilus influenzae, Staphylococcus aureus, Moraxella catarrhalis;* aspergillus in HIV patients
  - Complications: orbital cellulitis or abscess, meningitis, brain abscess

- **Differential Diagnosis**
  - Viral or allergic rhinitis
  - Dental abscess
  - Dacryocystitis
  - Carcinoma of sinus
  - Headache due to other causes, especially cluster headache

- **Treatment**
  - Oral and nasal decongestants, broad-spectrum antibiotics, nasal saline
  - Functional endoscopic sinus surgery or external sinus procedures for medically resistant sinusitis, nasal polyposis, sinusitis complications

- **Pearl**

Sphenoid sinusitis is the only cause in medicine of a nasal ridge headache radiating to the top of the skull.

Reference

Poole MD: A focus on acute sinusitis in adults: changes in disease management. Am J Med 1999;106:38S. [PMID: 10348062]

Allergic Rhinitis (Hay Fever)

- **Essentials of Diagnosis**
  - Seasonal or perennial occurrence of watery nasal discharge, sneezing, itching of eyes and nose
  - Pale, boggy mucous membranes with conjunctival injection
  - Eosinophilia of nasal secretions and occasionally of blood
  - Positive skin tests often present but of little value in most instances

- **Differential Diagnosis**
  - Upper respiratory viral infections

- **Treatment**
  - Desensitization occasionally beneficial, especially in younger patients
  - Oral antihistamines; oral or inhaled decongestants
  - Short-course systemic steroids for severe cases
  - Nasal corticosteroids and nasal cromolyn sodium often effective if used correctly

- **Pearl**

A Wright's flambé of secretions is the best way to demonstrate eosinophils: stain the smear, ignite it, decolorize it, and the cells will be seen readily at low power.

Reference

Corren J: Allergic rhinitis: treating the adult. J Allergy Clin Immunol 2000; 105(6 Part 2):S610. [PMID: 10856166]

Epiglottitis

- **Essentials of Diagnosis**
    - Sudden onset of stridor, odynophagia, dysphagia, and drooling
    - Muffled voice, toxic-appearing and febrile patient
    - Cherry-red, swollen epiglottis on indirect laryngoscopy; pharynx typically normal or slightly injected
    - Should be suspected when odynophagia is out of proportion to oropharyngeal findings

- **Differential Diagnosis**
    - Viral croup
    - Foreign body in larynx
    - Retropharyngeal abscess

- **Treatment**
    - Humidified oxygen with no manipulation of oropharynx or epiglottis
    - Airway observation in monitored setting, intubation with tracheotomy stand-by
    - Children usually need intubation—adults need close airway observation
    - Parenteral antibiotics active against *Haemophilus influenzae* and short burst of systemic corticosteroids

- **Pearl**

The patient with a severe sore throat and unimpressive pharyngeal examination by tongue blade has epiglottitis until proved otherwise.

Reference

Park KW et al: Airway management for adult patients with acute epiglottitis: a 12-year experience at an academic medical center (1984–1995). Anesthesiology 1998;88:254. [PMID: 9447879]

External Otitis

- **Essentials of Diagnosis**
  - Presents with otalgia, often accompanied by pruritus and purulent discharge
  - Usually caused by gram-negative rods or fungi
  - Often a history of water exposure or trauma to the ear canal
  - Movement of the auricle elicits pain; erythema and edema of the ear canal with a purulent exudate on examination
  - When visualized, tympanic membrane is red but moves normally with pneumatic otoscopy

- **Differential Diagnosis**
  - Malignant otitis externa (external otitis in an immunocompromised or diabetic patient with osteomyelitis of the temporal bone); pseudomonas causative in diabetes

- **Treatment**
  - Prevent additional moisture and mechanical injury to the ear canal
  - Otic drops containing a mixture of an aminoglycoside or quinolones and a corticosteroid
  - Purulent debris filling the canal should be removed; occasionally, a wick is needed to facilitate entry of the otic drops
  - Analgesics

- **Pearl**

A painful red ear in a diabetic is assumed to be malignant otitis externa until proved otherwise.

Reference

Ostrowski VB et al: Pathologic conditions of the external ear and auditory canal. Postgrad Med 1996;100:223. [PMID: 8795656]

Viral Rhinitis (Common Cold)

- ■ Essentials of Diagnosis
  - • Headache, nasal congestion, watery rhinorrhea, sneezing, scratchy throat, and malaise
  - • Due to a variety of viruses, including rhinovirus and adenovirus
  - • Examination of the nares reveals erythematous mucosa and watery discharge

- ■ Differential Diagnosis
  - • Acute sinusitis
  - • Allergic rhinitis
  - • Bacterial pharyngitis

- ■ Treatment
  - • Supportive treatment only
  - • Phenylephrine nasal sprays (should not be used for more than 5–7 days) and decongestants may be useful
  - • Secondary bacterial infection suggested by a change of rhinorrhea from clear to yellow or green; cultures are useful to guide antimicrobial therapy

- ■ Pearl

To date, no cure has been discovered for the common cold; physicians should not anticipate one.

Reference

Mossad SB: Treatment of the common cold. BMJ 1998;317:33. [PMID: 9651268]

Acute Sialadenitis
(Parotitis, Submandibular Gland Adenitis)

- **Essentials of Diagnosis**
  - Inflammation of parotid or submandibular gland due to salivary stasis and infection
  - Facial swelling and pain overlying the parotid or submandibular gland
  - Often seen in severe dehydration
  - Examination shows erythema and edema over affected gland and pus from affected duct
  - Leukocytosis
  - Complications: parotid or submandibular space abscess

- **Differential Diagnosis**
  - Salivary gland tumor
  - Facial cellulitis or dental abscess
  - Sjögren's syndrome
  - Mumps
  - Lymphoepithelial cysts in immunocompromised patients

- **Treatment**
  - Antibiotics with gram-positive coverage
  - Warm compresses
  - Hydration
  - Oral rinses

- **Pearl**

Look for this in marathon runners after the race on hot days; hyper-amylasemia clinches the diagnosis.

Reference

Silvers AR et al: Salivary glands. Radiol Clin North Am 1998;36:941. [PMID: 9747195]

22

Poisoning

Acetaminophen (Tylenol; Many Others)

■ Essentials of Diagnosis
- Nausea and vomiting after ingestion; may be no signs of toxicity until 24–48 hours after ingestion
- Serum acetaminophen levels measured 4 hours after ingestion or at initial evaluation if longer than 4 hours since ingestion; level should be obtained in all drug overdoses
- Hepatic and renal injury not apparent until after 36–72 hours
- Striking elevations in aminotransferases; in some cases, fulminant hepatic necrosis
- Patients may not realize that combination analgesics (eg, Tylenol No. 3, Vicodin, Darvocet) contain acetaminophen

■ Differential Diagnosis
- Other hepatotoxin ingestion (eg, *Amanita* mushrooms, carbon tetrachloride)
- Alcoholic liver disease
- Viral hepatitis
- Overdose of other drug

■ Treatment
- Activated charcoal
- Gastric lavage if less than 1 hour since ingestion
- Acetylcysteine (140 mg/kg orally, followed by 70 mg/kg every 4 hours) if serum level is higher than toxic line on standard nomogram

■ Pearl

A serum acetaminophen should be obtained in all overdoses: once hepatotoxicity ensues, therapy is valueless, and the depressed suicidal patient tends to ingest multiple drugs.

Reference

Salgia AD et al: When acetaminophen use becomes toxic. Treating acute accidental and intentional overdose. Postgrad Med 1999;105:81. [PMID: 102123088]

Amphetamines, Ecstasy, Cocaine

- **Essentials of Diagnosis**
  - Sympathomimetic clinical scenario: anxiety, tremulousness, agitation, tachycardia, hypertension, diaphoresis, dilated pupils, muscular hyperactivity, hyperthermia
  - With cocaine in particular, stroke and myocardial infarction from vasospasm
  - Psychosis, seizures
  - Metabolic acidosis may occur
  - Urine toxicology screen
  - Ecstasy (MDMA) associated with serotonin syndrome (see antidepressants) and malignant hyperthermia

- **Differential Diagnosis**
  - Anticholinergic poisoning
  - Functional psychosis
  - Exertional heat stroke
  - Other stimulant overdose (eg, ephedrine, phenylpropanolamine)

- **Treatment**
  - Activated charcoal for oral ingestions
  - Gastric lavage if less than 1 hour since ingestion
  - Chemistry panel and creatine kinase for metabolic acidosis, renal failure, and rhabdomyolysis
  - For agitation or psychosis: sedation with benzodiazepines (lorazepam or diazepam)
  - For hyperthermia: remove clothing, cool mist spray, cooling blanket
  - For hypertension: phentolamine, nifedipine, nitroprusside, or labetalol (not propranolol because it may generate unopposed alpha-adrenergic effects and worsen hypertension)
  - For tachyarrhythmias or tachycardia, use esmolol—the short half-life allows rapid dissipation of effect if necessary

- **Pearl**

Chest pain in a middle-class patient with running shoes and casual clothing equals cocaine-induced coronary vasospasm.

Reference

Ghuran A et al: Recreational drug misuse: issues for the cardiologist. Heart 2000;83;:627. [PMID: 10814617]

Antidepressants: Atypical Agents (Serotonin Syndrome)

- ### Essentials of Diagnosis
  - Trazodone, bupropion, venlafaxine, and the SSRIs (fluoxetine, sertraline, paroxetine, fluvoxamine, and citalopram); well-tolerated in pure overdoses, high toxic-to-therapeutic ratios
  - History of ingestion paramount
  - Serotonin syndrome: changes in cognition or behavior (confusion, agitation, coma), autonomic dysfunction (hyperthermia, diaphoresis, tachycardia, hypertension), and neuromuscular activity (myoclonus, hyperreflexia, muscle rigidity, tremor, ataxia)

- ### Differential Diagnosis
  - Alcohol withdrawal
  - Heat stroke
  - Hypoglycemia
  - Neuroleptic malignant syndrome

- ### Treatment
  - Activated charcoal
  - Gastric lavage if less than 1 hour since large ingestion or if a mixed drug ingestion
  - Cardiac monitoring and ECG based on specific agent
  - Benzodiazepines initially; bupropion, venlafaxine, and SSRIs associated with seizures
  - Serotonin syndrome typically self-limited; stop all offending agents
  - Cyproheptadine (an antiserotonergic agent) in serotonin syndrome (4–8 mg orally, repeated once in 2 hours if no response)

- ### Pearl

Serotonin syndrome is more frequently due to the combination of an SSRI and another serotonergic agent: rave participants increase the risk by taking an SSRI ("preloading") followed by ecstasy.

Reference

Carbone JR: The neuroleptic malignant and serotonin syndromes. Emerg Med Clin North Am 2000;18:317. [PMID: 10767887]

Antidepressants: Tricyclics

- **Essentials of Diagnosis**
  - Tricyclic antidepressants include amitriptyline, desipramine, doxepin, imipramine, and nortriptyline
  - Peripheral antimuscarinic effects: tachycardia, dry mouth, dry skin, muscle twitching, decreased bowel activity, dilated pupils; may be offset by TCA-mediated alpha-adrenergic receptor inhibition
  - Central antimuscarinic effects: agitation, delirium, confusion, hallucinations, slurred speech, ataxia, sedation, coma
  - Cardiotoxic effects from voltage-dependent sodium channel inhibition: PR and QRS interval widening, right axis deviation of terminal 40 ms (terminal R in aVR, S in lead I), depressed contractility, heart block, hypotension, ectopy; QT prolongation from potassium channel antagonism
  - Generalized seizures from GABA-A receptor antagonism
  - Toxicity can occur at therapeutic doses in combination with other drugs (antihistamines, antipsychotics)

- **Differential Diagnosis**
  - Other drug ingestions: carbamazepine, antihistamines, class Ia and Ic antiarrhythmics, propranolol, lithium
  - Cocaine toxicity
  - Hyperkalemia

- **Treatment**
  - Activated charcoal
  - Gastric lavage if less than 1 hour since ingestion
  - Urine screen for other ingestions; qualitative TCA screen
  - Electrocardiographic and cardiac monitoring
  - Sodium bicarbonate for QRS > 100 ms, refractory hypotension, or ventricular dysrhythmia (1–2 meq/kg boluses to goal serum pH 7.50–7.55, then infuse D_5W with three ampules sodium bicarbonate at 2–3 mL/kg/h)
  - Benzodiazepines for seizures

- **Pearl**

TCAs are responsible for more drug-related deaths than any other prescribed medications—and are the most difficult to treat.

Reference

Ujhelyi MR: Assessment of tricyclic antidepressant toxicity: looking for a needle in a pharmacologic haystack. Crit Care Med 1997;25:1634. [PMID: 9377874]

Arsenic

- **Essentials of Diagnosis**
  - Leading cause of acute metal poisoning; second leading cause of chronic metal toxicity
  - Symptoms appear within 1 hour after ingestion but may be delayed as long as 12 hours
  - Severe abdominal pain, vomiting, watery diarrhea, metallic taste, skeletal muscle cramps, dehydration, delirium, seizures, and shock in acute overdose
  - With chronic ingestion, hypotension, gastroenteritis, peripheral neuropathy (stocking-glove distribution), nonspecific malaise, skin rash, anemia, and leukopenia
  - Abdominal x-ray may demonstrate metallic ingestion
  - Differential may reveal relative eosinophilia; smear may show basophilic stippling of red cells
  - ECG shows prolonged QT interval, especially in chronic toxicity

- **Differential Diagnosis**
  - Septic shock
  - Other heavy metal toxicities, including thallium and mercury
  - Other peripheral neuropathies, including Guillain-Barré syndrome
  - Addison's disease
  - Hypo- and hyperthyroidism

- **Treatment**
  - Gastric lavage for acute large ingestion
  - Activated charcoal may adsorb other ingested toxins
  - Whole-bowel irrigation if radiopaque material visible on abdominal x-ray
  - Chelation therapy of dimercaprol in acute symptomatic ingestions
  - Oral succimer (DMSA) preferred and less toxic agent for stable patients with suspected chronic toxicity
  - Twenty-four-hour urinary arsenic levels

- **Pearl**

A gaseous form (arsine) produces acute hemolytic anemia; treatment differs from that of poisoning with inorganic compounds.

Reference

Graeme KA et al: Heavy metal toxicity, Part I: arsenic and mercury. J Emerg Med 1998;16:45. [PMID: 9472760]

22

Beta-Blockers

- ## Essentials of Diagnosis
  - Hypotension, bradycardia, atrioventricular block, cardiogenic shock
  - Altered mental status, psychosis, seizures, and coma may occur with propranolol, metoprolol, and other lipophilic agents
  - Onset of symptoms typically 1–3 hours, may be from 15 minutes to 10 hours
  - Bronchospasm or hypoglycemia infrequent

- ## Differential Diagnosis
  - Calcium antagonist overdose
  - Digitalis or other cardiac glycoside ingestion
  - Tricyclic antidepressant toxicity

- ## Treatment
  - Gastric lavage if less than 1 hour since ingestion
  - Activated charcoal
  - Electrocardiographic and cardiac monitoring
  - For bradycardia and hypotension, if refractory to normal saline bolus, then glucagon bolus (0.05–0.15 mg/kg) followed by intravenous infusion (0.075–0.15 mg/kg/h)
  - If glucagon insufficient or unavailable, then dopamine or norepinephrine infusion
  - Isoproterenol, magnesium, correction of hypokalemia, sodium bicarbonate, overdrive pacing, or aortic balloon pump
  - Supportive therapy for coma or seizures

- ## Pearl

Be wary of unopposed alpha-agonism in beta-blocker ingestion, especially in hypertensives who may have pheochromocytoma.

Reference

Lip GY et al: Poisoning with anti-hypertensive drugs: beta-adrenoceptor blocker drugs. J Hum Hypertens 1995;9:213. [PMID: 7595901]

Calcium Antagonists (Calcium Channel Blockers)

- **Essentials of Diagnosis**
  - Bradycardia, hypotension, atrioventricular block
  - Cardiac arrest or cardiogenic shock
  - Decreased cerebral perfusion leads to confusion or agitation, dizziness, lethargy, seizures

- **Differential Diagnosis**
  - Beta-blocker toxicity
  - Tricyclic antidepressant toxicity
  - Digitalis toxicity
  - Hypotensive, bradycardiac shock typically distinct from hyperdynamic shock of hypovolemia or sepsis

- **Treatment**
  - Gastric lavage if less than 1 hour since ingestion
  - Activated charcoal
  - Whole bowel irrigation and repeated charcoal for large overdose of sustained-release preparations
  - Electrocardiographic and cardiac monitoring
  - Monitor electrolytes for acidosis, hyperkalemia, hypocalcemia
  - Supportive therapy for coma, hypotension, and seizures
  - To reverse cardiotoxic effects: fluid boluses, then calcium chloride boluses to obtain ionized calcium of 2–3 meq/L; if ineffective, then glucagon (0.1 mg/kg intravenous bolus, then 0.1 mg/kg/h infusion); if refractory, then dopamine or norepinephrine
  - To improve rate and contractility, there may be roles for amrinone, atropine, high-dose insulin with dextrose, or aminopyridine; rescue methods include slow (50 beats/min) cardiac pacing, aortic balloon pump, hemoperfusion, and bypass

- **Pearl**

Verapamil is the most potent negative inotrope of the calcium blockers; beware of its use in cardiomyopathic patients with arrhythmias.

Reference

Proano L et al: Calcium channel blocker overdose. Am J Emerg Med 1995; 13:444. [PMID: 7605536]

Carbon Monoxide

- ■ Essentials of Diagnosis
  - May result from exposure to automobile exhaust, smoke inhalation, or improperly vented gas heater
  - Symptoms nonspecific and flu-like: fatigue, headache, dizziness, abdominal pain, nausea, confusion
  - With more severe intoxication, cherry-red skin, lethargy, seizures, coma
  - Secondary injury from ischemia: myocardial infarction, rhabdomyolysis, noncardiogenic pulmonary edema, renal failure
  - Survivors of severe poisoning may have permanent neurologic deficits
  - Elevated arterial or venous carboxyhemoglobin level; routine arterial blood gases, and pulse oximetry may indicate falsely normal oxygen saturation levels

- ■ Differential Diagnosis
  - Cyanide poisoning
  - Depressant drug ingestion
  - Myocardial ischemia
  - In chronic intoxication, headache of other cause

- ■ Treatment
  - Specific treatment depends on clinical symptoms
  - Remove from exposure
  - Maintain airway and assist ventilation; intubation may be necessary
  - 100% oxygen by nonrebreathing face mask
  - Hyperbaric oxygen if response limited or in the setting of loss of consciousness, myocardial ischemia, or a pregnant patient

- ■ Pearl

Elevated hematocrit and headache in an auto repairman or traffic policeman suggest the diagnosis.

Reference

Piantadosi CA: Diagnosis and treatment of carbon monoxide poisoning. Respir Care Clin N Am 1999;4:183. [PMID: 10333448]

Cardiac Glycosides (Digitalis)

- **Essentials of Diagnosis**
  - Accidental ingestion, single large ingestion, or chronic use
  - Age, coexisting disease, electrolyte disturbance (hypokalemia, hypomagnesemia, hypercalcemia), hypoxia, and other cardiac medications (including diuretics) increase potential for digitalis toxicity
  - Acute overdose: nausea, vomiting, severe hyperkalemia, visual disturbances, syncope, confusion, delirium, bradycardia, supraventricular or ventricular dysrhythmias, atrioventricular block
  - Chronic toxicity: nausea, vomiting, ventricular arrhythmias
  - Elevated serum digoxin level in acute overdose; level may be normal with chronic toxicity

- **Differential Diagnosis**
  - Cardiotoxic plant or animal ingestion: oleander, foxglove, lily of the valley, rhododendron, toad venom
  - Beta-blocker toxicity
  - Calcium blocker toxicity
  - Tricyclic antidepressant ingestion
  - Clonidine overdose
  - Organophosphate insecticide poisoning

- **Treatment**
  - Activated charcoal
  - Gastric lavage if less than 1 hour since ingestion
  - Electrocardiographic and cardiac monitoring
  - Maintain adequate airway and assist ventilation as necessary
  - Correct hypomagnesemia, hypoxia, hypoglycemia, hyperkalemia or hypokalemia; calcium is contraindicated, as it may generate ventricular arrhythmias
  - Lidocaine, phenytoin, magnesium for ventricular arrhythmias; avoid quinidine, procainamide, and bretylium
  - Atropine, pacemaker for bradycardia or atrioventricular block
  - Ventricular arrhythmias, unresponsive bradyarrhythmias, and hyperkalemia with digoxin toxicity are indications for using digoxin-specific antibodies (Digibind); base dosing on estimated ingestion

- **Pearl**

Digitalis may cause or treat any arrhythmia: if they're not on it, start it; if they're on it, stop it.

Reference

Hauptman PJ et al: Digitalis. Circulation 1999;99:1265. [PMID: 10069797]

Cyanide

- **Essentials of Diagnosis**
  - Laboratory or industrial exposure (plastics, solvents, glues, fabrics), smoke inhalation in fires
  - By-product of the breakdown of nitroprusside, ingestion of cyanogenic glycosides in some plant products (apricot pits, bitter almonds)
  - Absorbed rapidly by inhalation, through skin, or gastrointestinally
  - Symptoms shortly after inhalation or ingestion; some compounds (acetonitrile, a cosmetic nail remover) metabolize to hydrogen cyanide, and symptoms may be delayed
  - Dose dependent toxicity; headache, breathlessness, anxiousness, nausea to confusion, shock, seizures, death
  - Disrupts the ability of tissues to use oxygen; picture mimics hypoxia, including profound lactic acidosis
  - High oxygen saturation of venous blood; retinal vessels bright red
  - Odor of bitter almonds on patient's breath or vomitus

- **Differential Diagnosis**
  - Carbon monoxide poisoning
  - Hydrogen sulfide poisoning
  - Other sources of acidosis in suspected ingestion: methanol, ethylene glycol, salicylates, iron, metformin

- **Treatment**
  - Remove patient from the source of exposure, decontaminate skin; 100% oxygen by face mask; intensive care
  - For ingestion, gastric lavage, activated charcoal
  - Inhaled amyl nitrite or intravenous sodium nitrite plus sodium thiosulfate antidote; nitrites may exacerbate hypotension or cause massive methemoglobinemia
  - When the diagnosis is uncertain, significant hypotension contraindicates empirical nitrite use; sodium thiosulfate alone (with 100% oxygen) may be effective
  - Also hydroxocobalamin, dicobalt edetate, 4-dimethylaminophenol—all given with thiosulfate

- **Pearl**

In a patient brought in from a theater fire with lactic acidosis, this is the diagnosis.

Reference

Beasley DM et al: Cyanide poisoning: pathophysiology and treatment recommendations. Occup Med (Lond) 1998;48:427. [PMID: 10024740]

Isoniazid (INH)

- **Essentials of Diagnosis**
  - Classic clinical triad: profound metabolic acidosis, hyperglycemia, seizures
  - Slurred speech, ataxia, coma, and seizures refractory to benzodiazepine or barbiturate treatment
  - Anticholinergic signs
  - Chronic therapeutic use results in peripheral neuritis, tinnitus, memory impairment, and hypersensitivity reactions
  - Hepatic failure the most dangerous adverse reaction to chronic use
  - Substantial genetic variability in the rate at which people metabolize INH

- **Differential Diagnosis**
  - Salicylate, cyanide, carbon monoxide, or anticholinergic overdose
  - In the patient with seizures, acidosis, and coma, consider sepsis, diabetic ketoacidosis, head trauma
  - Hepatitis due to other cause

- **Treatment**
  - Gastric lavage for large ingestion
  - Activated charcoal
  - Pyridoxine (vitamin B_6, 1 g for each g INH ingested; 5 g slow intravenous empiric dose)
  - Benzodiazepines as adjunct in seizure control
  - Supportive therapy for coma, hypotension

- **Pearl**

Ten to 20 percent of patients using INH for chemoprophylaxis will have elevated serum aminotransferases; 1% overall will progress to overt hepatitis; the former have no symptoms, the latter have those of typical hepatitis.

Reference

Romero JA et al: Isoniazid overdose: recognition and management. Am Fam Physician 1998;57:749. [PMID: 9490997]

Lead

- ## Essentials of Diagnosis
  - Results from chronic exposure; sources include solder, batteries, homes built before 1974, artist's paint, gasoline
  - Symptoms and signs include colicky abdominal pain, gum lead line, constipation, headache, irritability, neuropathy, learning disorders in children, episodes of gout
  - Ataxia, confusion, obtundation, seizures
  - Peripheral blood smear may show basophilic stippling and hypochromic microcytic anemia; renal insufficiency common
  - Bone radiographs in children show lead bands; abdominal radiographs show radiopaque material in intestine
  - Blood lead > 10 µg/dL toxic, > 70 µg/dL severe
  - Elevation of free erythrocyte protoporphyrin in chronic exposure

- ## Differential Diagnosis
  - Other heavy metal toxicity (arsenic, mercury)
  - Tricyclic antidepressant, anticholinergic, ethylene glycol, or carbon monoxide exposure
  - Other sources of encephalopathy: alcohol withdrawal, sedative-hypnotic medications, meningitis, encephalitis, hypoglycemia
  - Medical causes of acute abdomen (eg, porphyria, sickle cell crisis)
  - For chronic toxicity: depression, iron deficiency anemia, learning disability
  - Idiopathic gout

- ## Treatment
  - Airway protection and ventilatory assistance as indicated; supportive therapy for coma and seizures
  - Activated charcoal for acute ingestion; consider whole bowel irrigation, endoscopy, or surgical removal if a large lead-containing object is visible on abdominal radiograph
  - Chelation therapy based on presentation and blood lead levels
  - Investigate the source and test other workers or family members who might have been exposed

- ## Pearl
  A cause of nonsurgical acute abdomen in the Southeast, where illegal whisky is made in car radiators.

Reference
Markowitz M: Lead poisoning: a disease for the next millennium. Curr Probl Pediatr 2000;30:62. [PMID: 10742920]

Lithium

- ■ Essentials of Diagnosis
  - Classic triad: painless rigidity, tremor, hyperreflexia
  - Multiple medications increase the risk of lithium toxicity (ACE inhibitors, benzodiazepines, caffeine, loop diuretics, NSAIDs, tricyclic antidepressants, haloperidol), as do renal failure, volume depletion, gastroenteritis, and decreased sodium intake
  - Worsening hand tremor, vertical or rotatory nystagmus, ataxia, dysarthria, polyuria (nephrogenic diabetes insipidus), delirium, stupor, rigidity, coma, seizures
  - Acute ingestions cause more gastrointestinal symptoms (nausea, vomiting, diarrhea, abdominal pain)
  - Elevated serum lithium levels (> 1.5 meq/L); acute ingestions lead to higher serum levels than chronic overdose
  - U waves, flattened or inverted T waves, ST depression, and bradycardia may be seen on ECG

- ■ Differential Diagnosis
  - Neurologic disease (cerebrovascular accident, postictal state, meningitis, parkinsonism, tardive dyskinesia)
  - Other psychotropic drug intoxication
  - Neuroleptic malignant syndrome
  - Delirium

- ■ Treatment
  - Gastric lavage if soon after ingestion; whole bowel irrigation for sustained-release preparations
  - Activated charcoal may be useful for other ingested medications; sodium polystyrene sulfonate (Kayexalate) may be useful to bind lithium
  - Aggressive normal saline hydration with close management of volume and electrolytes
  - Airway protection, ventilatory and hemodynamic support as indicated
  - Hemodialysis for severely symptomatic patients

- ■ Pearl

Consider lithium like sodium: it is handled identically by the kidney, and higher levels thus occur in volume depletion.

Reference

Timmer RT et al: Lithium intoxication. J Am Soc Nephrol 1999;10:666. [PMID: 10073618]

Methanol, Ethylene Glycol, & Isopropanol

- **Essentials of Diagnosis**
  - Methanol is found in solvents, record cleaning solutions, and paint removers; ethylene glycol in antifreeze; isopropanol (rubbing alcohol) in solvents, paint thinners
  - Elevated serum osmolality and osmolar gap occur initially, followed by development of anion gap metabolic acidosis
  - Methanol and ethylene glycol poisoning progress to confusion, convulsions, coma; ethylene glycol may produce tachycardia, hypocalcemia, with tetany, prolonged QT
  - Diplopia, blurred vision, visual field constriction, and blindness with methanol; oxalate crystalluria and renal failure with ethylene glycol; hemorrhagic gastritis and ketonemia without glycosuria or hyperglycemia with isopropanol
  - Urine may fluoresce under Wood's lamp in ethylene glycol ingestions

- **Differential Diagnosis**
  - Ethanol ingestion
  - Other causes of an anion gap acidosis (diabetic ketoacidosis, paraldehyde, isoniazid, salicylates, iron, lactic acidosis, uremia)
  - Hypoglycemia

- **Treatment**
  - Thiamine, folate, pyridoxine, and naloxone if indicated; check blood glucose, correct hypocalcemia and hypomagnesemia
  - Gastric lavage appropriate only immediately after ingestion; activated charcoal will not bind alcohols
  - Maintain adequate airway and assist ventilation
  - Supportive therapy for coma and seizures
  - Sodium bicarbonate in presence of metabolic acidosis due to methanol or ethylene glycol ingestion
  - Ethanol infusion to level of 100–150 mg/dL to prevent metabolism of methanol and ethylene glycol (not necessary for isopropanol); alternatively, fomepizole (4-methylpyrazole) may be used
  - Hemodialysis for severe toxicity

- **Pearl**

Ethylene glycol is colorless, not green; the color is an additive to discourage ingestion of anti-freeze.

Reference

Jones AL et al: Management of self poisoning. BMJ 1999;319:1313. [PMID: 10574863]

Methemoglobinemia

- **Essentials of Diagnosis**
  - More common in infants, especially with exposure to nitrogenous vegetables (spinach), well water with nitrates
  - Drugs that can oxidize normal ferrous (Fe^{2+}) hemoglobin to abnormal ferric (Fe^{3+}) hemoglobin (methemoglobin) include local anesthetics (lidocaine, benzocaine), aniline dyes, nitrates and nitrites, nitrogen oxides, chloroquine, trimethoprim, dapsone, and pyridium
  - Methemoglobin cannot bind oxygen
  - Dizziness, nausea, headache, dyspnea, anxiety, tachycardia, and weakness at low levels to myocardial ischemia, arrhythmias, decreased mentation, seizures, coma
  - Cyanosis unchanged by O_2; saturation fixed at 85% even in severe hypoxemia
  - Definitive diagnosis is by co-oximetry (may be from a venous sample); routine blood gas analysis may be falsely normal
  - Blood may appear chocolate brown (compare with normal blood); urine may also turn brown

- **Differential Diagnosis**
  - Hypoxia or ischemia
  - Sulfhemoglobinemia
  - Carbon monoxide or hydrogen sulfide poisoning

- **Treatment**
  - Gastric lavage and activated charcoal for recent, causative ingestion or if offending agent is not known
  - Discontinue offending agent; high flow oxygen
  - Intravenous methylene blue for symptomatic patients with high methemoglobin levels; patients with G6PD deficiency (higher incidence in black males and patients of Mediterranean ancestry) may develop hemolysis in response to methylene blue
  - If methylene blue therapy fails or is contraindicated, then exchange transfusion or hyperbaric oxygen

- **Pearl**

Patients with preexisting impairment of oxygen delivery (congestive heart failure, COPD, anemia) will be symptomatic at lower levels.

Reference

Wright RO et al: Methemoglobinemia: etiology, pharmacology, and clinical management. Ann Emerg Med 1999;34:646. [PMID: 10533013]

Opioids

- **Essentials of Diagnosis**
  - Euphoria, drowsiness, and constricted pupils in mild intoxication to somnolence, ataxia, hypotension, bradycardia, respiratory depression, apnea, coma, and death with more severe intoxication
  - Signs of intravenous drug abuse (needle marks, a tourniquet)
  - Some (propoxyphene, tramadol, dextromethorphan, meperidine) may cause seizures
  - Noncardiogenic pulmonary edema
  - Detectable in urine, though not all opioids produce positive results on general toxicology screens
  - Meperidine or dextromethorphan plus monoamine oxidase inhibitor may produce serotonin syndrome

- **Differential Diagnosis**
  - Alcohol or sedative-hypnotic overdose
  - Clonidine overdose
  - Phenothiazine overdose
  - Organophosphate or carbamate insecticide exposure
  - Gamma-hydroxybutyrate overdose
  - Congestive heart failure
  - Infectious or metabolic encephalopathy
  - Hypoglycemia, hypoxia, postictal state

- **Treatment**
  - Naloxone for suspected overdose
  - Gastric lavage for very large ingestions presenting within 1 hour
  - Activated charcoal for oral ingestion
  - Maintain adequate airway and assist ventilation, including intubation
  - Supportive therapy for coma, hypothermia, and hypotension
  - Benzodiazepines for seizures
  - Acetaminophen level

- **Pearl**

Be wary of unsuspected opioid toxicity in hospitalized patients taking acetaminophen with codeine and renal insufficiency.

Reference

Lehmann KA: Opioids: overview on action, interaction and toxicity. Support Care Cancer 1997;5:439. [PMID: 9406356]

Salicylates

- **Essentials of Diagnosis**
  - Many over-the-counter products contain salicylates, including Pepto-Bismol, various liniments, oil of wintergreen
  - Local gastric irritation, direct stimulation of central nervous system respiratory center, skeletal muscle metabolism, enhanced lipolysis, and uncoupled oxidative phosphorylation
  - Mild acute ingestion: nausea, vomiting, gastritis
  - Moderate intoxication: hyperpnea, diaphoresis, tachycardia, tinnitus, elevated anion gap metabolic acidosis
  - Severe intoxication: agitation, confusion, proteinuria, hyperventilation, seizures, pulmonary edema, cardiovascular collapse, hyperthermia, hypoprothrombinemia
  - Chronic pediatric ingestion: hyperventilation, volume depletion, acidosis, hypokalemia, metabolic acidosis, respiratory alkalosis; in adults: hyperventilation, confusion, tremor, paranoia, memory deficits

- **Differential Diagnosis**
  - Carbon monoxide poisoning
  - Any cause of anion gap metabolic acidosis (eg, methanol or ethylene glycol ingestion)

- **Treatment**
  - Elevated serum salicylate level; treatment should always consider both serum level and clinical condition
  - Gastrointestinal lavage or whole bowel irrigation for early, large, or sustained-release ingestions
  - Activated charcoal
  - Maintain adequate airway and assist ventilation
  - Supportive therapy for coma, hyperthermia, hypotension, and seizures; correct hypoglycemia and hypokalemia
  - Intravenous fluid resuscitation with normal saline; urinary alkalinization with sodium bicarbonate to enhance salicylate excretion
  - Hemodialysis for severe metabolic acidosis, markedly altered mental status, or clinical deterioration despite supportive care

- **Pearl**

The classic triad of salicylate poisoning: wide anion-gap acidosis, contraction metabolic alkalosis, respiratory alkalosis.

Reference

Sporer KA et al: Acetaminophen and salicylate serum levels in patients with suicidal ingestion or altered mental status. Am J Emerg Med 1996;14:443. [PMID: 8765104]

22

Theophylline

- ■ **Essentials of Diagnosis**
    - • Mild intoxication: nausea, vomiting, tachycardia, tremulousness
    - • Severe intoxication: tachyarrhythmias (premature atrial and ventricular contractions, multifocal atrial tachyarrhythmia, atrial fibrillation and flutter, runs of ventricular tachycardia), hypokalemia, hyperglycemia, metabolic acidosis, hallucinations, hypotension, seizures
    - • Chronic intoxication: vomiting, tachycardia, and seizures, but typically no hypokalemia or hyperglycemia
    - • Elevated serum theophylline concentration

- ■ **Differential Diagnosis**
    - • Caffeine overdose
    - • Iron toxicity
    - • Sympathomimetic poisoning
    - • Anticholinergic toxicity
    - • Thyroid storm
    - • Alcohol or other drug withdrawal

- ■ **Treatment**
    - • Gastric lavage or whole bowel irrigation early in large or sustained-release ingestions
    - • Activated charcoal; repeated doses may enhance elimination
    - • Ranitidine for vomiting
    - • Oxygen; maintain adequate airway and assist ventilation
    - • Monitor for arrhythmias; correct hypokalemia
    - • Treat seizures with benzodiazepines
    - • Hypotension and tachycardia may respond to beta-blockade (esmolol, labetalol)
    - • Hemodialysis or hemoperfusion for patients with status epilepticus or markedly elevated serum theophylline levels (> 100 mg/mL after acute overdose or > 60 mg/mL with chronic intoxication)

- ■ **Pearl**

Inappropriate sinus tachycardia in a patient with COPD may be the only clue to the diagnosis: once seizures occur, the prognosis worsens appreciably.

Reference

Vassallo R et al: Theophylline: recent advances in the understanding of its mode of action and uses in clinical practice. Mayo Clinic Proc 1998;73:346. [PMID: 9559039]

Index